Underst ... sia

UNDERSTANDING ANAESTHESIA

Second Edition

LEN E. S. CARRIE
M.B., Ch.B., F.F.A.R.C.S., D.A.

Consultant Anaesthetist
The Nuffield Department of Anaesthetics
John Radcliffe Hospital, Oxford
and
Clinical Lecturer, Oxford University

PETER J. SIMPSON
M.D., M.B., B.S., M.R.C.S., L.R.C.P.,
F.F.A.R.C.S.

Consultant Anaesthetist
Frenchay Hospital, Bristol
and
Senior Clinical Lecturer
Department of Anaesthesia, University of Bristol

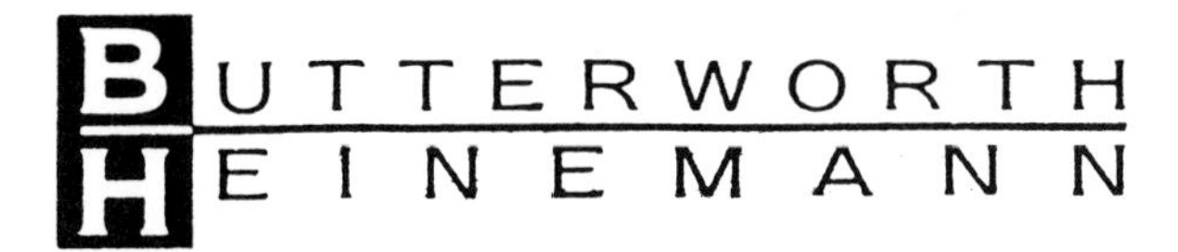

Butterworth-Heinemann Ltd
Halley Court, Jordan Hill, Oxford OX2 8EJ

PART OF REED INTERNATIONAL BOOKS

OXFORD LONDON GUILDFORD BOSTON
MUNICH NEW DELHI SINGAPORE SYDNEY
TOKYO TORONTO WELLINGTON

First published 1982
Second edition 1988
Reprinted 1989, 1990

British Library Cataloguing in Publication Data
Carrie, Len E.S.
Understanding anaesthesia.—2nd ed.
1. Anaesthesia
I. Title II. Simpson, Peter J.
617′.96 RD81

ISBN 0 7506 0122 1

Printed in Great Britain at the Alden Press, Oxford

Contents

Preface to Second Edition

In this Second Edition we have increased the scope of the book to make it more suitable for a wider audience. In particular we have enlarged the various chapters on equipment and monitoring to bring them in line with current practice. The whole book has been extensively reviewed and updated, particularly in the areas of anaesthetic pharmacology, where considerable changes have taken place in recent months. New drugs such as alfentanil, propofol, atracurium, vecuronium and isoflurane have been included, while others such as Althesin and propanidid have been omitted. The chapters on obstetric anaesthesia and local techniques have also been extensively revised to take account of recent advances in these areas. Newer techniques, such as microvascular and craniofacial surgery and the use of lasers, have been considered as have new developments in blood preservation, transfusion and colloidal replacement solutions.

We hope that this new edition represents an easily readable introduction to the practice of anaesthesia for all those involved in the speciality and that it will encourage them to consult more specialised texts as they become more experienced.

Preface to First Edition

This introduction to the principles and practice of anaesthesia has been written primarily to cover the curricula of postgraduate nurses and operating department assistants*, both of which put considerable emphasis on a knowledge of physiology and pharmacology. At the same time modern techniques of clinical measurement have been increasingly introduced into anaesthetic practice. We have therefore tried to include details of recent

*Joint Board of Clinical Nursing Studies (now English National Board), Course Number 182; City and Guilds Diploma Course for Operating Department Assistants.

advances in anaesthesia in addition to the appropriate basic science teaching and the historical and practical aspects of the speciality.

The early part of the book deals with the physiology and pharmacology relevant to anaesthesia, together with a general introduction to anaesthetic technique. Separate chapters deal with anaesthesia for particular surgical specialities and with regional anaesthetic techniques. The problems of intensive care, parenteral nutrition and chronic pain are also included to make the text as comprehensive as possible. Separate chapters towards the end deal with varying aspects of clinical measurement and equipment related to anaesthesia, sterilisation of apparatus, theatre pollution and electrical safety.

The book has grown considerably in length from what was originally planned, but we found it difficult to shorten it if the subject matter was still to be fully covered. The format of a large number of short chapters with a précis of the contents placed under each chapter heading was chosen to make reference easy.

Although originally written for postgraduate nurses and ODAs, we hope that the text is likely to be of benefit to a wider audience including junior anaesthetists, medical students and nurses in intensive care.

Acknowledgements

We are indebted to Drs Tony Fisher and Richard Fordham for contributing Chapters 36 and 38 and to Dr Gordon Paterson for help with Chapter 35. We are also grateful to Mr Richard Salt (formerly Principal Chief Technician in the Nuffield Department of Anaesthetics in the University of Oxford) and Mr Lawrence Hugill (Sterile Services Manager of the Central Sterile Services Department at the Slade Hospital in Oxford) for invaluable assistance with Chapters 8 and 46.

Lastly, we owe a special debt of gratitude to Miss Sue Crook who meticulously, but somehow always cheerfully, carried out (virtually single-handed) the formidable task of all the typing and secretarial work concerned with this book.

1 Anaesthesia: History and Introduction

History. Introduction.

HISTORY

Only a brief summary will be given here of some of the outstanding events in the history of anaesthesia; more detailed history is given in the relevant chapters.

Various dental extractions and operations had been carried out under nitrous oxide or ether anaesthesia in the few years before 1846, but modern anaesthesia is usually considered to date from 16 October 1846, when William T. G. Morton, a Boston dentist, successfully administered ether to a young man whose operation for a tumour on his neck was performed before an assembly of prominent medical men at the Massachusetts General Hospital.

Considering the slowness of communications in those days, the rate at which anaesthesia spread across the world was remarkable. By 19 December 1846 ether had been used in England for dental extractions, and by the following year John Snow, the first professional anaesthetist and one of the greatest names in early anaesthesia, had written a book about ether. Also in 1847, James Young Simpson, Professor of Midwifery in Edinburgh, introduced chloroform as an anaesthetic agent in obstetrics. Religious and other objections were finally overcome when Snow administered chloroform to Queen Victoria at the birth of Prince Leopold in 1853. Chloroform and ether were to remain the most popular anaesthetic agents for the next hundred years.

There had been isolated instances of the successful use of nitrous oxide as an anaesthetic agent, but an unsuccessful demonstration of its use in 1845 by Wells at the Massachusetts General Hospital, its weakness as an agent, and problems in devising equipment led to its virtual disappearance from the anaesthetic scene for some years. It began to regain popularity when Joseph Clover, another giant of early anaesthesia, used it as a relatively pleasant induction before ether anaesthesia. The first Boyle's machine was introduced in 1917.

Nitrous oxide was first used to relieve pain in childbirth by Klikovitch of St Petersburg in 1880, and became popular when Minnitt's nitrous oxide–air machine was introduced in 1934. These 'gas and air' mixtures are now obsolete and inhalational analgesia in labour is now usually provided by Entonox, premixed nitrous oxide and oxygen in one cylinder in the proportions 50:50, first produced by the British Oxygen Company in 1961. The overall importance of nitrous oxide in anaesthesia has greatly increased since the introduction of muscle relaxant drugs, because these agents provide excellent operating conditions under light, general anaesthesia.

Local analgesia dates from 1884 when Köller described the effect of cocaine applied topically to the eye. Spinal analgesia for a surgical operation was first carried out by Bier in 1899, and the first epidurals (which were in fact caudals) were carried out in 1901 by Sicard and Cathelin of France. The first time the lumbar approach to the epidural space was used was in 1921 by a Spaniard, Fidel Pagés. Continuous regional techniques date from the 1940s, Lemmon performing continuous spinal analgesia via a malleable needle and, in 1946, Tuohy performed the first continuous spinal via a catheter introduced through a needle specially designed for the purpose.

The first continuous lumbar epidurals were carried out by Hingson and Southworth of the United States also using malleable needles. In 1947, Curbelo of Havana was the first to carry out continuous epidural analgesia using a ureteric catheter, introduced with the help of a Tuohy needle.

Endotracheal intubation, as a means of resuscitation using tubes made usually of metal or a wire spiral covered with leather, had been used since the late 18th century. It was not until 1880 that MacEwen of Glasgow first used an endotracheal tube for administering an anaesthetic. The use of rubber tubes for endotracheal anaesthesia developed from the work of Magill and Rowbotham, who used this technique to facilitate head and neck surgery on casualties of the First World War.

One of the greatest advances in anaesthesia was the introduction of the neuromuscular blocking agents to provide relaxation for surgical operations. Griffith and Johnson of Montreal in 1942 used the first agent, curare. Decamethonium, a long-acting depolarising muscle relaxant, was first used in 1949, and suxamethonium followed in 1951.

The glass syringe and needle were introduced by Pravaz of Lyons and popularised by a Scot, Alexander Wood, in 1854. In the first part of the 20th century attempts were made to administer many agents (including chloroform and ether) intravenously. The first agent to make intravenous anaesthesia popular was hexobarbitone, introduced in 1932, and in 1934 Lundy of the Mayo Clinic introduced thiopentone into clinical use. Now, more than 50 years later, it remains the best and most popular of the intravenous induction agents.

INTRODUCTION

The word 'anaesthesia' is derived from the Greek and means 'without feeling'. 'Analgesia', also from the Greek, means 'without pain'. There is widespread acceptance of the term general anaesthesia, but debate sometimes arises as to whether local anaesthesia or local analgesia is the correct term to apply to the effect produced by local anaesthetic or local analgesic drugs. Whatever the correct etymological derivation, these terms have become fairly freely interchangeable. The terms 'regional anaesthesia' and 'regional analgesia' are now commonly used to describe nerve-blocking techniques.

The 'Triad' of Anaesthesia

Any general anaesthetic can usually be divided into three components—narcosis (sleep), analgesia (pain relief), and relaxation (muscular relaxation). Different surgical operations require different proportions of the three components. Once a patient is unconscious it is not always clear how much analgesia an agent is providing. However, some agents undoubtedly provide more analgesia than others, and this is more obvious when the agents are used in subnarcotic concentrations. Hence nitrous oxide and trichloroethylene, both excellent analgesics, can be used in this way to provide pain relief in obstetrics. Halothane, a poor analgesic, is ineffective when so used.

In the same way, halothane when vaporised by a gas which has no analgesic properties (e.g. oxygen or air) tends to provide poor operating conditions for even minor operations unless fairly high concentrations are used. The addition of nitrous oxide to the halothane and oxygen, however, provides a versatile and popular anaesthetic mixture with good proportions of analgesia and narcosis.

In the early days of anaesthesia, when single agents were used (e.g. chloroform, ether, or more recently cyclopropane), all the components of the triad had to be obtained from the single drug. The main problem was that muscular relaxation was provided by these single volatile agents only at the deeper levels of anaesthesia. The proportions of the narcotic and analgesic components were greatly in excess of those required for the operation; hence the patient sometimes took hours to regain full consciousness and often suffered from other distressing side-effects, in particular vomiting. The incidence of postoperative respiratory and venous thrombotic complications was high.

Modern anaesthetic agents allow the proportions of the three components of the triad to be more easily adjusted to individual requirements, with a corresponding improvement in the patient's operative and postoperative well-being. In particular, the introduction of muscle relaxant drugs has meant that excellent relaxation may be obtained simply by an injection from a syringe, while the patient is only lightly anaesthetised—a great improvement on the profound and often prolonged anaesthesia required to provide similar operating conditions when a single anaesthetic agent was used.

Before each patient arrives in the anaesthetic room it is good practice for the anaesthetist and those who are helping him to decide which components of the triad will provide the best conditions for the operation and what combination of drugs can best be used to provide them. For example, for many operations where profound muscle relaxation is not required the induction of anaesthesia is most pleasantly and smoothly performed by an intravenous agent like thiopentone. Maintenance of anaesthesia may then be performed with nitrous oxide, oxygen, and halothane with the patient breathing spontaneously—the nitrous oxide providing more analgesia and the halothane more narcosis than that provided by the sleep dose of thiopentone.

For an operation where muscle relaxation is required, anaesthesia may still be induced with thiopentone and endotracheal intubation carried out with the help of a depolarising or non-depolarising muscle relaxant. Maintenance of anaesthesia can then be provided with nitrous oxide, oxygen and an adjuvant, with further increments of muscle relaxant as required. This sequence will also provide good operating conditions for thoracic surgery, where muscle relaxation is not so important but controlled ventilation is required to prevent the lung collapsing once the pleural cavity has been opened.

Despite the basic importance of the components of the triad of anaesthesia it should be realised that they are not the only factors affecting the decision about which anaesthetic agents to use. For example, even with modern agents it may be difficult after long operations to ensure that the patient will wake up quickly if a spontaneous respiration technique is employed. The rapid return of the patient's protective reflexes at the end of anaesthesia is always important and sometimes, for example when recovery facilities are inadequate, may be vital to the patient's safety. For this reason an anaesthetist might use a muscle relaxant technique even when relaxation is not particularly necessary.

Another example of other factors affecting the choice of anaesthetic technique could occur in the elderly patient, where adequate operating conditions with a spontaneous respiration technique might be provided only by an anaesthetic mixture of such strength that hypotension was unavoidable. Again, the anaesthetist might provide an anaesthetic that was safer for the patient if he were to use a muscle relaxant technique.

This introduction indicates only some of the more important factors affecting the choice of anaesthetic technique. There are many others occurring in individual cases, but, with the wide choice of spontaneous respiration, controlled respiration and regional techniques available today, it should be possible to provide most patients with an anaesthetic which combines a high degree of safety with a low incidence of serious postanaesthetic complications.

2 Applied Anatomy and Physiology in Anaesthesia

Cardiovascular system. Respiratory system. Autonomic nervous system. Kidney. Fluid and acid–base balance.

CARDIOVASCULAR SYSTEM

Heart

The anatomical structure of the heart, as it lies in the thorax, is illustrated in Figure 2.1. The right and left sides of the heart are separate in normal circumstances, the blood flowing via the lungs to pass from the right side of the heart to the left. A small amount of blood in fact circulates through the bronchial as opposed to the pulmonary circulation, or drains from the coronary arteries into the coronary sinus and thence into the lumen of the ventricles, providing a small (1–2 %) shunt of de-oxygenated blood to the left side of the heart.

Normal cardiac contraction

Blood reaches the atria from the periphery via the superior and inferior venae cavae (SVC, IVC), flowing down a small pressure gradient. Venous return is enhanced both by the negative pressure created in the chest by active inspiration and by the peripheral muscle pump. Anaesthesia, involving intermittent positive pressure ventilation, may therefore diminish venous return and subsequently cardiac output. The atria act as a storage reservoir, allowing subsequent blood flow into the

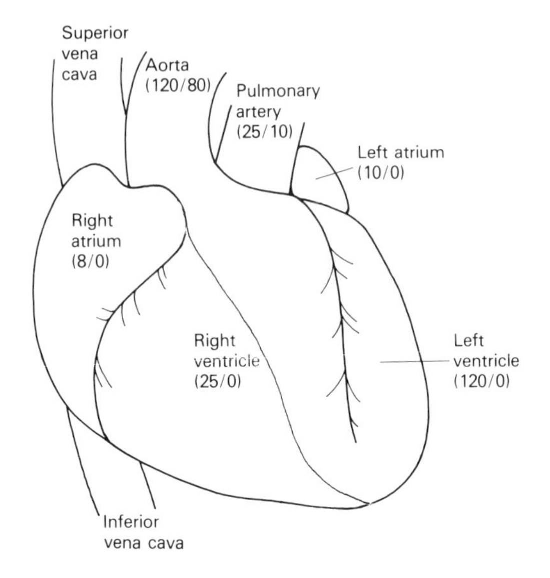

Fig. 2.1 The heart (systolic and diastolic pressure indicated in mmHg)

ventricles during diastole. Towards the end of diastole the atria themselves contract, providing an extra 10–30 % of ventricular filling. Atrial contraction is not essential, but significantly improves ventricular filling and therefore cardiac output. This is evident when considering the relatively low cardiac output associated with atrial fibrillation or heart block. During systole the ventricles contract, forcing blood into the pulmonary artery and the aorta, and during this period the ventricular muscle is compressed and therefore little or no blood flows down the coronary arteries which supply oxygenated blood to the heart muscle. Coronary blood flow, and therefore myocardial oxygenation only occurs during diastole. If the period of diastole is shortened by an increase in heart rate, myocardial oxygenation may be reduced, and if this tachycardia is accompanied by increased demands on the myocardium in the form of exercise or hypertension, in susceptible patients angina may be precipitated by the relative imbalance of oxygen supply and demand.

Figure 2.1 also illustrates the pressures developed in the various chambers of the heart and the aorta. The atria are relatively low-pressure organs, while the ventricles generate a high systolic pressure equal to that in the aorta or pulmonary artery, but the end distolic pressure is only marginally above zero. The right ventricle pumps out the same quantity of blood as the left, but at a much lower pressure, the right side of the heart pumping against the pulmonary vascular bed. Pulmonary hypertension may therefore be caused by an increase in resistance of the pulmonary vasculature which, in turn, may be associated with lung disease or hypoxia.

Control of heart rate

The heart is formed from excitable tissue, muscle differing only slightly from nervous tissue in its degree of excitability. It therefore possesses its own inherent rhythm, which will be apparent if the external influences on heart rate are removed. Normal conduction of the cardiac impulse originates in the sinoatrial node in the right atrium and proceeds across the atrium to the atrioventricular node and then down the bundle of His, which bifurcates to supply impulses to both the right and left ventricles. The normal heart rate generated from the sino-atrial node varies between 60 and 120 beats per minute in fit adults and young children, respectively. This beat is regular, varying only mildly with the respiratory cycle (sinus arrhythmia). The sinoatrial node, however, is influenced both from the brain via the vagus nerve, tending to slow the heart (bradycardia), and from sympathetic fibres or circulating catecholamines, both of which tend to produce an increase in heart rate (tachycardia). With normal conducting tissue this increase in heart rate is transmitted to the remainder of the atria and the ventricles. If a conduction defect exists, areas of the heart may produce their own inherent rhythm. If this develops from the atrioventricular node (nodal rhythm), the atrial rate may be maintained but efficient atrial contraction does not occur (Chapter 19). This may result in a relative inefficient filling of the ventricles. If there is a complete heart block between the atria and the ventricles, the ventricles will beat with their own inherent rhythm at a rate of 40 beats per minute. This may allow extra beats from other excitable areas of the heart to interpose themselves, producing supra-ventricular or ventricular ectopic beats. All these disorders of cardiac rhythm tend to reduce the efficiency of heart filling and therefore cardiac output.

Cardiac output

The volume of blood ejected from the heart in a fixed time is referred to as the cardiac output and is usually measured in litres per minute. This amount of blood is dependent both on the heart rate and on the volume of blood ejected from the left ventricle during each contraction. This last measurement is known as the stroke volume, the cardiac output being equal to the stroke volume multiplied by the heart rate. Cardiac output also influences the arterial blood pressure. The amount of blood rejected by the heart balanced against the resistance to flow offered by the peripheral circulation determines the pressure generated in the aorta and the major vessels. Arterial blood pressure, therefore, is equal to cardiac output multiplied by peripheral resistance.

Peripheral Resistance

The resistance in the peripheral circulation depends mainly on the degree of arteriolar vasodilation or constriction. The veins act as capacitance vessels—i.e. a reservoir for blood—but are not capable of extreme contraction. The arterioles are under the control of the sympathetic nervous system (ch. 14), arteriolar vasoconstriction occurring as a result of increased sympathetic activity. A reduction in sympathetic tone produces arteriolar vasodilation, the parasympathetic system playing no part in vasodilation. Vasodilation itself is effected simply by a reduction or abolition of sympathetic tone, as occurs when a patient faints.

The degree of peripheral vasodilation is also affected by the release of local metabolites, which may be produced in excess as a result of reduced tissue oxygenation and the production of lactic acid. Local acidosis or carbon dioxide release, together with accumulation of other metabolites, may produce arteriolar vasodilation and therefore an increase in peripheral perfusion but a reduction in peripheral resistance. Certain organs, such as the brain, the kidney and the coronary circulation, are able to control blood flow through their vascular beds, maintaining the flow at a constant level irrespective of fluctuation in arterial blood pressure. This is effected by local control of arteriolar diameter in response to tissue metabolism and, in the case of the brain for example, means that cerebral perfusion pressure does not change between mean arterial blood pressures of 60 mmHg and 150 mmHg. This phenomenon is known as autoregulation and is specialised in these organs. Nevertheless, most vascular beds are capable of a degree of autoregulation. Not all areas vasoconstrict at the same time. In sympathetic overactivity, when the subject needs to be ready to run away, vasoconstriction may be observed in the skin and splanchnic circulation; but vasodilation will occur in the muscle beds to supply extra blood flow to this area.

Control of Blood Pressure

The baroceptor mechanism is responsible for controlling blood pressure. Baroceptors are situated in the arterial wall of the aortic arch and in the region of the common carotid arteries, and are sensitive to changes in pressure within the lumen of the vessel. As the pressure rises the nerve impulse activity, passing from these areas to the medulla of the brain, increases. If the pressure falls, activity decreases. This nervous activity controls the output of the vasomotor centre, the area of the brain responsible for control of blood vessel diameter. Baroceptor activity inhibits the vasomotor centre. An increase in blood pressure, causing increased baroceptor activity, therefore inhibits the vasomotor centre producing vasodilation and a fall in blood pressure. Conversely, a reduction in baroceptor activity causes increased vasomotor centre activity and vasoconstriction. The vasomotor centre is also influenced by hypoxia, hypercarbia and higher centres in the brain. The baroceptors also influence the cardiac centre in the brain controlling heart rate via the vagus nerve. Increased baroceptor activity resulting from an increase in blood pressure tends to stimulate the vagus nerve and reduce heart rate, thereby lowering blood pressure. Hypovolaemia, on the other hand, is compensated for by peripheral vasoconstriction and an increase in heart rate.

RESPIRATORY SYSTEM

The lungs lie in the thoracic cavity on either side of the mediastinum. They consist of conducting airways and lung tissue, whose function is to allow diffusion of gases from the air into the bloodstream across the alveolar capillary membrane. Under ideal conditions this membrane is only two cells thick, allowing only minimal interruption to gas diffusion. The alveoli themselves greatly increase the area available for gas exchange and so make this process more efficient.

The lungs are surrounded by two layers of a membrane, the pleura. The visceral pleura is closely applied to the lung surface and the parietal pleura lines the chest wall. Under normal conditions these two layers are closely applied to one another and there is only a potential space between them. The outward pull of the chest wall opposing the inward pull of the elastic recoil of the lung creates a negative pressure within the pleural space which is responsible for holding the lung in an expanded position.

Anatomy of the bronchial tree and its relevance to endobronchial intubation and one-lung anaesthesia for thoracotomy is discussed in Chapter 35.

Breathing

At the end of a normal, quiet expiration the lungs are in the resting respiratory position, their elastic recoil being opposed by the chest wall and the negative pressure in the intrapleural space. Inspiration is an active process initiated by the expansion of the thoracic cage, which inevitably draws the lungs outwards by negative pressure and, as a result air flows down the bronchi. Initially, expansion of the thoracic cage is diaphragmatic, the intercostal muscles which enlarge the thoracic cage itself being used only when larger volumes of gas need to be exchanged as oxygen consumption rises in the body as a result of exercise. The diaphragm is supplied by the phrenic nerve from the third, fourth and fifth cervical nerves, while the individual intercostal nerves supply the various thoracic segments. For this reason a high thoracic extradural or spinal anaesthetic is unlikely to impair respiration seriously until it reaches the mid-cervical region. Patients with spinal cord transection are also able to breathe, provided that the level of cord damage is not above C3.

In contrast to inspiration, expiration is passive, depending solely on the elastic recoil of the lungs. Active expiration is possible by using extra muscles, such as those of the abdominal wall, to increase the upward movement of the diaphragm.

Normal Lung Volumes

The volumes of air contained in the lungs at different phases of the respiratory cycle are important in assessing lung function. These are illustrated in Figure 2.2, the most important being the tidal volume, i.e. the volume of air exchanged during normal quiet respiration, and the vital capacity which is the maximum amount of air that a patient is able to exchange.

An index of adequacy of lung function is obtained from a measurement of the volume of air which a patient is able to exhale forcibly (forced expiratory volume) in one second (FEV_1), expressed as a proportion of their total vital capacity. This FEV_1 to vital capacity ratio is normally over 80%. At the end of maximal expiration a small amount of air, the residual volume, still remains in the lungs, this being air trapped in the alveoli at the end of a maximal expiration.

Compliance

The expression 'compliance' is used to indicate the degree of

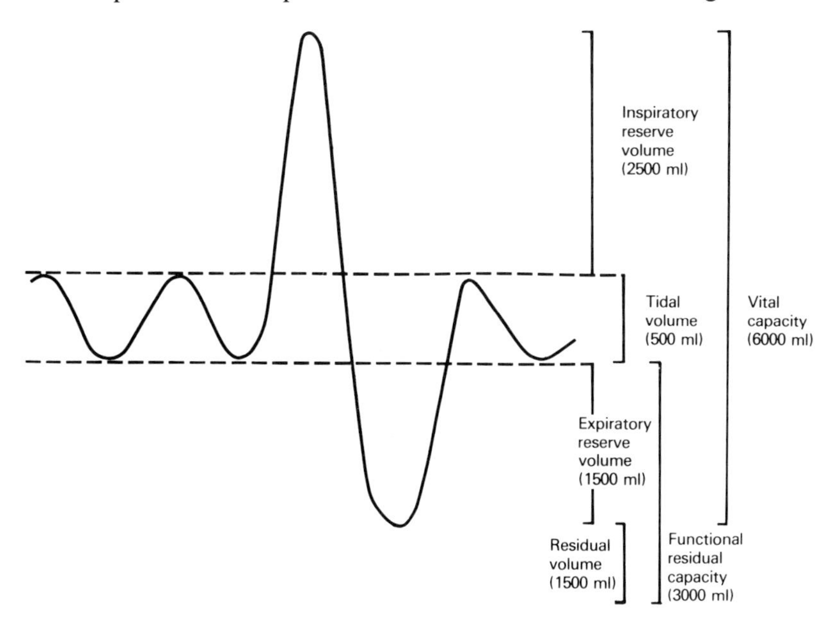

Fig. 2.2 Normal lung volumes

'stiffness' of the lungs. A compliant organ is one which is easy to distend and therefore a lung with high compliance is relatively easy to distend, while low compliance implies that the lung is stiff as a result of acute or chronic disease or infection. In lungs with low compliance a relatively large amount of energy may be needed to overcome the initial stiffness of the lungs when inspiration occurs, in the same way that a balloon is more difficult to blow up until it has begun to expand.

Gas Exchange

The volume of gas inspired in one minute is known as the minute volume. This is the product of the respiratory rate and the tidal volume and at rest is usually about 6–8 litres per minute in a 70 kg man. In extreme exercise this may increase by three to four times that amount. As the dead space in the lung (i.e. the volume of the airways not taking part in gaseous exchange) is a fixed portion of any breath (120–150 ml) an increase in respiratory rate will inevitably increase dead-space ventilation while an increase in tidal volume with no increase in respiratory rate will result in increased alveolar ventilation without any increased ventilation of the dead space. Deep breathing is therefore more advantageous to patients than rapid shallow respiration.

Once gas has reached the alveoli, oxygen and carbon dioxide are exchanged across the alveolar capillary membrane to equilibrate with the blood concentrations of these gases. Other gases, such as anaesthetics and nitrogen, also diffuse freely across this membrane, although in the case of nitrogen, which is not consumed in the body, the overall net flow of gas from one side to the other is zero. Diffusion depends on the pressure exerted by each individual gas on either side of this membrane, the overall result being that gas diffuses down concentration gradients from an area of high concentration to a low one. In the lungs, therefore, oxygen flows from the alveoli into the bloodstream and carbon dioxide passes in the reverse direction.

As we live at atmospheric pressure, the total pressure exerted by all the gases present in room air must equal atmospheric pressure, that is 760 mmHg. Likewise, the overall pressure exerted by the gases in the alveoli or in the blood must also equal 760 mmHg. The composition of gases in these various compartments is illustrated in Table 2.1.

Table 2.1 Physiological gas partial pressures (mmHg)

	Room air	Alveolus/arterial blood	Venous blood
Nitrogen	610	573	617
Oxygen	150	100	50
Carbon dioxide	–	40	46
Water vapour	–	47	47

Carriage of Oxygen in the Blood

Oxygen is carried in the blood in two ways: (1) in combination with haemoglobin or (2) dissolved in the plasma. A gram of normal haemoglobin will combine with 1·38 ml oxygen so that, with a normal haemoglobin concentration of 14 g per 100 ml blood, 20 ml oxygen will be carried in combination with haemoglobin in 100 ml blood. In this case the haemoglobin is said to be fully saturated with oxygen. The degree of saturation of haemoglobin and the amount of relative desaturation which occurs as the blood perfuses peripheral tissues and releases oxygen are dependent on the oxyhaemoglobin dissociation curve (Fig. 2.3).

Haemoglobin is fully saturated with oxygen when the arteries Po_2 is over 70 mmHg. Below this level saturation fall rapidly for only a small fall in arterial Po_2 thus enabling the haemoglobin to release oxygen to the tissues while maintaining them at an adequate partial pressure of oxygen. Certain factors tend to influence the readiness with which haemoglobin releases oxygen, such as temperature, acidosis, and Pco_2. This means that in certain conditions, when oxygen availability is at a premium, other factors in the body ensure adequate release from the haemoglobin.

Hypoxia

A lack of available oxygen within the body is known as hypoxia. Four main types are recognised, depending on the factors which cause them.

Hypoxic hypoxia

This is due either to a lack of available oxygen in the inspired air

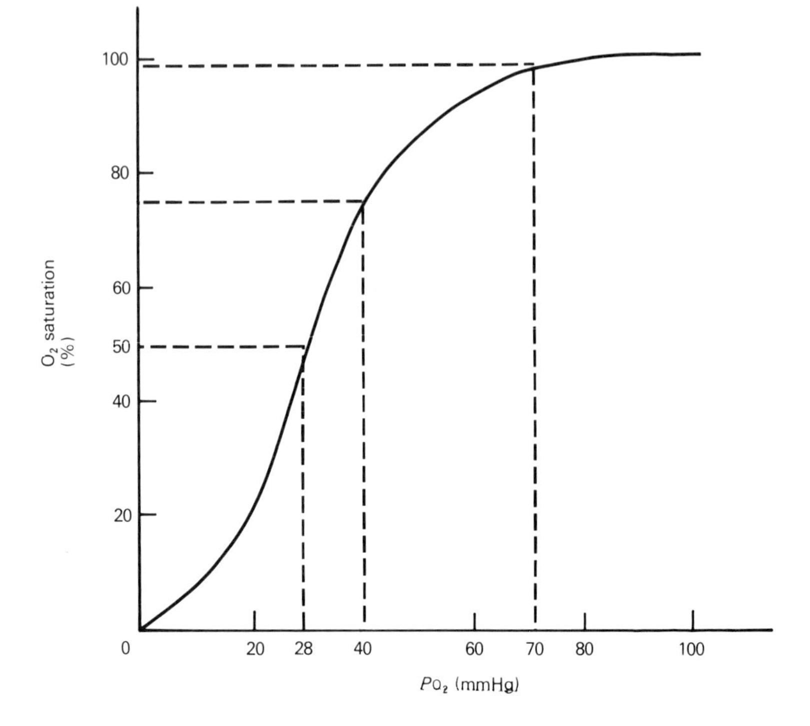

Fig. 2.3 Oxyhaemoglobin dissociation curve

or to difficulty in inspiration, both of which produce a low content of oxygen in the arterial blood.

Anaemic hypoxia

This is due to a reduction in the available haemoglobin and therefore the oxygen carriage is reduced.

Stagnant hypoxia

In cases of poor peripheral perfusion, when blood flow is sluggish through peripheral tissues as a result of vasoconstriction, hypoxia and cyanosis may occur as a result of excessive oxygen uptake from the available blood.

Histotoxic hypoxia

This results from cellular damage, when the cells are unable to use the oxygen supplied to them.

Carbon Dioxide Transport

Carbon dioxide is carried in the blood in three ways.

In solution in the plasma
Carbon dioxide combines with water to form carbonic acid which, in turn, dissociates into hydrogen and bicarbonate ions.

$$CO_2 + H_2O \rightleftarrows H_2CO_3 \rightleftarrows H^+ + HCO_3^-$$

As carbamino compounds
Carbon dioxide combines with proteins to form carbamino compounds, but this is responsible for only a small amount of carbon dioxide carriage.

In the form of bicarbonate
Carbon dioxide in solution passes from plasma into the red cells while in the peripheral tissues. Carbonic acid, which is formed in the red cells under the influence of an enzyme, carbonic anhydrase, then dissociates into hydrogen and bicarbonate ions. The haemoglobin within the red cell combines with the free hydrogen ions, thereby neutralising them and preventing a change in pH. The free bicarbonate then diffuses out of the red cell in exchange for chloride ions moving into the red cell, the bicarbonate then being carried within the plasma. This exchange of bicarbonate with chloride is known as the chloride shift and occurs in the peripheral tissues. A reverse process occurs in the lungs when chloride leaves the red cell and bicarbonate enters it to reform carbon dioxide, which is then excreted in the lungs (Fig. 2.4).

Venous blood contains a higher concentration of carbon dioxide than arterial blood (*see* Table 2.1) and on reaching the lungs gives off carbon dioxide which diffuses into the alveoli, thereby reducing the arterial CO_2 concentration. The influence of carbon dioxide carriage within the blood upon acid–base balance is dealt with on p. 34.

Control of Respiration

Although man is able to increase and decrease his respiratory rate and depth at will, normal respiration is not under voluntary

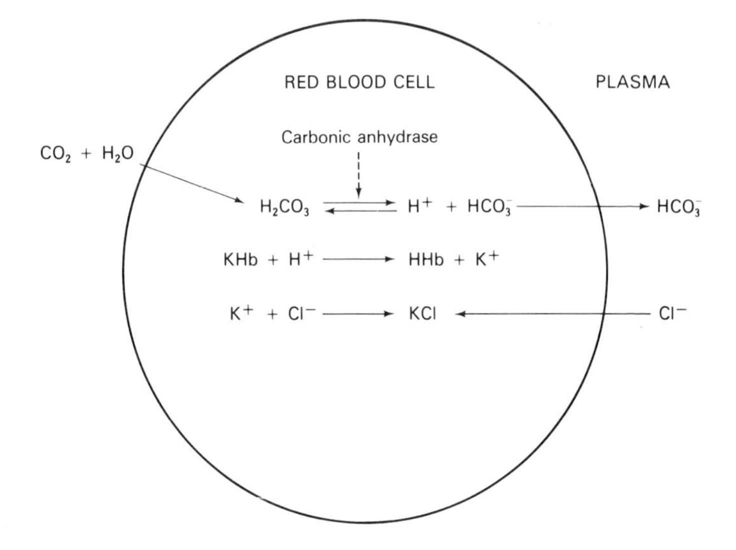

Fig. 2.4 'The chloride shift'—red cell CO_2 transport

control. In normal man the respiratory centre in the medulla of the brain is sensitive to changes in the blood carbon dioxide concentration which, in turn, influences hydrogen and bicarbonate ions and the concentration of these within the cerebrospinal fluid (CSF). It is probably changes in CSF pH or bicarbonate concentration that influence the respiratory centre and alter respiratory rate. Normal breathing is therefore dependent on CO_2 concentration and not on hypoxia. The peripheral chemoreceptors situated in the aortic and carotid bodies are sensitive to oxygen lack, and severe hypoxia will stimulate the respiratory centre via the chemoreceptors. This, however, is an abnormal response and very few severely ill bronchitics regularly respond to a hypoxic respiratory drive.

AUTONOMIC NERVOUS SYSTEM

The autonomic nervous system is divided into the parasympathetic and sympathetic nervous systems and is concerned with the innervation of smooth muscle (e.g. gut, bronchi, bladder, blood vessels and eye); the heart; and secreting glands.

Sympathetic Nervous System

The sympathetic fibres rise in the lateral horn of the grey matter of the spinal cord in the thoracolumbar region from T1 to L2. The preganglionic sympathetic fibres (Fig. 2.5) synapse with the postganglionic fibres in the ganglia of the sympathetic chain running along the length of the spinal cord on the anterolateral bodies of the vertebrae. The postganglionic fibres then run in a mixed nerve to their point of action.

Parasympathetic Nervous System

The parasympathetic system has a cranio-sacral outflow, fibres

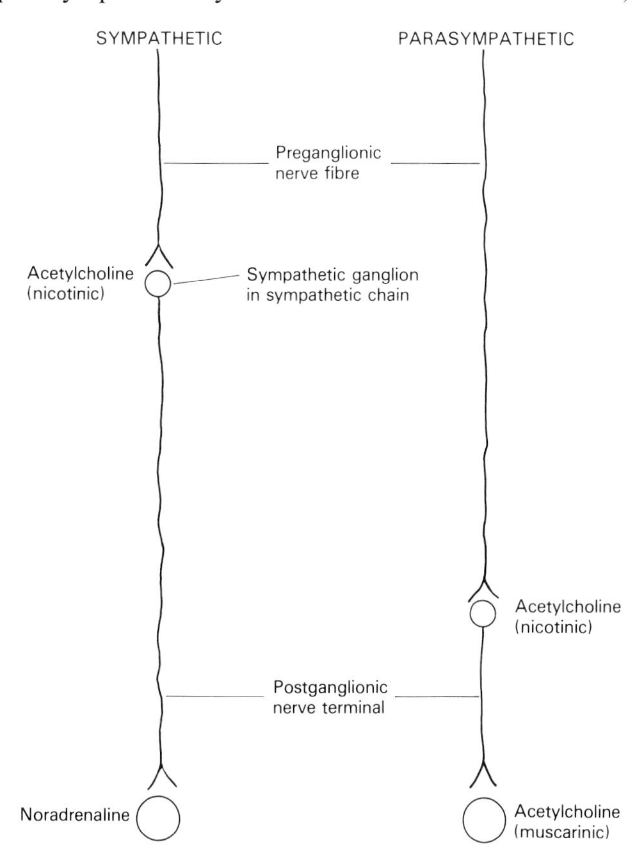

Fig. 2.5 Basic autonomic pharmacology

being found in cranial nerves 3, 7, 9 and 10, and in the second, third and fourth sacral segments of the spinal cord. In contrast with the sympathetic system, where the postganglionic fibre tends to be long, the postganglionic parasympathetic fibre is often short. Hence the preganglionic fibres synapse in ganglia in the immediate vicinity of the effector organ. The parasympathetic activity in the cranial nerves may be summarised as follows:

3rd nerve supplies the ciliary muscle and the iris of the eye
7th nerve supplies the submandibular and sublingual salivary glands
9th nerve supplies the parotid salivary gland
10th nerve (the vagus) supplies parasympathetic fibres to the thorax and abdomen affecting heart, bronchi, gut and pancreas.

Transmission in the Autonomic Nervous System

The two main transmitting substances concerned, acetylcholine and noradrenaline, are indicated in Figure 2.5. The actions of acetylcholine are normally divided into muscarinic and nicotinic, the muscarinic being synonymous with parasympathetic activity and the nicotinic being those at the skeletal neuromuscular junction and the autonomic ganglia. These names are derived from the similarity of the individual actions of acetylcholine to those of the naturally occurring substances, muscarine and nicotine.

Actions of the Sympathetic Nervous System

These may be summarised in the 'fight and flight' reaction (Fig. 2.6), so that increased sympathetic activity produces the following effects: increased heart rate and blood pressure; vasoconstriction of skin and vasodilation in skeletal muscle; bronchial dilation; and dilation of the pupil of the eye. Gastrointestinal motility is inhibited and the sphincters constrict. The sweat glands and erector pilae muscles are also activated.

Actions of the Parasympathetic Nervous System

These may be likened to a fat man sitting down after a heavy meal (Fig. 2.6), so that there is a decrease in heart rate and an

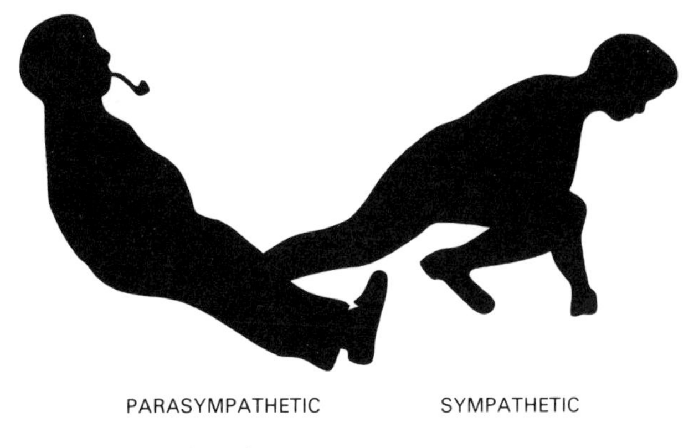

Fig. 2.6 The autonomic nervous system

increase in gastrointestinal activity with the digestive tract sphincters relaxing and the bladder emptying. Bronchoconstriction occurs together with an increase in salivary, gastric and pancreatic glandular activity. The pupils constrict and the bladder sphincters relax.

The actions of both systems indicate some of the natural antagonism which occurs. In addition, however, certain autonomic activity—for example, vasoconstriction of the skin which is produced by increased sympathetic activity—is not counteracted by parasympathetic stimulation. Vasodilation in skin is due simply to inhibition of sympathetic activity.

Acetylcholine Metabolism

Figure 2.5 indicates the sites at which acetylcholine acts as the transmitter substance, both in the synapse between pre- and post-ganglionic neurones and also, in the case of the parasympathetic system, at the nerve effector organ junction. In normal circumstances acetylcholine is metabolised by a naturally occurring enzyme, cholinesterase. An enzyme called plasma or pseudocholinesterase also exists, although its normal physiological function is uncertain. Acetylcholine is continually broken down by cholinesterase into choline and acetic acid. The amount of acetylcholine present may therefore be increased either by using an inhibitor of cholinesterase (i.e. an anticholinesterase, for example neostigmine or pyridostigmine) or by giving a drug that mimics the actions of acetylcholine.

The actions of acetylcholine may be broadly subdivided into muscarinic and nicotinic, the muscarinic being predominantly parasympathetic while the nicotinic actions are those at the skeletal neuromuscular junction and at the autonomic ganglia. The muscarinic (parasympathetic) effects of acetylcholine can be enhanced with drugs like carbachol or methacholine, both of which increase intestinal activity and bladder tone and increase exocrine secretions. Succinylcholine (suxamethonium chloride) resembles acetylcholine and for this reason acts in a similar way, firstly by stimulating the skeletal neuromuscular junction, causing fasciculation, and then by producing neuromuscular blockade as a result of excess stimulation. This effect can be mimicked by an excessive accumulation of acetylcholine, which may occur in patients given an overdose of anticholinesterase.

The effects of acetylcholine may be blocked by different drugs, depending on the site of action. The muscarinic effects of acetylcholine are blocked by atropine and hyosine, and both these drugs therefore tend to produce a dry mouth, an increase in heart rate and a reduction in gastrointestinal motility. Other drugs also possess atropine-like actions, for example pethidine and the phenothiazine drugs as chlorpromazine and promethazine. The nicotinic actions of acetylcholine are stimulatory at the skeletal neuromuscular junction and at the autonomic ganglia. Of these, the neuromuscular effects are antagonised by the non-depolarising muscle relaxants, for example d-tubocurarine, pancuronium, and alcuronium.

Adrenaline and Noradrenaline Metabolism

Noradrenaline is the main transmitter substance in the postganglionic sympathetic neurone. Figure 2.7 indicates the normal mechanisms of release, metabolism and re-uptake of noradrenaline in this situation. After its release, noradrenaline may be taken up again into the adrenergic neurone and then either metabolised by monoamine oxidase or restored in granules ready for use again as a transmitter substance. Alternatively, it may be directly metabolised by catechol-O-methyl transferase, an enzyme which exists in the synaptic cleft between the neurone and the effector organ. Monoamine oxidase acts only on free noradrenaline in the nerve terminal and not on that stored in the vesicles. Noradrenaline is synthesised in the body from amino acids, an intermediary metabolite being dopamine.

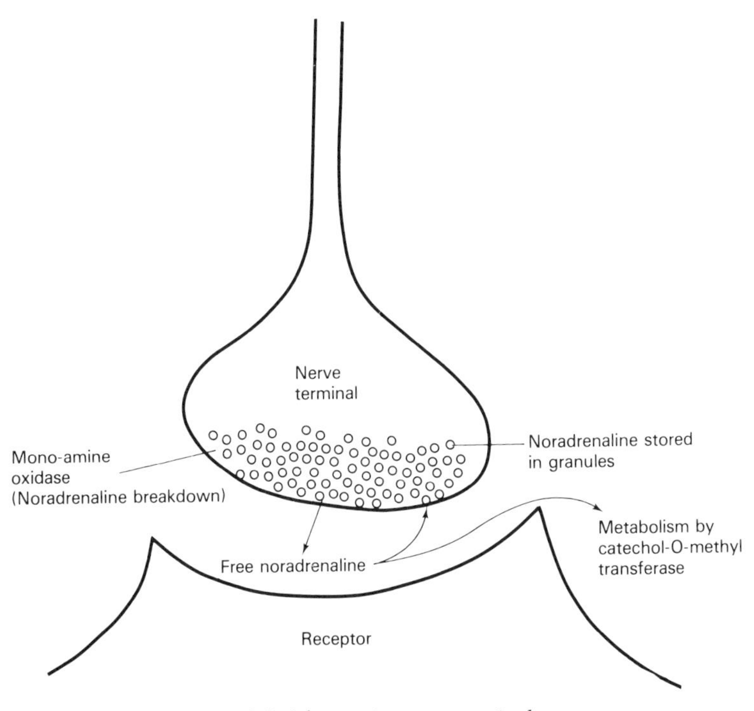

Fig. 2.7 Adrenergic nerve terminal

Alpha and Beta Theory of Adrenergic Transmission

The effects of adrenaline at various sites in the body have been classified in terms of two groups of separate receptors, alpha (α) and beta (β), the main actions being summarised in Table 2.2.

While adrenaline itself possesses both alpha and beta activity, other sympathomimetic amines possess relatively more of one or the other (Table 2.3). The beta effects are further subdivided into β_1 (effects on the heart) and β_2 (effects on the lung). The site of action of the α effects has also been subdivided into α_1 and α_2.

In normal clinical use the alpha effects of adrenaline most commonly observed are skin vasoconstriction causing an increase in blood pressure, while the beta effects are bronchodila-

Table 2.2 Main actions of adrenaline in the body

Adrenaline	
α	β
Force of cardiac contraction	Heart rate (β_1)
Peripheral vasoconstriction (skin + gut)	Bronchodilation (β_2)
	Muscle + kidney vasodilation

Table 2.3 Drugs affecting α and β adrenergic receptors

α-Stimulants	Adrenaline Noradrenaline (Dopamine)
β-Stimulants	Isoprenaline (β_1 and β_2) Salbutamol (β_2) Dopamine (β_1) Dobutamine
α-Blockers	Phentolamine Phenoxybenzamine
β-Blockers	Propranolol Practolol (β_1) Oxprenolol (β_1) Atenolol (β_1) Sotalol (β_1)

tion and an increase in heart rate. These differing effects of adrenaline are also blocked by different drugs, for example α-adrenergic blocking drugs, phentolamine, phenoxybenzamine and tolazoline, and β-blocking drugs, for example propranolol, practolol, oxprenolol. Although labetalol possesses both α- and β-blocking activity, the β-blocking effects would appear to be both longer lasting and considerably greater than the α-blocking effects.

KIDNEY

The kidneys are situated retroperitoneally on either side of the midline between T12 and L3. Together, at rest, they receive 25 %

of the cardiac output and serve several important functions. These are control of fluid and electrolyte concentrations within the body; regulation of blood pressure; and formation of red blood cells by secretion of the hormone erythropoietin.

The basic filtration unit of the kidney is the nephron, of which there are about one million in each kidney. Their structure is illustrated in Figure 2.8.

Basically, there are two distinct populations of nephrons, those whose Bowman's capsule is situated within the cortex itself and those whose capsule is near the renal medulla, the juxtamedullary group of nephrons, The cortical nephrons have short loops of Henle and are far more numerous than the juxtamedullary ones, whose long loops of Henle descend deep into the medulla along the pyramids, these being responsible for the development of a high concentration gradient for water reabsorption.

Blood Flow

One-tenth of the 1200 ml/min of kidney blood flow is filtered through the glomerulus, producing a daily filtration volume of 170 litres. The tubules are then responsible for selective reabsorption of almost all of this fluid. The filtration pressure within Bowman's capsule is equal to the arterial capillary blood pressure (70 mmHg), less both the osmotic pressure of the plasma proteins (25 mmHg) and the intratubular pressure (10 mmHg)—the net filtration pressure being of the order of 35 mmHg (Fig. 2.11c).

Renal Function

The main function of the tubular cells is to reabsorb selectively both fluid and electrolyte and to transfer them to the capillary network that surrounds the tubule and ultimately into the renal vein. Several processes exist within the tubule for the reabsorption of various constituents of the urine. The reabsorption of inorganic ions (e.g. sodium and potassium, and also substances such as glucose) is an active process requiring energy; these substances are reabsorbed at a rate that depends on the body's requirement. Reabsorption of water, on the other hand, is a

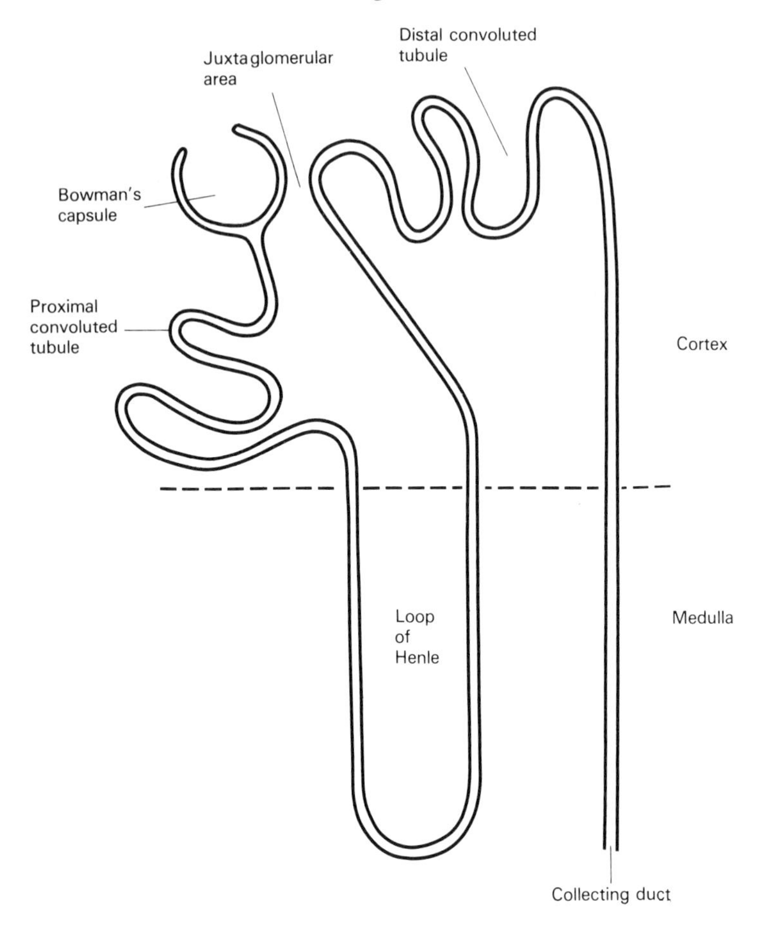

Fig. 2.8 Structure of cortical renal tubule

passive process and depends on the concentration gradient established by the active reabsorption of other ions. In this way, the proximal convoluted tubule is responsible for the coarse control of the urine volume and composition and it is left to the loop of Henle and the collecting duct, in the case of water reabsorption, and the distal convoluted tubule, in the case of ions, to produce the fine control over urine composition.

In addition to active and passive reabsorption from the tubules some substances are secreted by the tubules themselves, including some naturally occurring steroids and other glucuronides (products of metabolism) produced by the liver, hippuric acid and some drugs—for example, penicillin. Reabsorption of drugs from the tubule depends on their being in a fat-soluble form suitable for taking up the cells. This occurs only when the drug is in the un-ionised state. Acidic drugs are highly ionised in an alkaline medium and vice versa. In the case of an acidic drug, like aspirin, maintaining the urine alkaline—and therefore the aspirin—in an ionised form will prevent its reabsorption by the tubules. This explains the use of forced alkaline diuresis in the treatment of aspirin overdose. In normal circumstances the molecular weight of a substance determines whether or not it will diffuse across Bowman's capsule and into the tubule. The molecular threshold is about 70 000, which means that whereas substances like sodium, potassium, glucose, amino acids, urea, uric acid, creatinine and water are all small enough to pass into the tubular lumen, albumin, red cells, white cells and platelets are too large. Albumin with a molecular weight of 69 000 is just too large and this substance is the first to appear in the urine as an indication of kidney damage, however mild.

Loop of Henle

The loop of Henle and collecting duct systems are together responsible for the fine control of urine volume. This is achieved by the countercurrent mechanism, which depends on the fact that as the loop of Henle dips further into the medulla, more marked in the juxtamedullary than in the cortical nephrons, the surrounding tissue becomes progressively more concentrated. This increased concentration is effected by active reabsorption of sodium from the ascending loop of Henle, possibly under the influence of antidiuretic hormone. As more sodium is reabsorbed, the further down into the medulla the nephron passes the more concentrated the medullary tissue becomes. However, the ascending loop of Henle is normally impermeable to water, which is therefore reabsorbed only from the distal tubule and collecting ducts whose permeability to water reabsorption is under the control of antidiuretic hormone. As the collecting duct passes further down into the medulla, a greater volume of water is reabsorbed until ultimately the concentration of sodium in the urine equals that in the medullary tissue surrounding the tubule. This explains why the longer the juxtaglomerular loops of Henle are, the more water can be reabsorbed.

Distal Convoluted Tubule

Although the distal tubule is concerned only with the selective reabsorption of about one-eighth of the total ion content of the urine, it is this part of the nephron which produce fine control of urine volume and composition. As in the proximal tubule, active transport systems exist but, in addition, reabsorption is under the influence of two important hormones.

Aldosterone

A steroid hormone secreted by the zona glomerulosa of the adrenal cortex, stimulates reabsorption of sodium ions from the distal tubule in response to a low sodium concentration. In exchange for sodium, potassium ions are excreted and, conversely, reduced concentrations of aldosterone will reduce the extracellular sodium concentration. Water is also lost passively along the concentration gradient created by the sodium loss. Aldosterone secretion is stimulated by surgery, anxiety, trauma and haemorrhage and probably also by adrenocorticotrophic hormone (ACTH). In addition, aldosterone is released as part of the renin angiotensin system for maintaining blood pressure.

Antidiuretic Hormone (ADH, Vasopressin)

ADH is a peptide hormone produced by the posterior pituitary gland in response to two main stimuli:

1. A rise in the osmotic pressure of the plasma, which produces ADH release and therefore water retention. This is mediated via the osmoreceptors in the hypothalamus.
2. A fall in plasma volume detected by the volume receptors in the great thoracic veins and right atrium. In addition to these two primary stimuli, ADH release may be increased by stress, haemorrhage, shock, catecholamine release and also surgery and

certain anaesthetic agents, particularly ether, halothane and morphine.

Renin and Angiotensin System

In addition to its excretory role, the kidney exerts control over arterial blood pressure. This results from the juxtaglomerular apparatus sensing changes in renal arterial blood pressure. A fall in pressure promotes secretion of renin which converts an α-globulin (angiotensinogen) into angiotensin 1 which is, in turn, converted into angiotensin 2. Angiotensin 2 is a potent arteriolar vasoconstrictor that produces a widespread rise in systemic arterial blood pressure, thereby increasing renal perfusion pressure. It also stimulates the adrenal cortex to produce aldosterone which, in turn, increases extracellular fluid volume by sodium and water retention. Unilateral renal artery stenosis promotes renin secretion and is thought to be the cause of hypertension in this condition.

Autoregulation in the Renal Circulation

Quite apart from the renin angiotensin system, the renal circulation also exhibits the phenomenon of autoregulation. This is a property of the renal vasculature itself, and means that the kidney can maintain an adequate and constant blood flow despite changes in systemic arterial blood pressure within the range of 80–200 mmHg systolic. This is brought about by changes in renal vascular resistance in response to arterial pressure changes and is thought to be a local response of the vessels themselves and independent of hormonal influence. This phenomenon also exists in the cerebral and coronary circulations.

Erythropoietin

The rate of production of red blood cells by the bone marrow depends on the level of erythropoietin, a hormone which is formed by the action of a renal erythropoietic factor (REF) on a circulating globulin produced by the liver. The main stimulus to the release of this factor appears to hypoxia and, although it has been suggested that it is released from the juxtaglomerular apparatus, this is unrelated to the renin angiotensin system mentioned above. Hypoxia and haemorrhage stimulate erythropoietin production and, conversely, blood transfusion decreases the erythropoietic activity of the bone marrow.

FLUID AND ACID–BASE BALANCE

Man is about 70 % water, a 70 kg man having a fluid volume of about 45 litres (Fig. 2.9). This is divided between the intracellular and the extracellular space in a ratio of about 2:1, the intracellular fluid volume being 30 litres and the extracellular fluid volume 15 litres. The extracellular fluid is subdivided further into 12 litres of interstitial fluid and 3 litres of plasma.

The normal fluid balance of a 70 kg man involves the exchange of about 3000 ml of fluid per day. This is taken in by drinking, in food and in the metabolic activity of the body, particularly in the production of carbon dioxide and water from carbohydrate metabolism. Fluid is normally lost in the form of urine (1500 ml), through the skin (900 ml), in expired air (400 ml) and in the faeces (200 ml).

Fluid distributed throughout the body is an aqueous solution

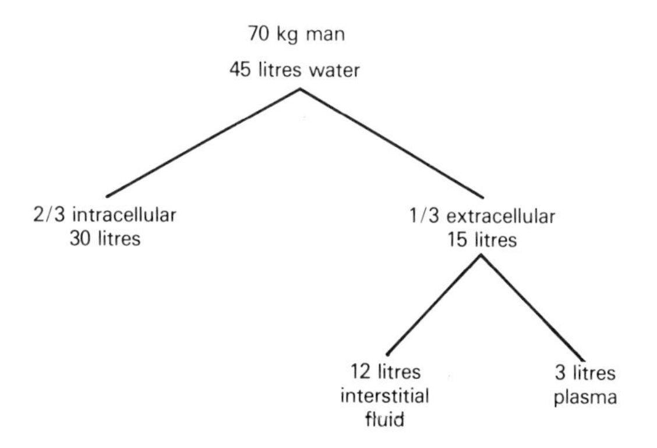

Fig. 2.9 Normal fluid balance of 70 kg man

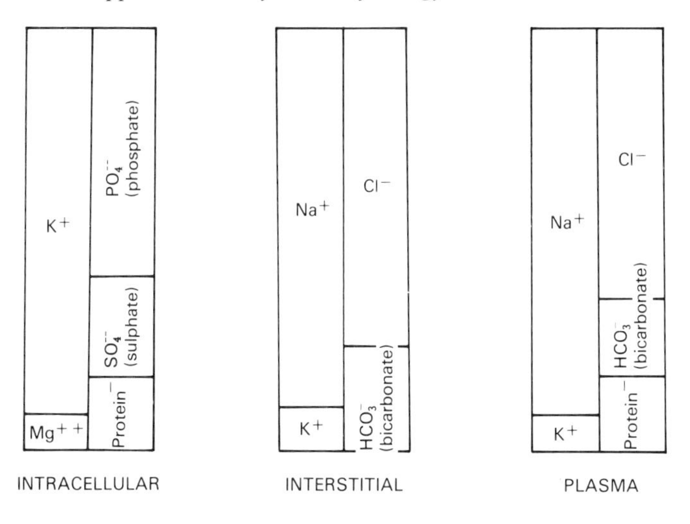

Fig. 2.10 Ionic distribution in body fluids

containing various amounts of positively and negatively charged ions (cations and anions). Their distribution is illustrated in Figure 2.10.

In addition to these there are some un-ionised substances—for example, glucose and urea. It is essential that a balance exists between anions and cations so that in plasma, for example, the numbers of sodium and potassium ions approximately balance the number of chloride and bicarbonate ions. Figure 2.10 shows that whereas potassium is present in far greater amounts within the cells, the intracellular sodium concentration is small and indeed sodium ions are excluded from the cells by an active process known as the 'sodium pump'. Only when cells are functioning inadequately or dead is sodium able to leak in and potassium to leak out. Sodium–potassium exchange is a temporary but integral part of nerve–impulse transmission.

Knowing that sodium is distributed only throughout the extracellular space—in other words 15 litres of body fluid—it is possible to estimate the degree of a total body sodium deficit. If, for example, the serum sodium concentration is 120 mmol instead of 140 mmol per litre, this implies that the body is deficient by 20 mmol per litre of body fluid, which contains sodium. In other words 20 × 15 mmol in all, i.e. 300 mmol sodium. A litre of normal saline contains 150 mmol, so in addition to his normal sodium requirement the patient requires

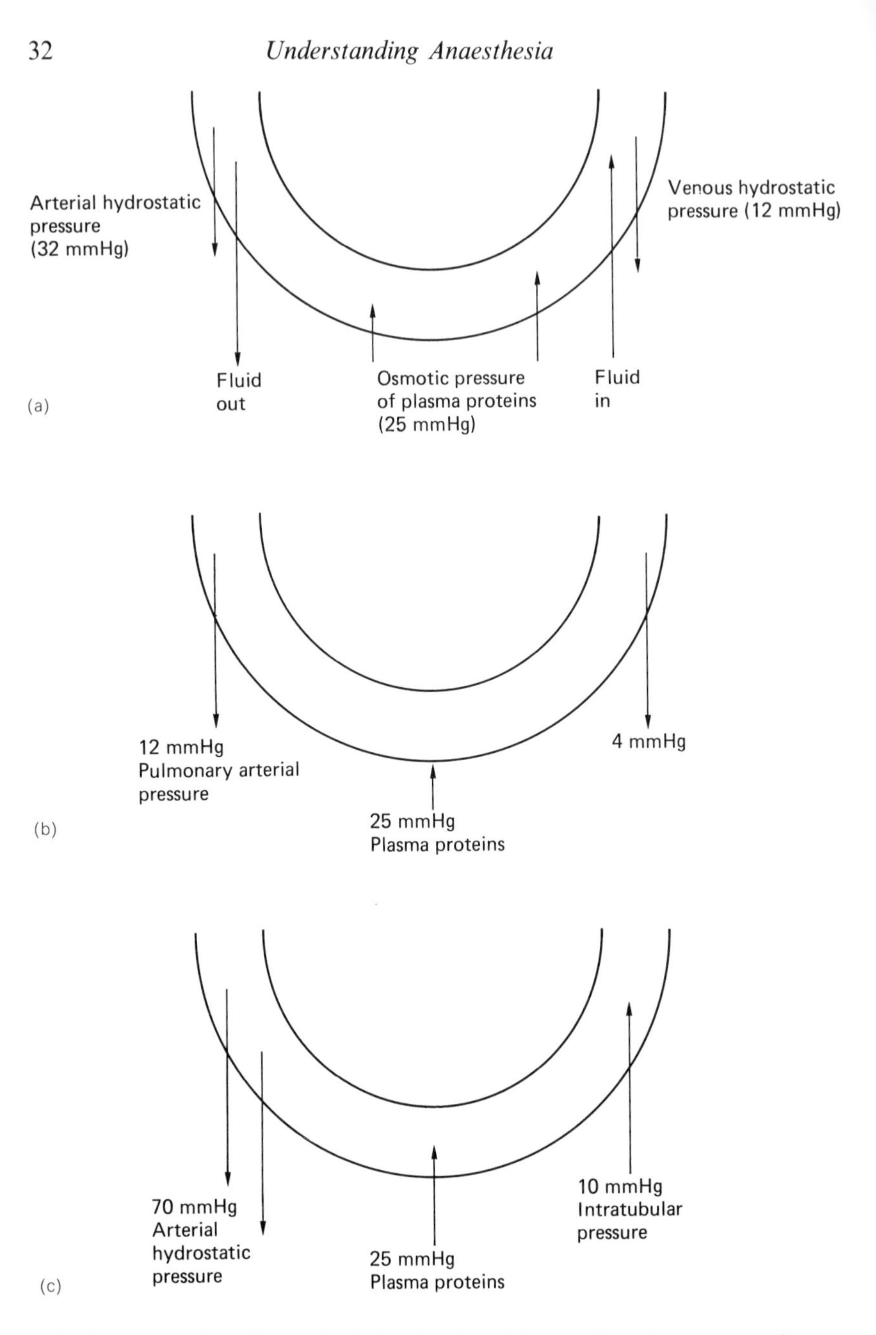

Fig. 2.11 Formation of tissue fluid: (a) Peripheral tissues, (b) pulmonary circulation, (c) glomerular filtration in the kidney

Table 2.4 Normal daily requirement of electrolytes

	mmol/day	g/day
Na^+	70–160	
K^+	50–80	
Ca^{++}	5–10	0·9–1·0
Sulphate		0·3–3·0
Phosphate		0·88
Nitrogen (amino acids)		15

2 litres of saline to restore his sodium depletion. Table 2.4 indicates the body's normal daily requirements for electrolytes.

Formation of Extracellular Fluid

The extracellular fluid compartment consists of both the plasma and the extravascular fluid in the ratio of about 3:12 litres. The ionic content of these two fluid compartments is similar, with the exception of plasma proteins, which are retained entirely intravascularly, and are responsible for the maintenance of intravascular fluid (*see* Fig. 2.10). They exert an osmotic pressure of about 25 mmHg, tending to retain fluid within the intravascular space. At the capillary level, Figure 2.11a illustrates how at the arterial end of the capillary the hydrostatic pressure, being greater than the osmotic pressure of the plasma proteins, tends to force fluid out of the capillaries, while at the venous end, where the osmotic pressure is greater than the hydrostatic pressure, the fluid re-enters the capillary.

In addition to this formation and removal by the blood vessels themselves the lymphatics are also present to reabsorb tissue fluid. A lack of plasma proteins, leading to a fall in the osmotic pressure, therefore tends to produce an increase in extravascular fluid (oedema), which may either occur in dependent parts such as the ankles or sacrum or, more seriously, in the lungs as pulmonary oedema. Under normal circumstances, the osmotic pressure of the plasma proteins (25 mmHg) greatly exceeds the net hydrostatic pressure in the pulmonary vascular bed (8 mmHg), but hypoproteinaemia or pulmonary hypertension will produce pulmonary oedema (Fig. 2.11b). Hence the maintenance of the colloidal osmotic pressure of the plasma is vital and may be augmented not only by giving plasma protein but also by other osmotically active substances, e.g. dextran, gelatin solutions and plasma protein fraction (PPF). The composition of plasma is illustrated in Figure 2.10. Apart from maintaining osmotic pressure, the main functions of the plasma proteins are to act as a temporary protein reserve to contribute towards blood viscosity and to act as buffers in maintaining acid–base balance.

Acid–Base Balance

Maintaining a constant ratio between acid and base (alkali) in the body is vital to the maintenance of normal pH within the physiological range of 7·38 to 7·42. This is mainly because many of the enzyme systems of the body function efficiently only at physiological pH; pH is an expression of the hydrogen ion (H^+) concentration or degree of acidity of the fluid, but because of the way in which it is derived a fall in pH (say, 7·4–7·2) represents a rise in hydrogen ion concentration and, since hydrogen ions are the active part of any acid, this produces an increase in acidosis. Conversely, a rise in pH represents a fall in hydrogen ion concentration and therefore an alkalosis. There are four, and only four, primary disorders of acid-base balance (Table 2.5) and these are either of respiratory or metabolic origin. The respiratory acid concerned is carbon dioxide which when combined with water forms carbonic acid. Failure to excrete carbon dioxide leads to respiratory acidosis, while overexcretion (e.g. overbreathing) leads to respiratory alkalosis. The most important metabolic acid is lactic acid, produced primarily by anaerobic cellular respiration. Lactic-acid accumulation produces a metabolic acidosis. Metabolic alkalosis is relatively rare and unimportant and is usually produced by abnormal ingestion of some alkali—e.g. aluminium hydroxide for peptic ulceration.

When faced with a primary problem of acid–base balance, the body's natural reaction is to try to compensate for this and the compensatory mechanisms represent the diametrically opposite acid-base state to that of the primary problem (Table 2.5). For example, a respiratory acidosis is compensated for by the body creating a metabolic alkalosis and a metabolic acidosis is com-

Table 2.5 Primary disorders of acid–base balance

Primary problem	Secondary compensation
Respiratory acidosis	Metabolic alkalosis
Respiratory alkalosis	Metabolic acidosis
Metabolic acidosis	Respiratory alkalosis
Metabolic alkalosis	Respiratory acidosis

pensated by the body producing a respiratory alkalosis. The following shows the fundamental biochemistry behind acid–base balance.

$$CO_2 + H_2O \rightleftarrows H_2CO_3\text{(carbonic acid)} \rightleftarrows H^+ + HCO_3^-\text{(bicarbonate, base, alkali)}$$

	LUNGS	KIDNEYS
	(fast compensation)	(slow compensation)

Carbon dioxide and water combine to form carbonic acid, a weak acid which dissociates within the body into hydrogen ions and bicarbonate ions. This reaction may proceed in either direction and the body has only two ways of correcting acid–base balance. The lungs can excrete or conserve carbon dioxide, a relatively rapid process because the brain can alter the respiratory rate to excrete or conserve carbon dioxide at very short notice. The kidneys, on the other hand, can excrete hydrogen ions (acid) or bicarbonate ions (HCO_3^-, alkali, base) selectively, but this is a relatively slow method of compensation requiring several hours to become established. The natural compensatory mechanism of the body is to use renal methods when the respiratory system is at fault, and the respiratory system when either the renal or other metabolic processes are at fault so that the kidneys eventually compensate for a respiratory acidosis by excreting abnormally large quantities of hydrogen ions.

Buffering Systems

Renal compensation takes several hours to become established, but it is vital that the pH of the body does not change. To prevent this there exists a system within the blood to buffer or minimise the pH change resulting from alterations in the concentrations of acid or base until the body is able to produce definitive compensation. It is remarkable and convenient that the principle buffering system which exists within the body again involves the carbon dioxide–bicarbonate system. The equation on p. 35 shows that carbon dioxide when dissolved in water produces hydrogen and bicarbonate ions. The following equation indicates the relationship between pH and the ratio of carbonic acid to bicarbonate, i.e. acid to base.

$$\text{pH} = \text{pK} + \log \frac{(\text{Base})}{(\text{Acid})} \quad \therefore \quad \text{pH} \quad \alpha \quad \frac{(\text{Bicarbonate})}{(\text{Carbonic acid})}$$

$$\text{pH} \quad \alpha \quad \frac{20}{1}$$

In normal circumstances the ratio of base to acid is about 20:1, so there is considerable reserve of base over acid that can neutralise the addition of any acid and thus prevent a change in pH. Provided that the kidneys definitively excrete the excess acid within the space of a few hours, thus allowing the bicarbonate reserve to be regenerated, this buffering system works excellently. In addition, man constantly produces both hydrogen and bicarbonate ions as part of normal cellular respiration, and if the kidneys selectively excrete hydrogen ions and conserve bicarbonate as necessary, the buffering system of the blood is maintained. Both the plasma proteins and haemoglobin are also able to absorb hydrogen ions temporarily, thus providing extra buffering capacity to the blood. This system therefore is capable of resisting change in pH in the short term until the body is able to excrete or conserve the relative acid or base to compensate for the metabolic insult.

Interpretation of Acid–Base/Blood Gas Results

Most laboratories supply their results in the following form:

pH
$P\text{CO}_2$
base deficit
standard bicarbonate
$P\text{O}_2$
oxygen saturation

In order to interpret acid–base balance it is vital to know whether the patient has been treated or is simply compensating for his own metabolic disorder. In an untreated patient the pH represents the primary problem, thus if the pH is acid the patient has a primary acidosis, though this may be either respiratory or metabolic in origin or a mixture of both. If the arterial $P\text{CO}_2$ is above normal in the case of a primary acidosis then the patient must have a respiratory acidosis, either on its own or as part of a mixed respiratory and metabolic acidosis. The $P\text{CO}_2$ therefore indicates the respiratory component of the acidosis.

The metabolic component is derived from the standard bicarbonate. By definition, the standard bicarbonate is the bicarbonate concentration of the blood when the $P\text{CO}_2$ of the blood has been corrected to normal, in other words so that there is no respiratory component to the bicarbonate concentration. The standard bicarbonate is normally 25 mmol per litre. The base refers to the amount of bicarbonate in excess of (base excess) or less than (base deficit) the standard figure of 25. If the base excess is -10, this represents a bicarbonate level of 15 mmol per litre. Since the bicarbonate we are considering is free bicarbonate, from the equations a fall in free bicarbonate must imply that a proportion of the remainder has been used to combine with free hydrogen ions; a fall in bicarbonate represents compensation for an acidosis. Hence the combination of standard bicarbonate and base deficit or excess indicates the degree of the metabolic component of the acidosis or alkalosis.

In addition to the interpretation of acid–base data, and sometimes more importantly, an arterial blood gas sample provides information as to the state of gas exchange within the lungs. This is done by measuring the $P\text{CO}_2$ and $P\text{O}_2$ levels (P representing the partial pressure of these gases in the arterial blood). Measurement of both these values within the normal range obviously indicates satisfactory lung function. Since oxygen diffuses across the alveolar membrane less readily than carbon dioxide, when this function is partially impaired, hypoxia, resulting from inadequate saturation of the haemoglobin (indicated by a fall from the normally 95–100 % oxygen saturation of haemoglobin), may well occur despite a normal level of $P\text{CO}_2$.

Measurement of arterial blood gases

In the past the only available electrode for acid–base and blood–gas measurement was a pH electrode and for this reason, although pH itself could be measured directly, $P\text{CO}_2$ had to be inferred from the actual pH of the blood. Nowadays, however, individual electrodes, sensitive either to pH, $P\text{CO}_2$ and $P\text{O}_2$, are commonly used in automatic blood–gas analysis.

3 Haematology and Blood Transfusion

Red blood cells. White blood cells. Platelets. Coagulation of blood. Fibrinolysis. Anticoagulants. Plasma. Prevention of deep venous thrombosis. Transfusion of blood. Blood grouping and crossmatching. Practical aspects of blood transfusion. Hazards of blood transfusion. Massive blood transfusion. Other blood products. Dextran. Gelatin solutions (Haemaccel, Gelofusine). Hetastarch (Hespan).

The circulating blood volume of a 70 kg adult is 5 litres, 1 litre of which is contained in the heart, arterial and capillary circulations, 1 litre within the pulmonary circulation and 3 litres in the venous circulation. Blood is a suspension of cells in plasma, the overall volume of the cells being about 45 % of the total blood volume.

RED BLOOD CELLS

The normal red blood cell count is 5 million per cubic millimetre, each cell having a life of about 120 days. A significant proportion of cells within a 3-week-old unit of transfused blood will therefore have reached the end of their useful lives. Red cells are formed from reticulo-endothelial cells in the bone marrow, the immediate precursor being the reticulocyte. In cases of high marrow activity after haemorrhage, a significant reticulocyte count may occur in the peripheral blood. The main function of the red blood cells is to transport oxygen in combination with the haemoglobin inside the cell. This is a protein of molecular weight 67 000 which combines with oxygen in the lungs and gives up oxygen in the peripheral tissues. (Further details of oxygen carriage are discussed in Chapter 2, p. 15) Cyanosis is the name given to the blue appearance of tissues resulting from de-oxygenated blood circulating through them. At least 5 g of reduced haemoglobin are necessary for cyanosis to be present; this condition is therefore extremely rare in anaemia and not pathological in situations of high red cell counts such as polycythaemia.

Red blood cells are removed from the circulation by the reticulo-endothelial system in the bone marrow, liver and spleen. The cellular protein and haemoglobin are broken down to amino acids, which are re-used in the body together with the iron which is stored as ferritin. The remainder of the haem molecule is converted to bilirubin and biliverdin, which combine with glucuronic acid in the liver and are excreted into the bowel. Interruption of bile pigment excretion leads to jaundice.

WHITE BLOOD CELLS

The normal white blood cell count is 5–10 000 cells/mm^3. Unlike the red cells, white cells exist in several different forms. The polymorphonuclear leucocytes (granulocytes) comprise about 70 % of the white cell count. These are subdivided according to their staining characteristics into basophils (1 %), eosinophils (3 %) and neutrophils (66 %). The neutrophils are phagocytes, able to engulf and remove foreign particles and bacteria from the blood, and are the main defence mechanism of the body against infection. Eosinophils are increased in allergic conditions such as asthma and hay fever and the basophils are thought to be circulating mast cells capable of releasing histamine.

The lymphocytes, comprising 25 % of the total white cell count, are divided into large and small types and are involved in the production of antibodies, which combine with and neutralise foreign substances known as antigens. Lymphocytes therefore provide a memory system of protection for the body against unwanted substances. The excessive formation of antibodies in this way is responsible for several hypersensitivity reactions to drugs (Chapter 24). In normal circumstances antibodies combine with foreign antigens to neutralise them and therefore prevent their effects, but in some conditions excessive antigen and antibody combination may release histamine or similar substances resulting in a hypersensitive reaction. These reactions sometimes occur in response to intravenous administration of certain anaesthetics, in particular induction agents and muscle relaxants.

The remaining white blood cells, 5–6 % of the total, are monocytes, another group of phagocytic cells.

PLATELETS

The normal platelet count is 250 000/mm^3, thrombocytopenia being the name given to a pathological reduction in the amount of platelets circulating in the peripheral blood. Their main function is to aggregate at the site of injury, causing a plug and preventing capillary bleeding. Their subsequent breakdown may release vasoconstrictive amines such as 5-hydroxytryptamine, producing local vasoconstriction and again preventing bleeding. Platelet consumption during severe bleeding may reduce their circulating numbers. This is common in massive blood transfusion when the normal clotting factors and the platelet count are both exhausted. Transfusion of fresh frozen plasma containing clotting factors and platelets themselves may be necessary to arrest haemorrhage. In normal circumstances a platelet count of 60 000 is sufficient to prevent pathological haemorrhage. The clumping of platelets forming a platelet plug is enhanced by two factors in the coagulation cascade of the body, and platelet breakdown yields a further platelet factor which is important in blood coagulation.

COAGULATION OF BLOOD

In normal circumstances a balance is maintained in the body between coagulation and clot breakdown (fibrinolysis). Blood

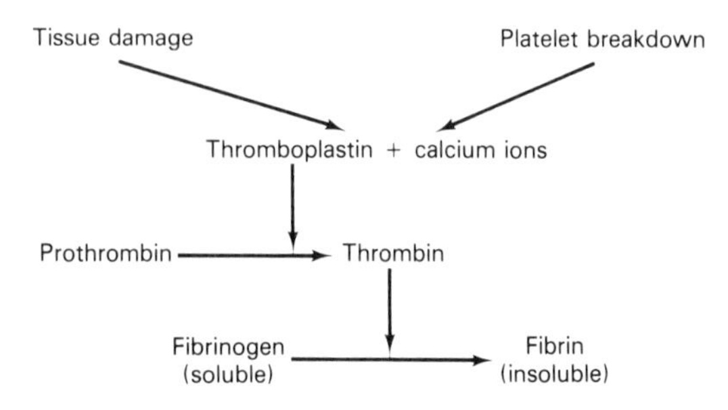

Fig. 3.1 Normal coagulation 'cascade'

clots are formed when the plasma protein fibrinogen changes into insoluble fibrin which, in turn, traps red cells and platelets to form a blood clot. The clotting factors are present in plasma, which will produce a clot without the presence of blood cells. Fibrinogen changes into insoluble fibrin under the influence of thrombin which in the presence of calcium ions, is produced by the action of thromboplastin on prothrombin (Fig. 3.1). Tissue damage (the extrinsic coagulation system) and platelet breakdown (intrinsic system) both release thromboplastin, which initiates the coagulation cascade. The presence of certain factors is also necessary for the system to work efficiently, and the absence of certain other factors produces coagulation disorders —for example, factor VIII, the anti-haemophilic factor is absent in haemophilia. Prothrombin is made in the liver and vitamin K is necessary for its production. Absence of vitamin K (e.g. in cases of liver damage and jaundice) may affect coagulation. Heparin, as a prothrombin antagonist, is itself indirectly antagonised by vitamin K.

FIBRINOLYSIS

The fibrinolytic system is the natural remover of unwanted blood clot and platelet aggregates, and acts by dissolving the fibrin network and producing fibrin degradation products. Activation of a circulating protein (plasminogen) is produced by tissue or blood activators, which in a similar cascade to the coagulation process enhance conversion of plasminogen to plasmin, the

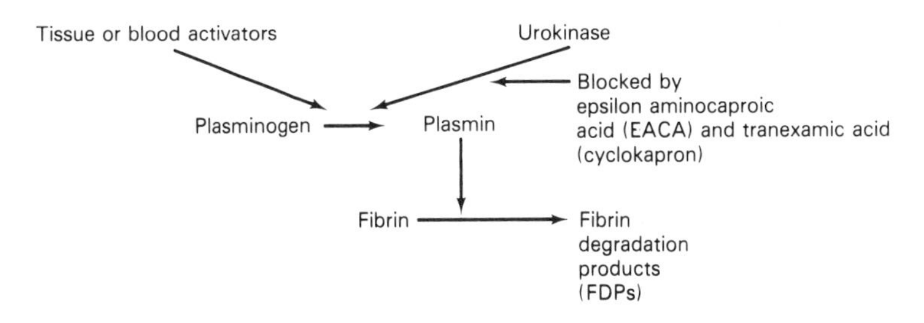

Fig. 3.2 Normal fibrinolytic 'cascade'

substance responsible for fibrin breakdown. Pathological fibrinolysis (Fig. 3.2) may occur in response to certain circulating fibrinolysins (e.g. urokinase released by the prostate) and may be prevented by antifibrinolytic agents such as epsilon aminocaproic acid (EACA) or tranexamic acid (cyclokapron).

Disseminated Intravascular Coagulation (DIC)

This disease of intravascular coagulation may be associated with many conditions, e.g. severe haemorrhage, pancreatitis, drug overdose, Mendelson's syndrome, or after major surgery and cardiopulmonary bypass. Abnormal coagulation occurs within the microcirculation using up the available clotting factors and reducing peripheral flow. This results in many of the presenting symptoms related to malfunction of organs such as lung, kidney, liver and brain. Subsequent proliferation of intravascular coagulation produces reduced efficiency of normal coagulation and profuse bleeding due to excessive consumption of fibrinogen and platelets. The correct treatment is to prevent further coagulation by anticoagulating the patient with heparin. This treatment may seem illogical, but it prevents further consumption of coagulation factors and allows restoration of normal clotting function.

ANTICOAGULANTS

These drugs are given to antagonise the normal clotting mechanisms in the blood, either to prevent pathological thrombosis after venous stasis and surgery or to prevent blood clot forming on, for example, artificial heart valves after operation. The two main anticoagulants are heparin and warfarin.

Heparin

Heparin is a naturally occurring anticoagulant—produced by mast cells—which forms a reversible combination with plasma proteins, the complex preventing the action of thrombin on fibrinogen. The action of heparin is antagonised by protamine but also naturally in the body by the enzyme heparinase. The duration of action of heparin is therefore only four to six hours and repeat doses or intravenous infusion are necessary to maintain full anticoagulation. Heparin is used to prevent thrombosis and embolism and has an immediate anticoagulant effect. Its use allows stabilisation of anticoagulation before more prolonged treatment with warfarin.

Warfarin

This anticoagulant acts by combination with vitamin K in the liver, inhibiting prothrombin synthesis. The onset of action is 24 to 48 hours before full anticoagulation is achieved. The action of warfarin is antagonised by vitamin K but, again, this is a slow process. Phenindione (Dindevan) acts as an anticoagulant in a similar way to warfarin.

Protamine

This ionic antagonist of heparin is used when rapid reversal of the anticoagulant effects are required. Normal physiological reversal of heparin anticoagulation takes between four and six hours and protamine is useful, for example, after cardiopulmonary bypass or renal dialysis when local heparinisation is used to prevent coagulation. Rapid infusion of protamine sulphate may cause myocardial depression and hypotension, so this drug should be given slowly by intravenous infusion rather than as a bolus dose.

PLASMA

Plasma comprises 55 % of the blood volume and is essentially a solution of electrolytes, mainly sodium chloride and bicarbonate in water, which also contains plasma proteins. Plasma is involved in the carriage of blood cells and oxygen, the maintenance of acid–base balance and the transfer of gaseous and metabolic waste products to the lungs and kidneys. Apart from its electrolyte content the plasma proteins form an essential part of this solution. Two of these proteins, albumin and globulin, are present in large quantities, while two others, prothrombin and fibrinogen, are present in smaller quantities. The globulin fraction of the plasma is largely responsible for maintaining immunity and antibody production (immunoglobulins), while the albumin is the protein most responsible for combination both with drugs and metabolic products.

Main Functions of Plasma Proteins

Maintenance of osmotic pressure
The presence of high molecular weight substances within the plasma produces an osmotic pressure intravascularly, tending to draw fluid into the blood vessels. This is essential for the prevention of oedema, hypoproteinaemia being associated with peripheral oedema and fluid leak into the tissues (*see* Fig. 2.11a).

Protein reserve
Although the body's need for protein cannot be met for more than a few hours by the metabolism of plasma proteins, these may provide a reserve during periods of excessive demands by the liver as a result of energetic exercise.

Buffering activity
The plasma proteins act as a buffer by combining with both acids and alkalis. As discussed in Chapter 2, the maintenance of normal plasma pH is essential to body function, and the plasma proteins provide an additional buffering system to that of the bicarbonate/carbonic acid system.

Viscosity
Due to its viscous nature the resistance to blood flow is governed by the plasma proteins and the cellular elements of the blood. Optimum blood viscosity is essential for adequate peripheral blood flow through tissues.

Carriage of Drugs within the Plasma

When drugs are injected or absorbed into the bloodstream they are almost entirely carried in the plasma to their sites of action. The active part of any drug is that which is in free solution within the plasma, while that in combination with plasma proteins is inactive. The degree of protein binding of drugs therefore governs their activity and, more important still, if two protein-bound drugs are administered simultaneously one may displace the other from the plasma proteins, thereby potentiating its action. An example of this is when a diabetic patient, established on oral hypoglycaemic drugs, is given aspirin, which is also protein-bound. This may displace the hypoglycaemic drug from the plasma proteins and produce excessive hypoglycaemia by increasing the relative amount of free drug within the plasma. There are several other examples of drug interaction due to competition for plasma protein binding and simultaneous drug therapy is often difficult to control and predict.

PREVENTION OF DEEP VENOUS THROMBOSIS (DVT)

The methods available are divided into pharmacological and mechanical, the latter being further divided into active and passive. The use of elasticated TED stockings reduces the volume of blood within the leg, preventing venous pooling and therefore thrombosis. Active intermittent calf compression using pneumatic leggings not only increases venous return and reduces pooling, but also activates fibrinolysis.

Pharmacological methods of DVT prevention include the infusion of dextran 70, 500 ml every 24 hours until the patient is fully mobile or subcutaneous heparin (Minihep), 5000 units every 8 or 12 hours over a similar period. Probably the most effective method, which should routinely be used for all high risk patients and those on the oral contraceptive pill is to combine TED stockings with a Minihep regimen.

TRANSFUSION OF BLOOD

The transfusion of blood and blood products is now widely used in anaesthetic practice, the availability of adequate supplies of whole blood being an essential part of major surgery. Although several other solutions are available for fluid and electrolyte replacement during surgery, none at present has the ability to carry oxygen in adequate amounts throughout the body. In some animals transfusions may be administered from one to another without blood grouping or crossmatching, but in man blood contains certain factors connected with the red cells which may make them incompatible with the cells from another individual; samples both from the donor and the recipient must therefore be checked for compatibility.

BLOOD GROUPING AND CROSSMATCHING

The four major blood groups identified in man are O, A, B and AB, present in 46 %, 42 %, 9 % and 3 % of the population, respectively. Patients belong to one or other group depending on the presence or absence of agglutinogens A and B on the surface of the red cells. Group A individuals have agglutinogen A on the surface of their red cells, while those with agglutinogen A and B belong to group AB and those with neither A nor B belong to group O.

Blood plasma contains agglutinins anti-A and anti-B which when combined with the appropriate agglutinogen, will cause agglutination of the red cells. Agglutinin anti-A is present in the plasma of group B and O, while anti-B is found in group A and group O. Group AB has neither anti-A nor anti-B agglutinins in the plasma and therefore does not possess any factor likely to cause blood group incompatibility by agglutination. Group AB patients are therefore known as universal recipients. Although group O blood contains both anti-A and anti-B, by the time these agglutinins are diluted after transfusion into a patient with normal blood volume, the amounts in the plasma will be insufficient to cause agglutination. Group O is therefore known as universal donor blood.

Routine crossmatching procedures include grouping the patient's blood, using sera containing anti-A or anti-B, and subsequently incubating samples of both donor and recipient blood together to look for signs of agglutination. Blood grouping also involves the detection and compatibility of various minor agglutinogens, C, D and E, the most important of which is D —the Rhesus factor. Patients with factor D (about 85 % of the population) are said to be Rhesus-positive. Unlike the ABC system, patients do not possess anti-D until they have been sensitised by exposure to blood containing factor D. If they are then Rhesus-negative they will manufacture anti-D which will produce agglutination upon subsequent exposure to factor D. This means that it is always possible to transfuse patients who are Rhesus-positive with Rhesus-negative blood, but if the patient has already been sensitised, the reverse is impossible. Universal donor blood is therefore not only group O, but also Rhesus-negative.

Since the agglutinogens A and B are present only on the surface of red cells, blood grouping and crossmatching is necessary only when transfusions of blood are being given. Plasma and other blood products may be given without crossmatching procedures without risk of agglutination.

PRACTICAL ASPECTS OF BLOOD TRANSFUSION

Storage

Whole blood should not be left at room temperature for longer than is necessary to complete the transfusion, this normally being within a maximum of five to six hours. Blood required for transfusion should either be placed in a refrigerator specifically designed for the purpose and maintained at 4°C, or transferred in specially designed cool containers for immediate use in theatre.

Checking

A systematic check of each unit of blood is vital before administration. This should be preceded by a check that the patient's blood group has been established, by reference to the identification label attached to the patient and not to the notes. The blood transfusion form must contain adequate data for identification with the patient concerned and simultaneously with the blood to be transfused. The correct procedure is for two people to cross-check the form with the patient, and then each bag of blood against the form. Of particular importance are the blood groups of both the patient and the crossmatched blood, the date of expiry of the blood (normally three weeks after collection), the patient's identification attached to the bag of blood and, finally, the appropriate number of the bag. Scrupulous attention to these details will avoid mistakes which may be fatal.

Administration of Blood

Blood is normally administered through a peripheral drip at a rate of 500 ml over a maximum of five to six hours. Considerable variation may occur, of course, when patients are being transfused in theatre or in response to considerable blood loss, and in this event not only must the blood be carefully checked but certain other precautions should also be taken. Since the blood will be cool the use of a warming coil and water bath to allow the transfusion to be given at body temperature will prevent cooling of the patient.

The use of microfilters in addition to the normal filter within the intravenous administration set will prevent considerable quantities of broken red cells and aggregates of white cells and platelets from reaching the patient and being deposited within the small capillaries of the lung. These filters are relatively cheap

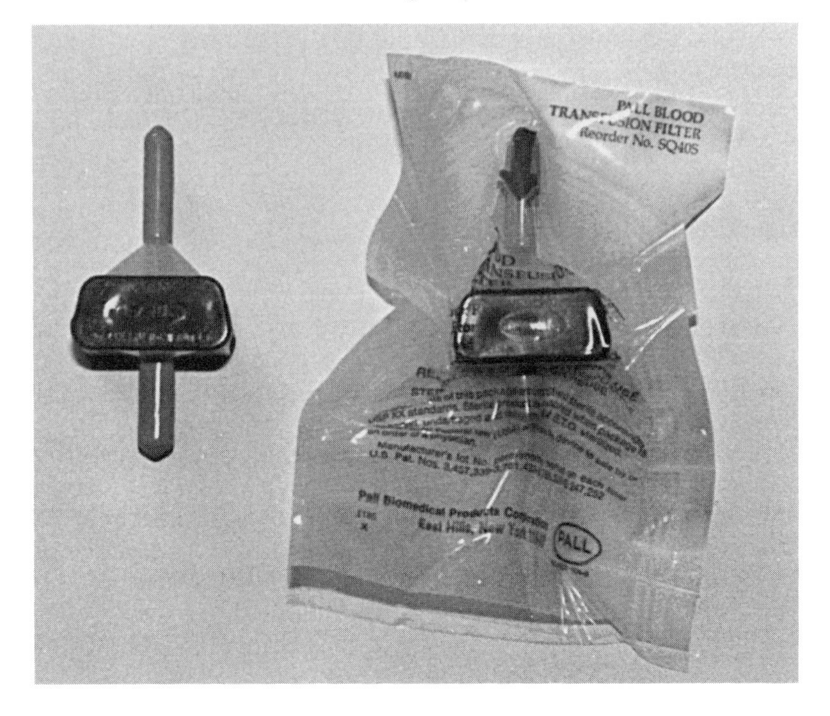

Fig. 3.3. Screen-type blood microfilter

and should be used wherever possible. Although opinions on the use of blood microfilters vary, their ability to reduce or prevent transfusion of microemboli is not in question. Two main types of filter exist. The screen filter e.g. Pall Ultipor (Fig. 3.3) is simply a mesh with a pore size of 20 μm, which tends to clog up with use, but is very efficient. Depth filters have an *average* pore size of 20 μm and rely on adsorption. They tend to become less efficient with use as their adsorptive capacity is reduced. It has been shown that pressurising blood through filters, particularly the screen types, results in significant histamine release, and this practice is not now recommended.

HAZARDS OF BLOOD TRANSFUSION

The scrupulous detail attached to every aspect of blood grouping and crossmatching by the National Blood Transfusion Service has minimised complications of blood transfusion caused by mismatching. Nevertheless, these do occur occasionally and may result in appreciable and serious degrees of intravascular coagulation if not detected early. Minor and relatively subclinical reactions to blood transfusion may occur more frequently, manifested usually as tachycardia, flushing, pyrexia or skin rashes. In this event, intravenous chlorpheniramine (Piriton), an antihistamine, may be used to alleviate symptoms. In all cases where transfusion reaction is suspected, the transfusion should be stopped and a sample of the patient's blood should be returned with the transfused blood to the laboratory. Serious agglutination and capillary blockage may cause severe pain—usually in the abdomen or loin—and subsequent haemolysis of the cells will produce haemoglobinuria and renal failure.

Blood transfusions may also lead to cross-infection, particularly of conditions such as hepatitis and syphilis, though these are prevented by modern screening methods within the National Blood Transfusion Service. All donated blood is now also routinely screened for HIV antibody, although this may still be negative in a recently infected individual in whom insufficient time for antibody production has passed. Other infective complications may arise around the transfusion site, but these are rarely serious.

MASSIVE BLOOD TRANSFUSION

With the exception of mismatching and infection, most complications of blood transfusion occur as a result of large quantities of blood being given too quickly. Massive blood transfusion is defined as the transfusion of half a patient's blood volume within an hour and may produce several complications. Stored blood inevitably contains not only intact red cells but broken cells, platelet aggregates, white cell aggregates and other debris. In addition, stored blood is depleted in 2–3 diphosphoglycerate (2–3 DPG) necessary for optimum oxygen carriage, and this takes several days to be restored. Blood is collected into bags which already contain an anticoagulant, either acid–citrate–dextrose (ACD) or citrate–phosphate–dextrose (CPD). In both cases the clotting factors in the blood will be depleted, as both platelets and fibrinogen are viable for only 24 to 48 hours after collection.

Hypothermia

Blood stored at 4°C needs to be warmed to body temperature by using a warming coil attached to the intravenous infusion set to avoid progressive hypothermia with large transfusions and, in particular, acute cooling of the heart.

Filtration

Microfilters prevent debris accumulating within the microcirculation of the lungs and are essential during massive transfusion.

Serum Potassium

Cellular breakdown within stored blood inevitably increases the serum potassium concentrations. Although these rarely produce pathological hyperkalaemia, ECG monitoring is essential to detect early signs, particularly peaked T-waves.

Citrate Toxicity

The citrate used as an anticoagulant in stored blood combines with calcium within the patient and may produce serious reductions in the serum calcium concentration. This occurs only with rapid and large blood transfusions but requires intravenous calcium therapy to prevent the effects of hypocalcaemia, particularly on the myocardium. During a massive transfusion 10 ml 10 % calcium gluconate should be administered with every fourth unit of blood.

Metabolic Acidosis

Anaerobic respiration in red cells in stored blood, together with the acid anticoagulants used, inevitably means that large transfusions will produce a metabolic acidosis. Patients may be able to compensate for this, but impaired cardiac function is an indication for correction with bicarbonate. This should not be done overenthusiastically because one of the end products of citrate metabolism within the liver is bicarbonate, and massive transfusion may produce a metabolic alkalosis on the first or second postoperative day.

Coagulation Disorders

The lack of normal clotting factors and platelets within stored blood may result in severe depletion and bleeding during surgery, particularly when the available factors are being consumed at a rapid rate. Pathological consumption of clotting factors in the form of disseminated intravascular coagulation may also occur as a side-effect of massive blood transfusion. Clotting factors may be replaced by the transfusion of fresh frozen plasma or platelets and this should always be contemplated towards the end of the operation or immediately afterwards when haemostasis has been achieved or when it is causing problems.

Circulatory Overload

Massive transfusion is best carried out in conjunction with central venous pressure monitoring to give some indication of the degree of transfusion required. Massive blood loss is often difficult to assess and, particularly in older people with poor cardiac reserve, acute heart failure and pulmonary oedema are easily precipitated after transfusion.

OTHER BLOOD PRODUCTS

Although the replacement of blood lost during surgery is best achieved with whole blood, many transfusion centres now issue either plasma-reduced blood or packed cells from which the plasma has been used to prepare other blood fractions such as platelets or clotting factors. The use of concentrated red cells is particularly advantageous when patients require pre-operative transfusions. They have a normal blood volume but a reduced red cell level and therefore haemoglobin concentration, and do not require transfusion of plasma as well as blood.

Due to the risks of transmitting infection, transfusion of dried plasma is now almost obsolete in the UK, but human plasma protein fraction (HPPF) or human albumin solution (HAS) are widely used. Essentially, both are pasteurised plasma, heated to 60 °C to destroy both potential infection and antigens but not to denature the plasma proteins. In this form it is particularly useful when the plasma volume requires expansion in place of an adequate or high red cell content.

SAGM Blood

It is now generally accepted that unless whole blood is specifically necessary, stored blood is supplied either in a plasma reduced form or as red cells resuspended in SAGM (saline–adenine–glucose–mannitol). This new additive is *not* an anticoagulant but will prolong the life of stored red cells, making them suitable for use for four or even five weeks after donation. The blood is still collected into citrate–phosphate–dextrose (CPD) as an anticoagulant and so the potential complications related to this will not be prevented. If surgical blood loss is to be replaced with SAGM blood, it may be necessary simultaneously to replace plasma losses with either HAS or a volume expander such as Haemaccel.

DEXTRAN

This polysaccharide (sugar) solution is used as a plasma volume expander. The numbers (40, 70, 110) after the name refer to the average molecular weight of the dextran molecules in thousands. Thus dextran 70 with a molecular weight of 70 000 resembles serum albumin. Normally, albumin is not excreted by the kidney (though in sickness albuminuria is an early feature), implying that the renal molecular threshold is about 65–70 000. The transfusion of dextran therefore results not only in expansion of the intravascular volume by 500 ml, but also, by increasing the osmotic pressure of the plasma, tends to draw additional fluid into the intravascular space. Dextran 70 will not be excreted through the kidneys until the molecules are broken down and become smaller. Dextran 40 will remain within the circulation for a shorter time, but because it is less viscous than plasma containing plasma proteins, will reduce blood viscosity, and is used to increase peripheral blood flow in vascular disease. Dextran 70 also has an antiplatelet action that prevents aggregation, and is therefore used in the prophylaxis of deep venous thrombosis. The dextrans, however, do not contain oxygen, can only be given up to a maximum of 1 litre per day and interfere with blood crossmatching. They may produce hypersensitivity reactions, especially in patients with an allergic tendency, e.g. asthmatics. Their use should be confined to those who need blood-volume expansion without red cells or as an emergency when blood is not available.

GELATIN SOLUTIONS (HAEMACCEL, GELOFUSINE)

Haemaccel and Gelofusine are gelatin solutions of average molecular weight 30 000, and are often used in place of dextran. Their molecular size means that they are not retained within the blood vessels for as long as dextran 70 but are useful as plasma volume expanders. They are also increasingly used in conjunction with SAGM suspended red blood cells for the replacement of whole blood loss during surgery. Haemaccel has a longer shelf life than dextran, so is more useful in major accident packs where prolonged storage may be required. Hypersensitivity reactions of similar frequency to dextran have been reported and these agents should therefore be used with caution.

HETASTARCH (HESPAN)

This hydroxyethyl starch solution has recently become available in the UK. Its large molecular weight (450 000) makes it considerably longer acting than either the dextran or gelatin solutions. It may have considerable advantages in the treatment of massive haemorrhage in a patient with multiple injuries but, by remaining in the circulation for a long time, may delay the subsequent administration of blood, if circulatory overload is to be avoided.

4 Premedication

Aims of premedication. Groups of drugs used. Premedication for different age groups. Emla cream 5%.

In the first part of this chapter the aims of premedication are listed, and its place in modern anaesthesia examined in detail. Next some of the groups of drugs used for premedication are discussed and, finally, a possible scheme of premedication for the various age groups is presented.

AIMS OF PREMEDICATION

Drying of Salivary and Bronchial Secretions

The drying up of salivary secretions has long been considered as one of the main purposes of premedication. Drugs that have this action are called 'antisialogogues'. These agents also tend to have a similar effect on bronchial secretions.

Antisialogogue drugs were introduced in the days when anaesthesia was laboriously induced by inhalational methods. Some agents (e.g. di-ethyl ether), if not expertly administered, could cause copious outpouring of secretions. This made it difficult to get the patient down to deeper planes of anaesthesia and the whole procedure could be stormy, tedious and frightening.

Not only has the introduction of intravenous anaesthetic agents and muscle relaxants made the induction of anaesthesia speedier and smoother, but some modern inhalational agents (e.g. halothane) tend to dry up secretions. Some patients find the dry mouth caused by the premedication uncomfortable by the time they arrive in the anaesthetic room and, in the postoperative period, this antisialogogue effect may for a time make sputum viscid and difficult to expectorate.

In modern anaesthetic conditions, then, if antisialogogues are not essential, why are they still so routinely prescribed? The fact that it is a habit of many years may be to some extent responsible, but there are times when the drying of secretions is important and, because these are not all predictable, many anaesthetists still routinely prescribe a drying agent. For example, before operations on the mouth and nose a reduction in secretions is desirable as their sudden outpouring may obscure the surgical field. In the same way, prolonged use of the laryngoscope when intubation is difficult may lead to excessive salivation. Less predictably, some patients, when given an intravenous induction, almost immediately develop laryngeal stridor or begin to cough. Whether this is initiated by secretions getting on to the vocal cords or through an irritant effect of the intravenous agent is difficult to establish but the problem is perpetuated by the excessive production of salivary and bronchial secretions which results. This problem arises more commonly in smokers and bronchitics, who have irritable respiratory tracts, but it can occur in anyone. It is largely for these reasons that an antisialogogue is still commonly prescribed as part of the premedication.

Reduction of Anxiety

The most important factor in reducing patient anxiety is not the administration of drugs but the pre-operative visit by the anaesthetist. Nevertheless, many patients prefer to have some sedation before arriving in the anaesthetic room and a wide variety of drugs are used for this purpose. The degree of sedation (or, indeed, whether it is advisable at all) depends on many factors, including the general state of the patient, whether the case is an emergency, whether the anaesthetic is to deliver a baby, how important it is that the patient regains consciousness quickly after the anaesthetic and whether the patient is intending to go home the same day.

Prevention of Vagal Reflexes

The term 'vagal inhibition' is often used to describe a syndrome in which there is overaction of the cardiac vagus resulting in bradycardia or even asystole. Many different surgical and anaesthetic stimuli are thought to be capable of providing the afferent side of this reflex arc, including traction on any intra-abdominal mesentery, dilation of the anus, traction on the extra-ocular eye muscles and stimulation of the upper respiratory tract with laryngoscope, endotracheal tube, sucker, or even high concentrations of anaesthetic vapours. It is more likely to happen if the patient already has a bradycardia as is often associated with the taking of β-adrenergic blocking drugs or other antihypertensive treatment, or the administration of halothane or enflurane. It is also more likely if there is some associated detrimental factor, especially hypoxia or hypercarbia.

Atropine administered subcutaneously or intramuscularly, in doses usually used for premedication, produces blood levels that are so low as to be almost ineffective in blocking these vagal reflexes. To produce any worthwhile vagal blocking effect atropine must, in an adult, be given intravenously in a dose of 0·6 mg upwards.

Aid to Anaesthesia

All general anaesthesia consists of narcosis, analgesia and muscular relaxation. The analgesia provided by a narcotic given in the premedication thus forms part of the anaesthetic. There are other ways in which narcotics or pethidine may help to provide smooth general anaesthesia: (1) by reducing twitching and hiccups associated with some intravenous induction agents; (2) by reducing the tachypnoea produced by some volatile agents, e.g. halothane, enflurane and especially trichloroethylene; and (3) by making awareness under light muscle relaxant anaesthesia less likely. However, most drugs providing sedation in premedication have a fairly long action and they are likely to have an effect long after the anaesthetic has been discontinued. This must be borne in mind if a rapid return to full consciousness is essential.

Other Uses for Premedication

Occasionally other drugs are given with the premedication, although they are not usually regarded as true premedicant agents. These include steroids in patients who are already on (or have recently been on) steroid therapy, bronchodilators in asthmatics, insulin in diabetics, antibiotics in patients with valvular heart disease to prevent subacute bacterial endocarditis and antacid therapy as prophylaxis against Mendelson's syndrome.

GROUPS OF DRUGS USED

Antisialogogues

Atropine sulphate
Atropine, probably the commonest agent used to dry secretions, has been in use since before the end of the 19th century. Its theoretical disadvantage is that it is a central nervous system stimulant, but this effect is not usually impressive. Indeed, in higher doses it may produce some drowsiness which explains why it does not seem to antagonise sedative drugs, with which it is given as premedication for children.

Hyoscine hydrobromide (Scopolamine)
This other commonly used antisialogogue differs from atropine in being a central nervous system depressant, causing drowsiness and amnesia. It is also an anti-emetic. With a narcotic it provides much better pre-anaesthetic sedation than atropine, but being a more powerful drying agent is more likely to give the patient an uncomfortably dry mouth.

Glycopyrrolate (Robinul)
This synthetic, long-acting anticholinergic drug was introduced in 1960. It has an equivalent drying action to that of atropine and hyoscine, but produces less tachycardia and does not stimulate the central nervous system.

Drugs to Produce Sedation

Narcotics

Some anaesthetists consider it irrational to give narcotic agents to patients who have no pain. However, their ability to produce sedation and euphoria has stood the test of time. The agents most commonly used are morphine, papaveretum and pethidine. Of these agents pethidine has the least sedative effect and for premedication is probably best combined with hyoscine. Pethidine has some slight bronchodilator action (as opposed to morphine and papaveretum which may cause bronchoconstriction), and is therefore the agent of choice in asthmatics. These agents all cause central vasomotor and respiratory depression, effects which can cause spectacular hypotension and depression of respiration if they are given in full dosage to the frail or elderly. These drugs also tend to produce nausea and vomiting, effects that are occasionally seen by the time the patient arrives at the anaesthetic room.

Antihistamines

Many of these are phenothiazine derivatives and those used in premedication include promethazine (Phenergan), promazine (Sparine) and trimeprazine (Vallergan). Apart from their antihistaminic action these drugs (1) produce sedation, (2) potentiate and prolong the action of narcotics, (3) are anti-emetic, (4) tend to dilate the bronchi and (5) have some atropine-like action in drying salivary secretions. Their main disadvantages are that their duration of action tends to be long and they may cause hypotension. A proprietary mixture of promethazine 50 mg and pethidine 100 mg (Pamergan P100) is available.

Benzodiazepines

This rapidly expanding group of drugs was introduced in the 1960s. Many benzodiazepines are used by the public at large as tranquillisers or sedatives. They include diazepam (Valium), nitrazepam (Mogadon), lorazepam (Ativan) and temazepam (Normison). Of these agents, diazepam and lorazepam are the most popular for premedication when, in addition to their sedative and tranquillising properties, they tend to produce amnesia. For premedication they are usually given by mouth and have the advantage that owing to their long duration of action the timing of administration is not critical. Postoperatively, this long duration of action may not always be an advantage. Their main disadvantages are that they are not so reliably effective as the narcotics and as they provide no analgesia, their use increases the patient's likely requirement for intravenous analgesia during the anaesthetic.

Butyrophenones

Examples of the butyrophenones are droperidol (Droleptan) and haloperidol (Serenace). They are called 'neuroleptic' drugs and induce a state of mild sedation, apathy and mental detachment. Unfortunately, these effects may be deceptive, patients stating that they have been mentally terrified but unable to show their emotions. A better effect is produced if an analgesic agent such as fentanyl or phenoperidine is used in addition to the butyrophenone drug, the combination then being referred to as 'neuroleptanalgesia'. These combinations have gained more popularity on the Continent than in the UK.

Barbiturates

Barbiturates are much less used for premedication than formerly. Although they are probably the most reliable of drugs at producing sleep, especially in children, they have a marked tendency to produce postoperative restlessness, especially in the presence of pain.

PREMEDICATION FOR DIFFERENT AGE GROUPS

It is emphasised that the following is only one of many possible schemes of premedication, that there is much permissible overlap between the age groups and that adjustments should be made for particular factors—e.g. debilitated patients or emergencies.

Neonate–2 Years

Subcutaneous or intramuscular atropine alone is commonly given to this age group. For a premature baby, 0·1 mg is sufficient; for an average weight neonate up to a baby weighing

10 kg, 0·2 mg should be given; from 10—20 kg, 0·4 mg; and above that weight the full adult dose of 0·6 mg may be given. Some anaesthetists avoid giving atropine to neonates. This is certainly advisable if they have a pyrexia, as atropine's action in preventing sweating tends to raise the temperature further.

2–8 Years

In most children the phenothiazine, trimeprazine tartrate, given by mouth in a dose of 2–4 mg/kg (1–2 mg per pound) is an effective premedication. Although it has some antisialogogue action of its own it is probably best to add oral atropine in a dose of 0·6–1·2 mg in operations on the mouth and nose.

Trimeprazine is conveniently made up as a syrup which contains 6 mg per ml. The two agents should be given by mouth at least two hours pre-operatively as the trimeprazine is not always fully effective before this time has elapsed. Small children may go to sleep with this dosage, or if not are usually awake but cooperative. Because of the increase in volume of syrup with the bigger children it is wise to put an upper limit on the dose of trimeprazine at 72–78 mg (12–13 ml). This means that bigger children will be given less than 4 mg/kg, but this does not matter because it is easier to talk to and gain the confidence of older children at the pre-operative visit, which is the most essential part of any child's premedication. Except after painful operations, children tend to stay lightly asleep for the rest of the day.

Rectal premedication

This method has declined in popularity but there may still be a place for its use in frightened children coming for anaesthesia, especially recurrently. Rectal thiopentone and methohexitone have been used, but absorption may be so rapid that the child is virtually anaesthetised, and should be carefully supervised in case he cannot maintain his own airway. More recently, diazepam has been used and is available in special rectal tubes containing 5 mg or 10 mg (Stesolid rectal tubes). The recommended dose is: 1–3 years, one 5 mg tube; over 3 years, one 10 mg tube.

8–65 Years

The 'adult' premedication mixtures of papaveretum and hyoscine, or pethidine and hyoscine may be used in this entire age group. The adult dose of the former is up to papaveretum 20 mg, and hyoscine 0·4 mg for a man, and papaveretum 15 mg and hyoscine 0·3 mg for a woman. For the latter mixture, the dose is pethidine 100 mg and hyoscine 0·4 mg for both men and women, although the dosage may be reduced to pethidine 75 mg and hyoscine 0·3 mg in women.

For the youngest children in this group these premedications should be scaled down according to body weight. The dose of papaveretum in the first mixture should be adjusted to give 2 mg/6 kg and in the second preparation the pethidine content adjusted to give 10 mg/6 kg. A useful advantage of the pethidine/hyoscine mixture is that it is provided in a standard ampoule of 2 ml which makes subdivision for the nursing staff easier than subdivision of the 1 ml papaveretum/hyoscine ampoule.

Some anaesthetists favour phenothiazine-containing premedication for the 8–65s. He may prescribe the drugs in combination as he thinks fit, or as the Pamergan mixture. In children, less than a whole ampoule would be given.

65+ Years

Because of wide variations in the ageing process, the age of 65 years is only a rough guide as to where the age group should begin. If narcotics are to be used the dose should be reduced as the patient becomes older and more frail. In addition, hyoscine tends to produce disorientation in older people and the dose should be reduced or atropine substituted. In all but the most robust of patients over 70 it is probably wise to give only atropine or withhold premedication altogether. Older people are in any case more phlegmatic, so that the undesirability of using powerful depressant drugs coincides with a lack of the psychological need for heavy sedation.

EMLA CREAM 5%

This cream, introduced by Astra in 1986, is a eutectic mixture containing lignocaine base 25 mg and prilocaine base 25 mg in each gram. It is the first cream which when applied to the surface of the skin reliably reduces or abolishes the pain of needle puncture. The technique is to apply a thick layer of Emla cream for 60–120 minutes beneath an occlusive and waterproof dressing. Its greatest use is in the 2–5 age group, although it may be used and is effective in older patients, including adults. It is not recommended for use in infants.

5 Intravenous Induction Agents

Thiopentone. Methohexitone. Propofol. Etomidate. Ketamine. Continuous intravenous anaesthesia. Hazards of intravenous induction agents.

Intravenous induction of anaesthesia is almost invariably used in adults, although gas induction is almost always possible except where this is unacceptable to the patient. The aim of an intravenous anaesthetic induction agent is to take the patient from a conscious state into surgical anaesthesia within a few seconds and to maintain him there for several minutes until the maintenance anaesthetic has taken over. The action of intravenous induction agents depends largely on a bolus dose being injected fairly rapidly and reaching the brain, the brain level being proportional to the plasma level of the drug. Diffusion of the drug from plasma into brain occurs mainly because of the concentration gradient. The plasma level rises rapidly due to fast injection; if the injection rate is too slow anaesthesia may not be induced. Thiopentone (the 'truth drug') for example, is effective in subanaesthetic doses by simply allowing the patients to talk in an uninhibited fashion. The plasma level of an intravenous agent then falls due to dilution, redistribution, protein binding and metabolism. As the brain level falls, the effect of the drug wears off and the patient wakes up.

THIOPENTONE

Thiopentone (Pentothal, Intraval) is an ultra-short-acting barbiturate that produces a smooth induction of anaesthesia within one arm–brain circulation time. Its action, which lasts between 5 and 10 minutes, is terminated by rapid dilution and redistribution. The metabolism and subsequent excretion of thiopentone, however, is prolonged due to its redistribution into body fat and may take up to 48 hours. Thiopentone may produce severe hypotension primarily as a result of peripheral vasodilation which may be complicated by myocardial depression, particularly in sick, hypovolaemic patients. Thiopentone also causes respiratory depression and apnoea by decreasing the respiratory centre's sensitivity to carbon dioxide and may also cause laryngeal spasm and bronchospasm, particularly in asthmatics. Although usually given intravenously, rectal thiopentone may be given to children to induce anaesthesia, and intravenous thiopentone as an infusion has been used to control convulsions in epilepsy. Thiopentone should not be given to patients who are sensitive to barbiturates or to those suffering from porphyria (Chapter 17).

METHOHEXITONE

Methohexitone (Brietal) is another ultra-short-acting barbiturate with a shorter duration of action than thiopentone. In common with many of the shorter-acting induction agents, methohexitone administration may be associated with several excitatory phenomena such as coughing, hiccoughing, salivation, extraneous movement, hypertonus and apnoea. Nevertheless, when brief anaesthesia is important, methohexitone is extremely useful. Its actions are similar to thiopentone, but its cardiovascular depression is less pronounced. The actions of methohexitone are likewise terminated by redistribution and metabolism, excretion occurring over 24 hours. Methohexitone should not be given to epileptics because it may precipitate convulsions.

PROPOFOL

Propofol (Diprivan) is a non-barbiturate induction agent which provides a smooth induction, largely free from many of the side-effects seen with methohexitone. It is cardiovascularly stable, producing only a small reduction in blood pressure, but may produce significant respiratory depression if used by continuous infusion in a spontaneously breathing patient. Hypersensitivity reactions have not so far been reported but since Diprivan is suspended in soya-bean emulsion (see Intralipid), the large volumes necessary in some patients may produce problems with hyperlipidaemia.

ETOMIDATE

Etomidate (Hypnomidate) is another non-barbiturate intravenous induction agent, widely used on the Continent, mainly because of its lack of severe depressant effects on the cardiovascular system. Excitatory side-effects are common and it seems to have no distinct advantages over other agents. Pain on injection is common, and thrombophlebitis may sometimes occur, particularly when injected into a small vein. Etomidate has been shown to produce adrenal suppression and low levels of serum cortisol when used as a continuous infusion in intensive care. For this reason its use has now been restricted to single doses for induction of anaesthesia.

KETAMINE

Ketamine (Ketalar) is a dissociative anaesthetic agent, given either intravenously or intramuscularly. It is said to preserve the pharyngeal and laryngeal reflexes, thus protecting the airway during anaesthesia. Ketamine is particularly useful for patients with airway problems requiring sedation for repeated operation (e.g. burns and radiotherapy), its high level of analgesia then being of extreme benefit. Ketamine is a cardiovascular stimulant producing noradrenaline release, resulting in hypertension and tachycardia, and should not be used in hypertensive patients. It may produce hallucinations and nightmares while waking in some patients, particularly those who have not been premedicated; patients recovering from ketamine anaesthesia should therefore be left undisturbed to reduce the incidence of side-effects.

CONTINUOUS INTRAVENOUS ANAESTHESIA

Although these agents are commonly used at present only to induce anaesthesia, there is no reason why continuous administration of an induction agent, e.g. etomidate, methohexitone or Diprivan in the form of an intravenous infusion, could not be used to maintain anaesthesia. Considerable research is being undertaken into intravenous anaesthesia, particularly its advantages in its lack of pollution and adequacy of sedation. Intermittent bolus injections of Diprivan or etomidate are already used, particularly in minor gynaecological surgical anaesthesia and bronchoscopy. It is probably better to use a rapidly metabolised agent, like Diprivan, to avoid the cumulative effect of a drug like thiopentone.

Unfortunately two of the most suitable drugs for this technique, Althesin and etomidate, are no longer available. Diprivan is undoubtedly the agent of choice at present, although excessively large infusion volumes may be required.

HAZARDS OF INTRAVENOUS INDUCTION AGENTS

The most severe hazards associated with intravenous induction of anaesthesia are probably cardiovascular collapse associated either with hypovolaemic shock, or in patients with cardiovascular disease. Relative overdose of these agents is a common problem in sick and elderly patients, and also in young patients, particularly those who are shocked as a result of blood or fluid loss. Hypotension is posturally sensitive, particularly with thiopentone when the effects are largely due to peripheral vasodilation and therefore usually respond to rapid fluid administration. Intravenous induction agents may produce apnoea and should not be used in patients with obstructed or difficult airways in whom ventilation may be impossible. Hypersensitivity reactions have been reported to all the intravenous induction agents, particularly Althesin, propanidid and thiopentone, although the mechanism is uncertain. Specific hazards are associated with individual sensitivity to barbiturates and diseases like porphyria (Chapter 17).

Extravascular Injection

Extravascular injection of intravenous induction agents may produce severe irritation, particularly with thiopentone, which is an extremely alkaline agent and may produce localised tissue necrosis. Accidental extravascular injection should be followed by injection of hyaluronidase into the area to encourage diffusion and absorption.

Intra-arterial Injection

Accidental intra-arterial injection of thiopentone, particularly in the antecubital fossa, may produce severe symptoms of arterial obstruction within the microcirculation of the hand, and indeed permanent ischaemia has been reported. This appears to be related to the alkaline nature of the solution forming crystals within the small vessels and obstructing blood flow within the hand. Accidental intra-arterial injection should be followed by injection of a vasodilator and, if necessary, a sympathetic block of the affected limb with the intention of producing a maximum degree of vasodilation.

6 Uptake and Distribution of Volatile and Intraveneous Anaesthetic Agents

Volatile anaesthetic agents. Intraveneous anaesthetic agents.

VOLATILE ANAESTHETIC AGENTS

Physical Properties

There are several physical properties that influence the efficiency of a particular compound as an anaesthetic agent. It is particularly important to be able to produce a high concentration of the agent at atmospheric pressure since it has been shown that one needs to be able to achieve ten times the normal anaesthetic maintenance concentration of a volatile agent to make it useful for both induction and maintenance of anaesthesia. The saturated vapour pressure (SVP) provides such an index since it indicates the maximum proportion of atmospheric pressure which can be occupied by a saturated vapour of the substance. Thus halothane with an SVP of 247 mmHg theoretically allows a maximum concentration of 33% to be achieved, thus fulfilling the requirements of a useful anaesthetic agent, the normal maintenance halothane concentration being 0·75–1%.

Trichloroethylene, on the other hand, with an SVP of only 60 mmHg does not fulfil these requirements: induction with trichloroethylene is both difficult and prolonged. Other physical properties of the agent, such as its solubility in rubber or metal, may also influence the uptake.

Lungs

The most important factor in uptake of a volatile anaesthetic agent is its alveolar concentration which, in turn, depends on minute volume ventilation. The lungs are not normally resistant to the free diffusion of anaesthetic agents and lung disease is therefore relatively unimportant. The inspired agent is diluted by and must equilibrate with the air that remains in the lungs as functional residual capacity (FRC).

Minimum alveolar concentration (MAC)
MAC indicates the minimum alveolar concentration of an agent required to produce lack of reflex response to skin incision in man. Some common values are: halothane 0·765%; ether 1·92%; trichloroethylene 0·17%; enflurane 1·68%; isoflurane 1·15%. Once the volatile anaesthetic agent is present in adequate quantity within the alveolus, further uptake depends on its passing into the circulation.

Uptake into Circulation

The rate of uptake from the alveolus into the blood depends on the following.

Concentration gradient across alveolar membrane
This gradient is between the inspired concentration and the venous concentration of the agent, the latter being dependent on tissue uptake.

Solubility of agent in blood
This is governed by the blood–gas solubility coefficient. Some typical values are: nitrous oxide 0·47; halothane 2·36; trichloroethylene 9·15; and ether 12·1. The higher the blood–gas

solubility coefficient the more soluble is the agent in blood. If the solubility is low, only small quantities of the agent will leave the alveolus and dissolve in the blood and therefore the alveolar concentration will rise rapidly. Since it is this concentration which determines the arterial tension of the agent, this blood tension will rise rapidly and determine the concentration gradients to other tissues and particularly the brain. Agents that are relatively insoluble in blood (e.g. nitrous oxide) rapidly produce high blood tensions and therefore a high concentration gradient from blood to brain and high brain levels. This is synonymous with rapid induction and, since recovery is a direct reversal of this process, with rapid recovery also. Conversely, agents with a high blood solubility (e.g. ether) take a long time to achieve adequate blood tension and subsequently brain tension. To a certain extent this may be compensated for by a high inspired concentration, but recovery is inevitably prolonged.

Pulmonary blood flow

As the pulmonary blood flow rises, more of the agent is removed from the alveolus and therefore the arterial blood tension takes longer to rise, and induction takes longer. Conversely, with a decrease in pulmonary blood flow, induction is rapid since alveolar and therefore arterial tensions rise quickly. Pulmonary blood flow in this situation is synonymous with cardiac output.

Changes in ventilation

These have little effect in the case of insoluble agents since the alveolar concentration is always high. Soluble agents, on the other hand, are influenced by increased ventilation because, as a result of this, alveolar concentration may suddenly rise.

Tissue Uptake

This is dependent on the following.

Concentration gradient

This gradient is between the blood and tissues, and therefore on the alveolar concentration. Once equilibrium is reached no further uptake occurs.

Tissue Blood Solubility

Most anaesthetic agents are equally soluble in tissue and blood with the exception of halothane, which is three times more soluble in brain and muscle than in blood and extremely soluble in fat. This last property is common among anaesthetic agents (e.g. halothane), and fats are known to store inhalational anaesthetics.

Tissue blood flow
It is convenient to divide the tissues into four groups:

Vessel-rich group: Brain, liver, heart and kidney, receiving a total of 70–75% of the cardiac output. The concentration of anaesthetic agent will rise rapidly in all these organs, equilibrium being reached within about 10 minutes.

Intermediate group: Skeletal muscle and skin: 20% of the cardiac output.

Fat group: This is 5% of the cardiac output.

Vessel-poor group: Bones, etc: less than 1% of the cardiac output. Equilibration in the fat and vessel-poor groups takes place extremely slowly.

Concentration Effect

If two anaesthetics are given simultaneously, say nitrous oxide and halothane, one (N_2O) being present in high concentration, then as this is removed into the blood the other gases in the alveolus rapidly assume greater proportions. The rate of this effect obviously depends on the uptake of the high concentration gas into the blood and is therefore most pronounced with a very soluble anaesthetic agent (e.g. ether) and the factors are lessened if the halothane itself is already present in a high concentration.

Diffusion hypoxia (Fink phenomenon)
At the end of an anaesthetic, nitrous oxide is exhaled and if at this point the patient is allowed to breathe air, the lungs will, for a while, contain a mixture of nitrous oxide, nitrogen, oxygen,

carbon dioxide and water, thus lowering the overall concentration of oxygen and producing relative hypoxia. In addition, as the nitrous oxide is breathed out, the total exhaled volume is greater than the inspired volume and therefore the alveolar carbon dioxide concentration falls. This leads to a fall in arterial carbon dioxide concentration, which depresses ventilation and accentuates the hypoxia already produced.

Metabolism and Distribution

As discussed (p. 73), the vast majority of volatile anaesthetic agents are excreted unchanged in the expired air. Nevertheless, a small proportion of almost every agent is metabolised within the liver and these metabolites are subsequently excreted in the bile and urine. The common metabolites and their potential toxicity are indicated in Table 6.1.

Table 6.1 Common metabolites and their potential toxicity

Agent	Metabolites	Potential toxicity
Halothane	Trifluracetic acid Trifluracetaldehyde Bromide and chloride ions	Hepatotoxic
Methoxyflurane	Free fluoride ions	Nephrotoxic
Trichloroethylene (with hot soda-lime)	Dichloracetylene	Ototoxic

INTRAVENOUS ANAESTHETIC AGENTS

Uptake

Uptake depends on a number of important factors.

1. The rate of injection.
2. Concentration of the agent.
3. The volume injected.
4. The site of injection, e.g. artery, vein (central or peripheral).
5. The circulation time.

The circulation time itself is dependent on the cardiac output, which itself is influenced by premedication, other drugs and the age and general fitness of the patient. The lower the cardiac output the longer the arm to brain circulation time.

Distribution

The distribution of intravenous anaesthetic agents is the main factor to influence the waking time after a single intravenous dose. The action of intravenous agents depends on rapid administration of a large dose producing a high blood-to-brain concentration gradient. This level is then rapidly reduced by dilution within the bloodstream over a few minutes and then decays more slowly as the agent is distributed to other body tissues in a similar way to the volatile anaesthetic agents. Redistribution to fat is a slow process since the fat blood flow is too small to account for this being the major route by which the action of intravenous agents is terminated. The ultra-short-acting barbiturates (e.g. thiopentone and methohexitone) are metabolised relatively slowly at the rate of about 10 to 15% of the total dose per hour.

A high proportion of the total dose of intravenous induction agents is protein-bound and therefore inactivated, the degree of binding depending on the pH of the plasma. A fall in pH leads to a fall in the unbound plasma concentration of thiopentone and, conversely, a given dose of thiopentone will last longer if a patient is hyperventilated. This effect is similar with methohexitone. In contrast to the barbiturate intravenous agents, which are only relatively slowly metabolised over many hours, other agents (e.g. Diprivan) are metabolised in the liver so rapidly that it is this metabolism that terminates their action. The inactive metabolites are conjugated and then excreted in the bile and subsequently the faeces and urine.

Ketamine is rapidly metabolised within the liver to alcohols, which are subsequently excreted in the urine. Although the commonly used intravenous induction agents do not produce active metabolites, diazepam, which is sometimes used as an induction agent, although broken down relatively rapidly in the liver, may still produce a prolonged effect from its active metabolites, particularly desmethyldiazepam and temazepam, though this effect is more prominent if the drug is given in repeated doses (Chapter 27). Accumulation of the intravenous induction agents after repeated administration is not a problem in those agents that are rapidly metabolised, but may produce pronounced effects in barbiturates, thiopentone and methohexitone, which accumulate in the body and are only slowly metabolised (Chapter 5).

7 Gases Used in Anaesthesia

Oxygen. Carbon dioxide. Nitrous oxide. Entonox. Cyclopropane

OXYGEN

History

In 1674 John Mayow of Oxford demonstrated the existence of oxygen (O_2) when he showed that both fire and respiration could continue until 1/5th part of the air in an enclosed chamber had been used up. However, Mayow's work was little known and credit for the realisation of the importance of this gas as a normal constituent of air is usually given to Joseph Priestley, a Unitarian minister, as a result of work he carried out in about 1775. He called oxygen 'dephlogisticated air'.

Commercial Preparation

Oxygen is usually produced commercially by a method known as the fractional distillation of liquid air. This method uses the fact that as the temperature of liquid air gradually rises its component gases are given off individually because of the difference in their boiling points. The boiling point of oxygen is −182·5°C.

Properties

Oxygen makes up 20·9% of normal air. It has a molecular weight of 32. It does not itself ignite, but in its presence combustible material (e.g. wood or cloth) burn much more vigorously. Thus dust, oil or grease may ignite in the heat caused by the compression wave produced when an oxygen cylinder is suddenly turned on. Precautions against this eventuality include (1) cautiously and slightly opening the cylinder valve before attaching it to the anaesthetic machine to blow out any dust, (2) opening the rotameter needle valves beforehand to 'leak' the sudden pressure rise off downstream, and (3) banning of all oil and grease from areas when oxygen is likely to be released under pressure. It has a specific gravity of 1·105 compared with air, which is 1·0.

CARBON DIOXIDE

History

Carbon dioxide (CO_2) was isolated by Joseph Black in 1757. Henry Hill Hickman, in 1824, published the results of his production of anaesthesia in animals by using this gas. He failed in his attempts to introduce it as an anaesthetic in man. Its significance in human physiology was not realised until the work of Haldane in England in 1926. This led to a widespread realisation of the dangers of carbon dioxide accumulation under anaesthesia and a fashion developed for producing hypocarbia, i.e. a reduction of the blood P_{CO_2} below its normal level, under anaesthesia. In recent years it has become apparent that this too has its disadvantages and usually attempts are now made to maintain approximate normocarbia.

Commercial Preparation

Carbon dioxide is usually produced commercially by the action of heat on calcium or magnesium carbonates.

$$\underset{\text{calcium carbonate}}{CaCO_3} \longrightarrow \underset{\text{calcium oxide}}{CaO} + \underset{\text{carbon dioxide}}{CO_2}$$

Properties

Carbon dioxide is a colourless gas which in high concentration has a pungent smell. Its molecular weight is 44 and its specific gravity 1·500. It occurs as a natural constituent of the air but only in a concentration of 0·03%. It is non-inflammable and does not support combustion, hence its use as the insufflating gas at laparoscopy.

Anaesthetic Uses of Carbon Dioxide

Many anaesthetists consider that carbon dioxide on anaesthetic machines is provided for convenience rather than necessity, and that because of its dangers it should not be routinely available. Its potential uses are as follows.

1. At induction of anaesthesia with a patient breathing spontaneously, the introduction of low concentrations of carbon dioxide into the anaesthetic mixture increases the rate and depth of respiration and thus speeds the induction.
2. The increased depth of respiration which carbon dioxide may produce at induction of anaesthesia also helps the introduction of an endotracheal tube when attempting the technique of blind nasal intubation.
3. At the end of an anaesthetic, when intermittent positive pressure respiration (IPPR) has been used, hypocarbia will result in a period of apnoea until the P_{CO_2} returns to normal levels. Carbon dioxide may conveniently be introduced into the reservoir bag at the end of the anaesthetic to speed the return of spontaneous respiration.

NITROUS OXIDE

History

In 1772 Joseph Priestley first prepared nitrous oxide (N_2O), and in 1800 Sir Humphrey Davy first demonstrated its anaesthetic properties. In 1844 in the USA an itinerant chemist, Gardner

Quincy Colton, demonstrated its anaesthetic properties to an audience which included a dentist named Horace Wells. The latter realised its potential use in dental practice, but after some success his attempt to show its use as a surgical anaesthetic at the Massachusetts General Hospital was something of a débâcle. It was rapidly superseded by ether and did not regain popularity for nearly 20 years.

Joseph Clover first used nitrous oxide to provide a relatively pleasant induction to ether anaesthesia and Boyle's machine was introduced in 1917. This permitted the vaporisation of ether in a stream of nitrous oxide and oxygen. Today, nitrous oxide with oxygen provides the basis for the vast majority of inhalational anaesthetics in countries where advanced anaesthetic equipment is available.

Commercial Preparation

Nitrous oxide is prepared by heating ammonium nitrate in large iron retorts at 240°C.

$$\underset{\text{(Ammonium nitrate)}}{NH_4NO_3} \longrightarrow \underset{\text{(Water)}}{2H_2O} + \underset{\text{(Nitrous oxide)}}{N_2O}$$

Properties

Nitrous oxide is a sweet-smelling, non-irritant, colourless gas, with a molecular weight of 44 and a specific gravity of 1·5. It is neither inflammable nor explosive, but like oxygen supports combustion of other oxidisable materials if an initial temperature high enough to decompose nitrous oxide into nitrogen and oxygen is supplied (450°C).

Nitrous oxide is an excellent analgesic (hence its use to relieve pain in labour), but is a weak anaesthetic agent. Consequently it may be impossible to produce full anaesthesia in a robust adult with nitrous oxide and oxygen alone without using a hypoxic mixture, i.e. a nitrous oxide percentage of over 80%. Similarly, when using muscle relaxant anaesthesia, nitrous oxide should almost always be supplemented with an inhalational or intravenous agent. Otherwise there is the real possibility, except with the frail or very ill, that the patient may develop some awareness under the anaesthetic (Chapter 24).

Nitrous oxide is generally regarded as non-toxic, but there have been occasional reports of reversible agranulocytosis after prolonged administration of the gas in intensive care. Another possible adverse effect of nitrous oxide occurs when there are collections of air in closed body cavities (e.g. pneumothorax). In these circumstances the nitrogen component of the air in the cavity returns to the circulation more slowly than the nitrous oxide escapes into the cavity. The result may be a dangerous increase in the volume of gas contained in the cavity.

ENTONOX

'Entonox' is the British Oxygen Company (BOC) name for pre-mixed gases in one cylinder containing 50% nitrous oxide and 50% oxygen. It is curious that this mixture is gaseous as its normal cylinder presure of 2000 p.s.i. The pressure at which nitrous oxide liquefies varies with the temperature, but around room temperature of 20°C it liquefies at 750 p.s.i. Oxygen, on the other hand, at its usual cylinder pressure of 2000 p.s.i. is in the gaseous form. However, when oxygen is bubbled through liquid nitrous oxide in a cylinder, the latter vaporises and a gaseous mixture of nitrous oxide and oxygen is formed. By continuing to introduce oxygen into the cylinder, various proportions of nitrous oxide and oxygen can be made and the mixture of nitrous oxide and oxygen in equal proportions known as Entonox is supplied in cylinders at a pressure of 2000 p.s.i.

Entonox cylinders vary from a portable 500 litre size to large 5000 litre cylinders intended for pipeline use. At normal environmental temperatures the nitrous oxide and oxygen remain in the gaseous phase, but if the temperature falls below −7°C some nitrous oxide liquefies and separates from the oxygen. In these circumstances, if the cylinder is used vertically with the valve at the top it is possible when the cylinder is nearing exhaustion to obtain a hypoxic mixture of almost pure nitrous oxide. Fortunately, the nitrous oxide can be restored to the gaseous phase by inverting the cylinder three times after it has been rewarmed.

Entonox is most popular as a convenient and effective method of pain relief in obstetrics, but may also be useful in other circumstances, e.g. for postoperative pain relief and changing burns dressings. It can also be used as the single, vaporising gas for small, portable anaesthetic machines.

CYCLOPROPANE

History

The anaesthetic properties of cyclopropane were first discovered by Lucas and Henderson of Toronto in 1929, but its use as a clinical anaesthetic agent was developed by Waters and his colleagues at Madison, Wisconsin, in the years just after 1930.

Commercial Preparation

Cyclopropane may be formed from trimethylene glycol, or simply by purification of the gas, which occurs naturally in the United States.

Properties

The gas is colourless, sweet-smelling and non-irritant except in high concentrations. Its molecular weight is 42 and the specific gravity 1·42. It is easily liquefied and usually provided in orange cylinders at a pressure of 75 p.s.i. It is probably the most explosive agent in common clinical practice and because of this, and because it is so expensive, it is always used in a closed circuit. For these reasons it has never become widely used in the UK, but in the USA, where it is less expensive and circle systems are in more common use, it is more popular.

Cyclopropane is a powerful anaesthetic agent, so that it is always possible to give a high concentration of oxygen; 50% cyclopropane in oxygen will rapidly induce anaesthesia and a range of 10–30% cyclopropane produces from light to deep anaesthesia.

During spontaneous respiration anaesthesia, cyclopropane produces respiratory depression in relation to the depth of anaesthesia, and in higher concentrations the myocardium is depressed. Cyclopropane also has a reputation for producing ventricular dysrhythmias. The reason for this is believed to be that cyclopropane increases the concentration of circulating catecholamines and simultaneously sensitises the myocardium to their effects. Factors that predispose to these abnormalities of cardiac rhythm are (1) high concentrations of cyclopropane, (2) hypercarbia, (3) hypoxia and (4) increased amounts of circulating catecholamines; factors that are identical to those which produce a high incidence of ventricular dysrhythmias with halothane. The risks with cyclopropane are even greater than those with halothane and it is unwise to inject adrenaline-containing solutions during cyclopropane anaesthesia.

'Cyclopropane shock' is a term applied to cardiovascular collapse that sometimes occurs during recovery from cyclopropane anaesthesia. Both cyclopropane and the hypercarbia, with which this type of anaesthesia is usually associated, stimulate the sympathetic nervous system. Withdrawal of these two stimuli at the end of the operation is believed to be the cause of this syndrome.

Cyclopropane also produces a somewhat high incidence of postanaesthetic nausea and vomiting. For these various reasons, cyclopropane has fallen from favour for maintenance of anaesthesia, but it still has its advocates for induction of anaesthesia in ill patients and children, provided it can be guaranteed that the operating theatre is free from static sparks.

8 Anaesthetic Gas Supply: The Anaesthetic Machine

British Standards Institution. Units of pressure. Identification colours of cylinders. Gas cylinders. Cylinder testing. Cylinder valves. Pin-index valve. Information carried on gas cylinders and valves. Gas pipelines. Pressure regulators or pressure reducing valves. Pressure gauges. Flowmeters. Oxygen failure warning devices. Testing the anaesthetic machine. Suction.

This chapter discusses the transport and supply of anaesthetic gases from their source in cylinders or a pipeline through the anaesthetic machine to its outlet. Chapter 9 describes the various anaesthetic circuits, by which the anaesthetic gases are carried from that point to the patient.

The most popular anaesthetic machine in common use is often referred to as Boyle's machine, although it is much changed from the original model introduced in 1917 by Edmund Boyle, a London anaesthetist. Basically, it remains a trolley with a working surface, special positions (yokes) for attaching anaesthetic gas cylinders or pipelines, pressure regulators for reducing the high pressure from most gas cylinders and means of metering the anaesthetic gases and vaporising bottles (now sometimes very sophisticated) for vaporising volatile anaesthetic liquids.

BRITISH STANDARDS INSTITUTION

This institution produces pamphlets called British Standards (or

BS) which cover hundreds of engineering and industrial products and techniques; several have been produced in the UK covering all aspects of medical gas cylinders and cylinder valves.

UNITS OF PRESSURE

Unfortunately despite attempts at standardisation, a profusion of units of pressure still exists. In this book the units cited will usually be those most commonly found in that particular situation, e.g. in this chapter, pounds to the square inch (p.s.i.) and bar are those found on most gas cylinders and cylinder valves. Other units are millimetres of mercury (mm Hg), kilopascals (kPa), atmospheres, kilograms/square centimetre (kg/cm^2) and centimetres of water (cm H_2O). For conversion factors the reader is referred to the Appendix.

IDENTIFICATION COLOURS OF CYLINDERS

The colour coding of the cylinder contents is also laid down in a British Standard, but unfortunately as yet there is no international agreement on this coding. The British Standard cylinder colour code is shown in Table 8.1. In some cases the valve end of the cylinder has special identification colours. In the case of gas mixtures, these colours are applied in four segments, two of each colour (e.g. Entonox).

Table 8.1 British Standard cylinder colour code

Name of gas	Symbol	Valve end colour	Body colour
Oxygen	O_2	White	Black
Nitrous oxide	N_2O	Blue	Blue
Cyclopropane	C_3H_6	Orange	Orange
Carbon dioxide	CO_2	Grey	Grey
Helium	He	Brown	Brown
Nitrogen	N_2	Black	Grey
Oxygen and carbon dioxide	$O_2 + CO_2$	White and grey	Black
Oxygen and helium mixtures	O_2 + He	White and brown	Black
Air (medical)	AIR	White and black	Grey
Oxygen and nitrous oxide mixture	$O_2 + N_2O$	White and blue	Blue

GAS CYLINDERS

These are usually made of steel, the types of steel being referred to as high carbon, low carbon and manganese for hospital use, or chrome-molybdenum for lightweight, portable cylinders. These terms refer to some of the constituents added to the iron in the manufacture of the steel, the percentage of the components being laid down in a British Standard.

CYLINDER TESTING

During the manufacture of the cylinders sample strips are taken from one of each batch of 100 cylinders and subjected to tensile (or stretching), impact and bend tests. Each completed cylinder also undergoes hydraulic pressure testing by a high 'proof' pressure of 3000 p.s.i. applied internally. The details of these tests are all described in British Standards.

In addition to these tests on new cylinders, hydraulic pressure testing should be repeated every five years. The date of testing is indicated either by symbols stamped on the shoulder of the cylinder or on the valve (see below) or by a colour-coded disc fixed round the neck of the cylinder.

CYLINDER VALVES

The cylinder valve is screwed into the neck of the cylinder. It is usually made of chromium-plated brass or bronze. There are two types in common use—the bull-nosed and the pin-index. A third type—the handwheel valve—is usually reserved for very large cylinders. In the past, pin-index valves have been used only on small medical gas cylinders as and when practicable, but in future they will be used irrespective of size. Full cylinders are supplied with a red plastic seal which prevents dust or grit from entering the valve outlet. It is nevertheless recommended that after removing the seal, but before attaching the cylinder to the machine, the valve be momentarily opened and closed to blow away any foreign matter which would otherwise be blown into the regulator. It is important to ensure that the handler's face is averted.

Once the cylinder is securely attached to the anaesthetic or other apparatus, the cylinder valve is opened by slowly turning the valve spindle two complete turns anti-clockwise with the valve key or handwheel provided.

PIN-INDEX VALVE

Pin-index valves are designed in such a way that it is possible to connect only the correct gas cylinder to the appropriate yoke on the anaesthetic machine (Fig. 8.1).

The upper of the three holes in the pin-index valve is the gas outlet. The lower two holes are placed on the circumference of a circle whose centre is the centre of the gas outlet hole and whose radius is 14·3 mm (9/16 in.). The positions of these holes are precisely laid down for each of the common medical gases by a British Standard. The only gas which does not have two lower hole positions is the nitrous oxide/oxygen mixture (Entonox), which has one central hole.

These pin-index holes are blind, having no internal connection

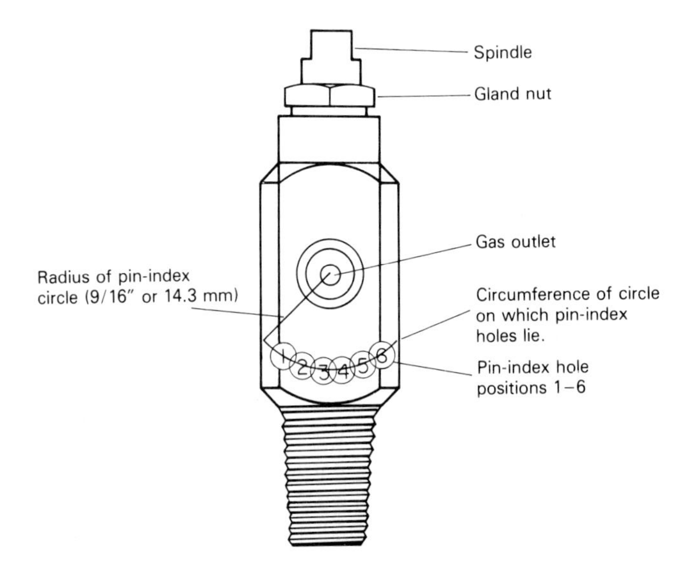

Fig. 8.1 Pin-index valve

within the cylinder valve. They correspond with pins in the appropriate position for the same gas in the yoke of the anaesthetic machine.

A sealing washer (Bodok seal) is essential between the pin-index valve and the valve yoke.

INFORMATION CARRIED ON GAS CYLINDERS AND VALVES

Some interesting and useful symbols and figures are carried on gas cylinders and valves. Some of these tend to be obscured by successive layers of paint and by batch number labels applied by the manufacturers, but among other information it should be possible to find the following.

Identification of Gas

The name or chemical symbol of the gas or gas mixture is indelibly stamped on the cylinder valve and painted on the cylinder, which also bears a label with the same information, and, for gas mixtures, the proportion of the constituents. This is, of course, in addition to the identification of the cylinder contents by colour coding.

Cylinder Size

The cylinder size is identified by a capital letter code (e.g. A, B, C) stencilled on the cylinder or shown on a label. The capacity of the cylinder is also marked on the valve end of the cylinder.

Tare Weight

The tare or empty weight of the cylinder plus valve is stamped on all cylinders containing liquefiable gases, i.e. nitrous oxide, carbon dioxide and cyclopropane. The cylinder contents for these gases can be measured accurately by weighing the cylinder and deducting the tare weight. The weight of 100 litres of the gas is given on a label on the cylinder, e.g. 100 l N_2O weighs 0·182 kg.

Maximum Permissible Working Pressure

This is stamped on the cylinder valve. The pressure might easily be exceeded if the cylinder were stored in the sun or beside a radiator.

Hydraulic Test Date

This has already been mentioned under 'Cylinder testing' (p. 87). When the date is stamped on the cylinder valve or cylinder shoulder it is represented by the last two figures of the date and the quarter of the year indicated by one of the figures 1 to 4 with a circle round it. Thus 81 3 ᗺB means that the cylinder was tested in the third quarter of 1981. Beside the date mark is stamped a test mark in the form of initials or a hieroglyphic to indicate the BOC testing centre where the test was carried out, e.g. BR = Brentford, ᗺB = Edmonton.

GAS PIPELINES

The alternative to using small cylinders of medical gases mounted on the anaesthetic machine is to have much larger cylinders housed in a central store, with the gases being transported throughout the hospital by pipelines. The commonest gases supplied in this way are oxygen and nitrous oxide, although it is becoming common in modern maternity hospitals to have piped Entonox. The third pipeline in most operating theatres is a suction line.

Essentially, the gas store consists of large cylinders of the gases, there usually being two banks of each type of gas. Only one bank supplies the pipeline at any one time. As that bank becomes exhausted, the fall in pressure automatically causes a switchover to the other bank and triggers an alarm. The usual hospital medical gas pipeline pressure is 60 p.s.i. (4 bars).

For hospitals using large amounts of oxygen, e.g. over 5000 cu. ft per week, it is usual for the oxygen to be supplied and stored in liquid form.

PRESSURE REGULATORS OR PRESSURE REDUCING VALVES

Probably the most important function of pressure regulators is to provide gases to the flowmeters at a constant pressure. Otherwise, as the pressure in the cylinder gradually falls, constant readjustment of the needle valve leading to the flowmeter would be required to maintain a constant flowrate. In addition, the gases were formerly carried from the cylinder to the anaesthetic machines by rubber tubing and this was only possible if the pressure was first greatly reduced. For instance, the old Adam's valve (the roughly inverted cone-shaped valve which sat on top of the cylinder) reduced the pressure to 6 p.s.i.

On modern anaesthetic machines the pressure regulators usually reduce the pressure to 60 p.s.i. and, instead of being sited on top of the cylinder, are usually tucked under the working surface of the machine.

PRESSURE GAUGES

These indicate the pressure in the gas cylinder to which they are attached or the gas pipeline pressure. The commonest type of pressure gauge is the Bourdon gauge (Fig. 8.2) which acts in the same way as the popular children's party toy of a curled tube of paper which straightens when blown into (Fig. 8.3).

In the Bourdon pressure gauge the curled tube is made of metal and requires great pressure to produce a slight straightening movement. The closed end of the tube is linked to a pointer which indicates the pressure.

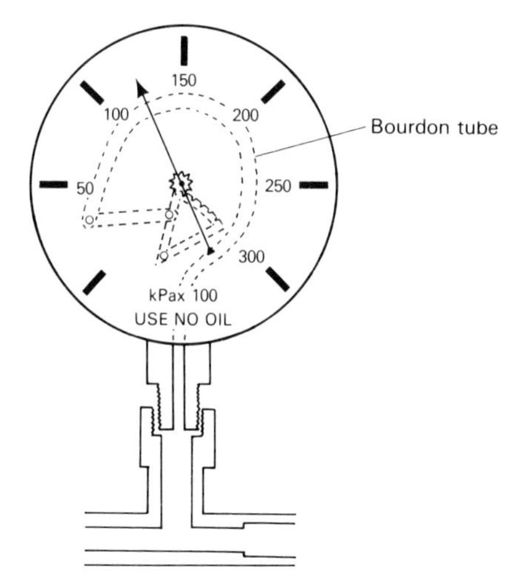

Fig. 8.2 Bourdon pressure gauge

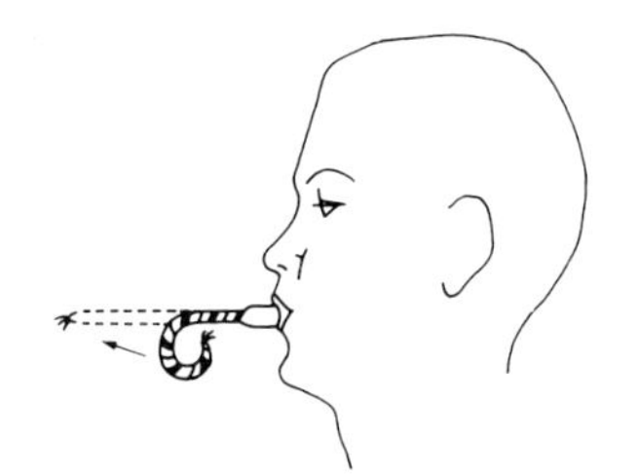

Fig. 8.3 Principle of Bourdon gauge

FLOWMETERS

Flowmeters may be divided into two groups: (1) constant pressure/variable orifice flowmeters; and (2) variable pressure/constant orifice flowmeters. (Examples are illustrated in Figs. 8.4 and 8.5.)

Constant Pressure Variable Orifice

The commonest example of this group is the Rotameter (Fig.

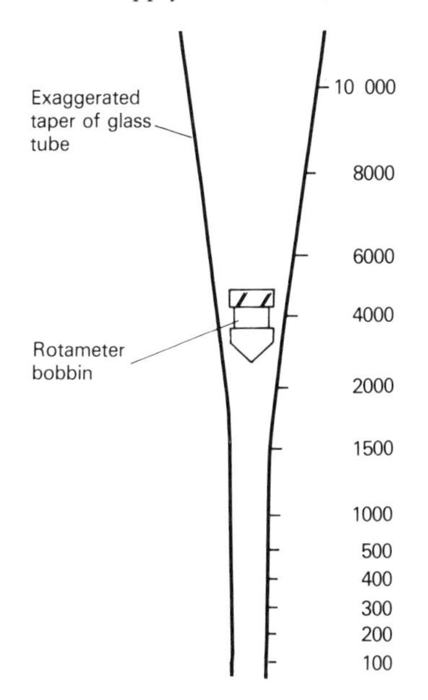

Fig. 8.4 Rotameter

8.4), the most popular flowmeter in use in anaesthetics. This consists of a glass tube mounted vertically within which a rotating bobbin is free to move. Although invisible to the naked eye, the tube tapers very gradually so that it is wider at the top than at the bottom. This means that there is an annular orifice between the bobbin and the walls of the glass tube, and this orifice increases in size as the bobbin moves up the tube.

The anaesthetic gas enters the lower part of the tube through a simple needle valve. This causes the bobbin to rise up within the tube, the gas escaping through the annular orifice. The bobbin settles at a level where its weight is balanced by the pressure drop across the orifice. As the needle valve is opened admitting more gas into the lower part of the tube the bobbin is forced higher in the tube as the higher gas flow requires a larger orifice to maintain the pressure drop at a constant level, i.e. that required to support the bobbin.

The rotation of the bobbin is caused by the gas blowing through oblique cuts made in the rim of the bobbin. Provided that the glass tube is mounted vertically, and provided that there is no dirt in it, the bobbin spins freely in the centre of the tube without touching the side. This eliminates any error which might be caused by friction and makes the rotameter more accurate.

The glass tube is calibrated to show the gas flow, the measurement being taken from the top of the bobbin. Not only are the tubes non-interchangeable for different gases but also each is calibrated with its own bobbin and must not be used for any other.

Variable Pressure/Constant Orifice

Figure 8.5 shows the Bourdon pressure gauge (described above) being used as a flowmeter of this group. The gas flowing through the orifice 'A' causes a build-up of pressure proximal to the orifice and this tends to straighten the Bourdon tube. The diameter of the orifice is constant, so the rise in pressure proximal to it increases with the flow rate. The gauge is calibrated for flow instead of pressure. As variable pressure/constant orifice flowmeters depend for their accuracy on a particular size of orifice, they are readily affected by partial occlusion of the orifice by dirt.

Because of differences in the densities and viscosities of different gases a flowmeter which is calibrated for one gas will not read correctly when another gas is passed through it.

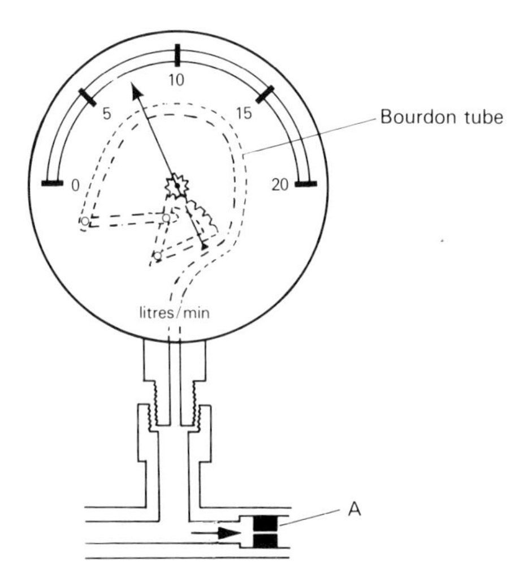

Fig. 8.5 Bourdon gauge used as flowmeter

On the Boyle's machine the flowmeters are grouped in a bank on the top left of the machine. After passing through them the gases mix in the hollow tube on the top rear of the machine. There they may be used to vaporise volatile anaesthetic liquids (Chapter 10) before passing to the outlet from the anaesthetic machine.

OXYGEN FAILURE WARNING DEVICES

It has been recommended that the ideal warning device should have the following features:

1. Be operated only by the oxygen supply.
2. Not be operated by mains or battery power.
3. There should be a warning of impending failure, and a further warning that failure has occurred.
4. The signals are audible and of sufficient length, volume and character.
5. When the device is triggered:

   (a) Other gases and vapours should cease to flow.
   (b) The breathing circuit is opened to the atmosphere.
   (c) The inspired oxygen concentration should be at least equal to that of air, and build-up of carbon dioxide should not occur whether respiration is spontaneous or controlled.

At present no device is available that fulfils all these requirements for pipeline as well as cylinder use. The anaesthetic staff should know the limitations of the particular devices used on their machines.

TESTING THE ANAESTHETIC MACHINE

Because of the variety of oxygen failure warning devices,

pressure relief valves, ventilators and circuits which may be used, it is not possible to give one description of a method of testing the entire anaesthetic apparatus which is to be used for a particular anaesthetic. However, the following is a description of the basic testing of the anaesthetic machine which the anaesthetist should carry out at the beginning of each list. It is assumed that the machine has both a pipeline and single cylinder supplies of nitrous oxide and oxygen and a cylinder supply of carbon dioxide.

The pipeline hoses for nitrous oxide and oxygen are disconnected from their outlets, the cylinders turned off and all the flowmeter controls turned on. Ensure that any flow through the flowmeters ceases.

The oxygen cylinder is then turned on and it is established that flow occurs only through the oxygen flowmeter. Check that the cylinder has adequate contents. Turn the cylinder off, and after the flow of oxygen through the flowmeter stops, connect the oxygen pipeline supply and again check that the flow occurs only through the oxygen flowmeter. Unplug the pipeline hose, check that the oxygen flow ceases, then reconnect the hose. A short, sharp pull on the hose ('the tug test') ensures that the connection is firm, after which the flow through the flowmeter is checked again,

Repeat this procedure with the nitrous oxide cylinder and pipeline.

After turning on the carbon dioxide cylinder to ensure that flow occurs from it through the carbon dioxide flowmeter, check that the cylinders have 'full' labels and leave the cylinder key on one of the cylinder valves.

Turn off all the flowmeter controls and ensure that the bobbins return to the bottom of the tubes.

Finally, turn on the oxygen bypass both to check it and to flush the system of nitrous oxide and carbon dioxide.

SUCTION

Suction apparatus is one of the most important pieces of equipment to the anaesthetist. The suction may be delivered by pipeline, where the suction is usually created by a powerful electrical pump, or by movable apparatus. The latter group consists of (1) electrically driven pumps (which usually require mains electricity), (2) Venturi-operated suction apparatus (which usually requires air or oxygen under pressure), or (3) hand (or more commonly foot) operated suction, which is the only truly portable kind.

It is important that suction should not only reach adequate subatmospheric pressures, but that these pressures can be reached quickly if required. At times it is also necessary to be able to control the pressures to lower levels, as in applying suction to a neonate's respiratory tract. In most instances it is essential that a large enough volume can be moved by the apparatus. For example, suction that can achieve a high pressure but only shift a few millilitres per minute would be useless at removing a large volume of vomit.

The degree of pressure attainable by pipeline suction should be of the order of 500 mmHg subatmospheric (2/3 of an atmosphere). This is fairly powerful and lesser pressures are acceptable from the other types of apparatus.

9 Anaesthetic Circuits or Breathing Systems

Principles of anaesthetic circuits. Classification of anaesthetic circuits.

This chapter on the transport of anaesthetic gases to the patient describes the apparatus from the gas outlet on the anaesthetic machine to the point of delivery to the patient. This part of the apparatus is usually referred to as the 'anaesthetic circuit' or 'anaesthetic breathing system'. While the latter term is more accurate, the former is still used colloquially and both will be used in this chapter.

Confusion in the classification of anaesthetic circuits arises partly from inconsistencies in nomenclature (especially of the terms 'semi-open' and 'semi-closed', which are used in different classifications for the same circuit) and partly from the number of variations in some of the types of circuit. For example, over 60 variations of the circle system may be produced by changing the position in the circle of some of its component parts, such as fresh gas flow entry point, soda-lime canister, expiratory valve and non-return valves. Before classifying anaesthetic circuits, some of their important principles will be enumerated.

PRINCIPLES OF ANAESTHETIC CIRCUITS

1. There must be an adequate inspired oxygen concentration. With some anaesthetic systems this may be supplied simply by room air.

2. There must be efficient elimination of carbon dioxide.
3. The circuit must not greatly increase the dead space.
4. The apparatus should not greatly increase the resistance to inspiration or expiration, the exception being the occasional application of a positive end-expiratory pressure.
5. The circuit should be simple, safe and reliable.

Dead Space

All anaesthetic circuits have a dead space which is inherent in the apparatus, whether the final connection to the patient is by a face mask, endotracheal or tracheostomy tube. A mask adds to the patient's dead space but the tubes reduce it considerably by bypassing the anatomical dead space of the nose and mouth. The extent of the apparatus dead space may be obvious, e.g. in the case of a non-rebreathing valve it extends from the patient as far as the expiratory port and in a T-piece system it extends to the point of entry of the fresh gas supply, provided that this is adequate. In the case of a circle system it extends as far as the connection to the corrugated tubing. In some of the more complex Mapleson D systems it may be less obvious because contamination of fresh gas by expired gases may occur.

The problem of apparatus dead space is particularly acute in paediatric anaesthesia (Chapter 38).

Apparatus Resistance

All apparatus tends to produce some resistance to respiration. In parts of anaesthetic circuits where the patient has to do the work of breathing, whether on the inspiratory or expiratory side, the anaesthetic tubing should be of large diameter. The narrowest part of the breathing system (which is always critical as regards the amount of effort required from the patient) is usually the endotracheal tube and connector. The next most likely source of resistance is provided by the valves in the system. Once again, the problem of resistance is most important in paediatric anaesthesia.

CLASSIFICATION OF ANAESTHETIC CIRCUITS

There is no general agreement about the classification of anaesthetic circuits, but the following classification divides the systems into three main groups: (1) open 'circuits', (2) circuits with an 'adequate' fresh gas flow, i.e. sufficient for carbon dioxide elimination, and (3) circuits with an 'inadequate' fresh gas flow which rely on soda-lime for elimination of carbon dioxide.

Groups (2) and (3) contain various subgroups. Instead of trying to master the characteristics of all these subgroups, examples of the most popular systems in the UK are emphasised below.

The efficiency of individual circuits in fulfilling the basic principles given above, especially as regards providing adequate oxygen and eliminating carbon dioxide, may vary considerably, depending on whether the system is being used for spontaneous or controlled respiration.

Open Circuits

The main example of this technique is the application of a volatile anaesthetic agent, such as diethyl ether, by a drop technique onto a gauze mask (e.g. a Schimmelbusch mask) or simply onto a handkerchief (the original 'rag and bottle' technique). Provided that the mask is held clear of the face, the oxygen supply is derived from the room air and there is no rebreathing as the expired gases escape freely into the atmosphere. Another example of this technique is the gaseous anaesthetic surreptitiously introduced onto the pillow of a small child.

Provided that the mask is held off the patient's face this system has no resistance and no dead space.

Circuits with Adequate Fresh Gas Flow

Circuits using non-rebreathing valves

The first example of this group of circuits incorporates a non-rebreathing valve, such as the Ambu-E valve (Fig. 9.1). The

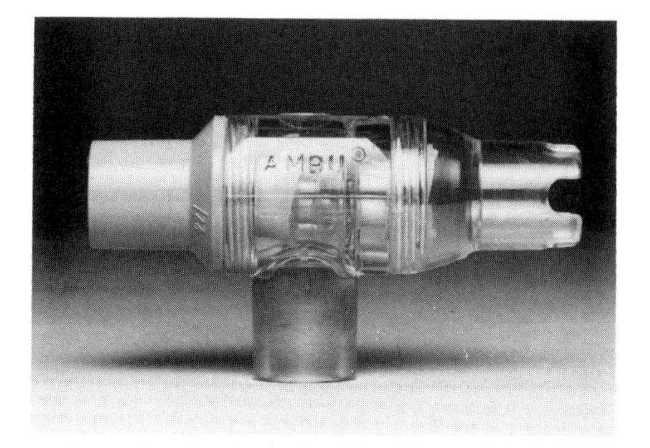

Fig. 9.1 Ambu-E valve

inspiratory side of this system incorporates a reservoir bag to deal with the peaks of the patient's inspiratory flow rate. The bag should not be referred to as a 'rebreathing' bag as this is not its function. The purpose of the bag is to continue filling with fresh gases during the patient's expiratory and expiratory pause phases so that it can deal with the patient's inspiratory peak flow which can easily reach 25–30 litres/min in the case of an adult. On inspiration, the valve cycles into the inspiratory position so that the patient is supplied with pure fresh gases. The expiratory port then opens and the patient breathes out into the atmosphere. These valves facilitate the precise adjustment of the anaesthetic mixture as there is no contamination of the fresh gas flow by expired gases. Indeed, the patient's minute volume may be calculated by adjusting the fresh gas flow so that the reservoir bag neither fills nor empties. A disadvantage of these valves is that they tend to stick if there is a build-up of moisture, or if the fresh gas flow appreciably exceeds the minute volume. This last problem may be avoided by incorporating an overflow valve, e.g. a Heidbrink valve on the inspiratory side. This circuit is also relatively expensive in its use of gases and vapours.

Semi-closed circuits

This group of circuits is commonly described by the useful but non-descriptive classification of Mapleson circuits A–F, as shown in Figure 9.2. This group contains many of the most popular anaesthetic circuits used in the UK. Instead of

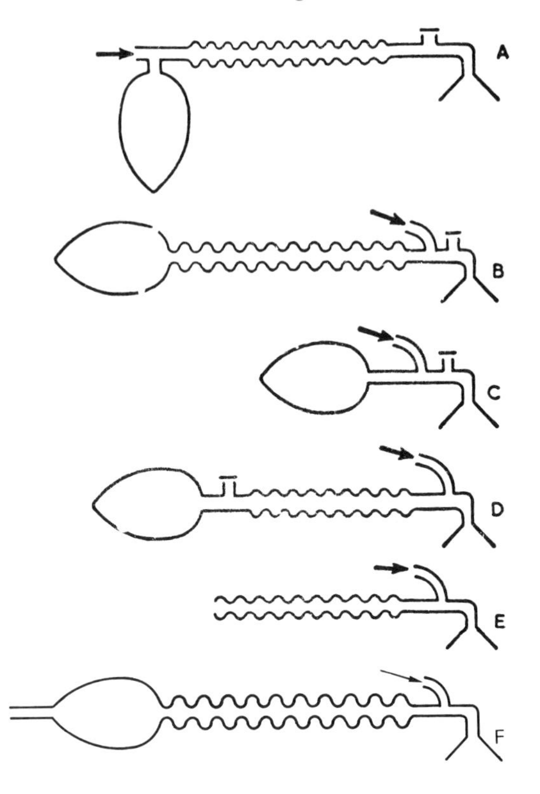

Fig. 9.2 Mapleson classification

describing each of the Mapleson circuits in detail it is proposed to describe some of the more frequently used circuits and indicate to which of the Mapleson systems they belong.

Magill circuit (Fig. 9.3). This is the Mapleson A circuit . The valve is a Heidbrink valve and there is a reservoir bag. Its popularity has declined because of the relatively cumbersome nature of the valve when it is modified to take a scavenging attachment. At the beginning of expiration the corrugated tubing fills first with the dead space gas and then with alveolar gas. As this expired gas flow meets the fresh gases the pressure under the expiratory valve increases. When the pressure reaches 2 cm water, the valve flap lifts and alveolar gas is vented into the atmosphere. Towards the end of expiration the pressure in the tubing begins to fall and the fresh gases begin to flow towards the patient again, flushing any remaining alveolar gas out through

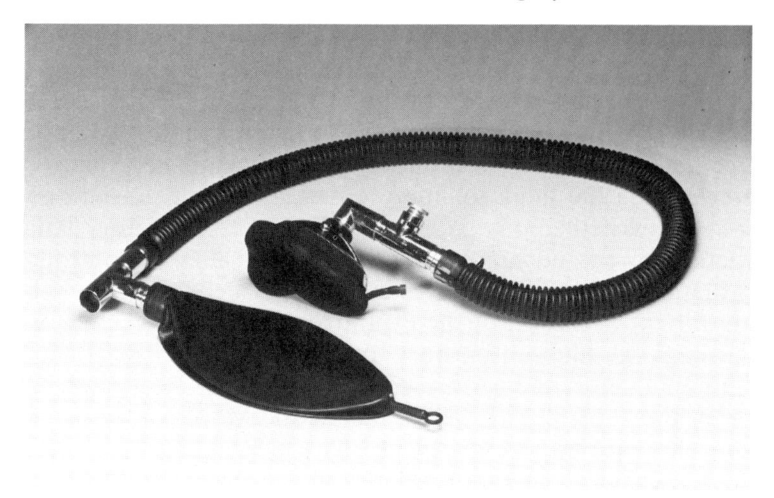

Fig. 9.3 Magill circuit

the valve. With a high fresh gas flow, dead space gas from the tubing and even fresh gas may be vented through the valve before it closes, but even if they are breathed in by the patient neither contains carbon dioxide. Hence this circuit preferentially eliminates alveolar gas, and rebreathing does not occur until the fresh gas flow falls below the alveolar ventilation, i.e. about 70 % of the minute volume. To use this circuit for controlled ventilation the Heidbrink valve has to be partially screwed down. Venting of gases through the valve occurs only when the reservoir bag is squeezed, i.e. during the inspiratory phase so that it is mainly fresh gas which is eliminated. For this reason the Magill circuit is an inefficient circuit for controlled ventilation.

Ayre's T-piece. This corresponds to the Mapleson E system and variations on this circuit are used widely in paediatrics. When this circuit is being used for spontaneous respiration, during expiration fresh gas and expired gases from the patient pass down the expiratory limb. During the expiratory pause these mixed gases are flushed further down the limb by fresh gas. Whether any of the expired gases are re-inspired depends on the rate of fresh gas flow and duration of the expiratory pause. The adverse effect of any rebreathing is reduced by the fact that as it will occur only at the end of inspiration, rebreathed gases tend to reach only as far as the patient's dead space, so they do not contaminate the alveolar gas. A fresh gas flow of about twice the minute volume is adequate to prevent significant rebreathing. If the fresh gas flow exceeds the peak inspiratory flow rate, no rebreathing will occur. This requires a fresh gas flow of about three times the minute volume. If the volume of the expiratory limb exceeds the tidal volume the patient will not inspire any room air. Whether this happens with shorter expiratory limbs depends on the adequacy of the fresh gas flow. Controlled ventilation with the T-piece system is performed most simply by intermittent occlusion of the expiratory limb. This may expose the lungs to high inspiratory pressures and IPPR is more commonly and safely performed by the Jackson–Rees modification of the T-piece (Fig. 9.4), which is the Mapleson F system. Controlled respiration is achieved by squeezing an open-ended bag inserted in the expiratory limb, the desired amount of lung inflation being achieved by adjusting the size of the orifice in the end of the bag, usually with the anaesthetist's little finger. The characteristics of the system are the same as during spontaneous respiration, contamination of inspired gases with the mixed gases from the bag not occurring provided that the expiratory limb has

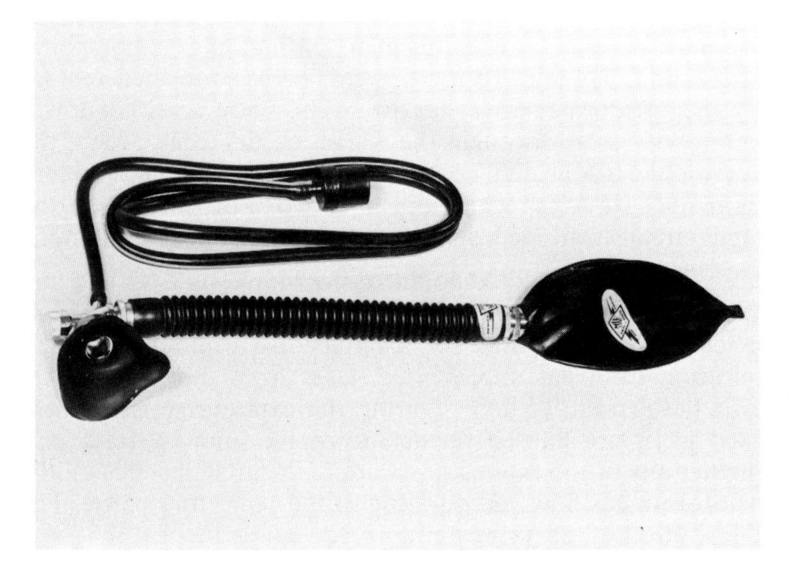

Fig. 9.4 Jackson–Rees modification of T-pieces

a volume at least equal to the tidal volume and provided that the fresh gas flow is adequate. Ventilation of the expiratory limb with air is the principle used by several paediatric ventilators, the air not reaching as far as the patient provided that the expiratory limb is of sufficient length. This is also the principle underlying controlled respiration with the Bain circuit (see below).

Coaxial circuits (Bain; Lack). Although first used by Macintosh and Pask in the early 1940s, interest has only recently been re-aroused in these types of circuit. The most popular of these is the Bain circuit (Figs 9.5 and 9.6a). In this system, fresh gases are led along the narrow inner tube to the region of the face mask or endotracheal tube. The expired gases pass along the outer tube before being vented through the expiratory valve. It may be seen that this corresponds to the Mapleson D system which, for spontaneous respiration, has characteristics similar to the Mapleson E or T-piece systems already described. Thus a fresh gas flow of about twice the minute volume is required to prevent rebreathing. However, the Bain circuit is more useful as a means of controlled respiration. It has been shown that a fresh gas flow of 70 ml/kg body weight is sufficient to maintain normocarbia, while a fresh gas flow of 100 ml/kg body weight will produce relatively mild hypocarbia. This occurs over a wide range of minute volumes, provided that this exceeds the fresh gas flow. Controlled respiration with the Bain circuit is achieved by manual compression of the reservoir bag after partially closing the expiratory valve, or by totally closing the expiratory valve and ventilating the expiratory limb with air after removing the reservoir bag (as described above for T-piece systems). It is important to insert an additional metre of corrugated tubing between the ventilator tubing and the end of the expiratory limb of the Bain circuit to prevent the anaesthetic gases being diluted with air.

The normocarbia produced by IPPR using the Bain circuit has advantages over the hypocarbia produced by many other systems of controlled respiration in that it causes less reduction of cardiac output and spontaneous respiration is resumed more rapidly at the end of the operation. Other advantages are that the tubing is light, long (1·8 m) and flexible and the change from spontaneous to controlled ventilation is easily made during head and neck surgery because the valve is remote from the patient. Pollution control is easy with a modified expiratory valve and, as mentioned above, controlled ventilation may be carried out by the simplest of ventilators applied to the expiratory limb. The only type of ventilator that is unsuitable is one driven by the fresh gas supply from the anaesthetic machine (e.g. Manley).

Apart from its relative inefficiency as a method of spontaneous respiration, the main disadvantages of the Bain's circuit lie in the fragility of the plastic tubing and the difficulty of detecting leaks in, or separation of, the small-bore fresh gas tube. This latter has become less of a problem with the introduction of semi-transparent outer tubing. However, before use a simple test should be made to confirm that both inner and outer tubes are intact. The outer tube is tested by closing the expiratory valve, occluding the patient end of the Bain circuit with the thumb and turning on a fresh gas flow of about 6 litres/min. If the outer tube is intact the reservoir bag will inflate and gentle manual compression will confirm that there are no leaks from the outer tube. The little finger is then inserted inside the end of the expiratory tube to occlude the patient end of the inner (fresh gas) tube. If the inner tube is intact, this occlusion of the fresh gas flow will cause the rotameters to dip below their previous reading or the pressure relief valve to blow off—if such a valve is included in the system. It is essential to remove the little finger as soon as the rotameters begin to drop, otherwise delicate pieces of apparatus such as

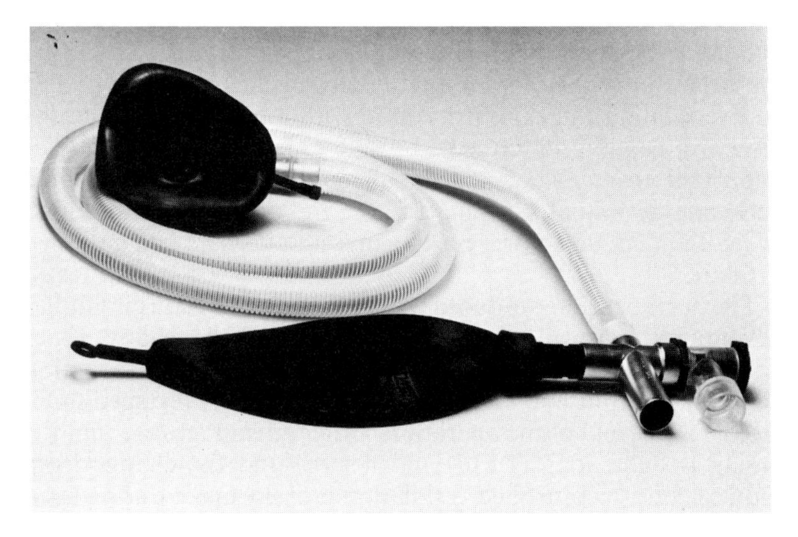

Fig. 9.5 Penlon coaxial version of Bain circuit

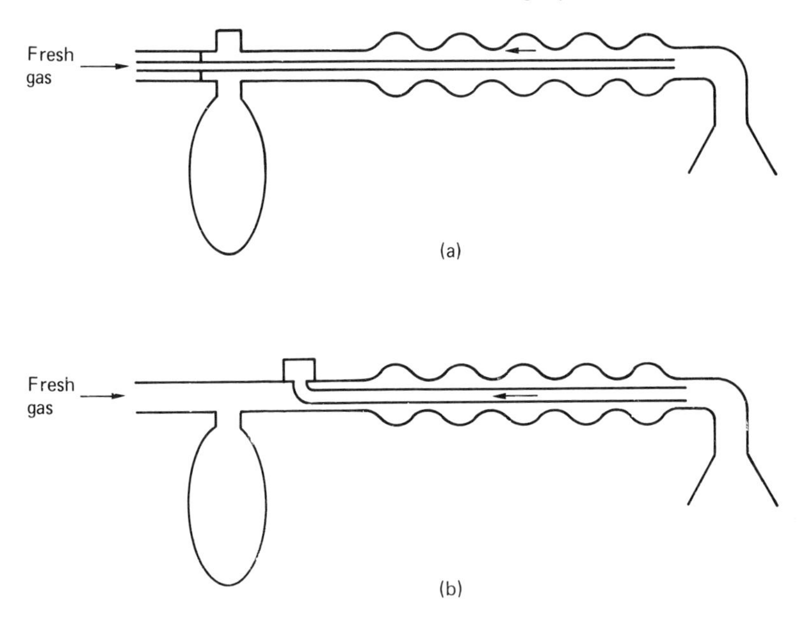

Fig. 9.6 Diagrammatic representation of (a) the Bain, and (b) the Lack circuits

temperature-compensated vaporisers may be damaged if exposed to the full pipeline pressure of 60 p.s.i.

The Lack circuit (Fig. 9.6b) is a coaxial circuit in which the fresh gases are carried to the patient through the outer tube (the reservoir bag is also on the inspiratory side), expiration occurring down the inner tube to the expiratory valve which is remote from the patient. It is a Mapleson A system, like the Magill circuit, and like the latter requires relatively modest fresh gas flows (approximately equal to minute volume) during spontaneous respiration to prevent rebreathing. It is thus more efficient than the Bain circuit for spontaneous respiration, while retaining the Bain's advantages of easy scavenging and a valve remote from the patient.

Circle systems without CO_2-absorption

This type of system is of relatively recent origin. The aim of these systems (used mainly with controlled respiration) is to avoid the hypocarbia that almost inevitably occurs during IPPR with circle systems incorporating carbon dioxide absorption. It has been found that with relatively large tidal volumes (10–15 ml/kg body weight) only mild hypocarbia occurs with fresh gas flows of the order of those for the Bain circuit. It is important to keep the expiratory valve and the point of addition of fresh gases to the circuit well separated to prevent the expulsion of too high a proportion of the fresh gases unused from the system.

Entrainment in T-piece systems (injectors). In this T-piece modification, the inspiratory limb is not at right angles to the patient and expiratory limbs, but is angled towards the patient's limb, or even parallel to it. Intermittent injection of oxygen at high pressure through a needle sized fresh gas flow orifice pointing in this direction entrains a larger volume of air through the expiratory limb. Stopping the oxygen flow allows the patient to breathe out. This has proved to be a convenient method of maintaining oxygenation of patients during bronchoscopy.

Insufflation. This form of anaesthesia has been usually confined to ear, nose and throat departments. Formerly a hollow hook placed in the corner of the mouth, or the side tube of a Boyle–Davis gag were used to insufflate anaesthetic mixtures, usually during tonsillectomy. This technique may be regarded as a variety of T-piece, the expiratory limb being represented by the patient's mouth and pharynx. Though popular, this was a relatively crude and uncontrolled method of anaesthesia, and nowadays the atmospheric pollution produced would be unacceptable. A slightly more refined technique is sometimes used for microlaryngoscopy. The anaesthetic mixture is delivered through a small tube (e.g. a suction catheter) whose tip lies somewhere within the trachea. High fresh gas flows delivered at this point are not desirable, so a relatively modest flow of a concentrated anaesthetic mixture is used, the patient diluting this mixture during inspiration with room air. Control is again erratic and, as pollution is considerable, a technique using endotracheal anaesthesia is preferable—if this is acceptable to the surgeon.

Circuits with an Inadequate Fresh Gas Flow

These systems derive from the theory that if sufficient oxygen is added to the system to provide the patient's basal requirements, and if some method of carbon dioxide absorption is used, the same anaesthetic mixture can be breathed over and over again.

The main justification for these circuits is economy in the use of anaesthetic gases and vapours. Other advantages are the conservation of expired heat and moisture, and less pollution of the theatre atmosphere. In a truly 'closed' system there is less risk of an explosion with explosive anaesthetic mixtures. The greater popularity of the very explosive and relatively expensive cyclopropane gas, in the USA, at least partially explains the commoner use of circle systems there.

Soda-lime

Soda-lime is the substance most commonly used to absorb CO_2. The composition of soda-lime, which varies slightly from manufacturer to manufacturer, is roughly:

Calcium hydroxide	94 %
Sodium hydroxide	5 %
Potassium hydroxide	1 %

Inert silicates are added to prevent powdering of the granules, which are of the size referred to as 4–8 mesh. The size of the granules is important to allow a large enough surface area for absorption and to prevent high resistance to gas flow. To the granules are added about 14 % of moisture content, which is essential for the reaction with CO_2 to take place.

A mixture of barium and calcium hydroxides (Baralyme) is the only commonly used alternative to soda-lime.

The reaction of CO_2 with soda-lime is shown in the formulae below. The calcium hydroxide is responsible for the major part of the CO_2 absorption, but combination occurs first with the more active sodium and potassium hydroxide to form sodium or potassium carbonate which then react with the calcium hydroxide, the sodium and potassium hydroxides being reconstituted in the process.

$$CO_2 + H_2O \rightarrow H_2CO_3$$

$$H_2CO_3 + \underset{\text{(sodium hydroxide)}}{2\ NaOH}\ \underset{\text{(potassium hydroxide)}}{(\text{or } 2\,KOH)} \rightarrow \underset{\text{(sodium carbonate)}}{Na_2CO_3}\ \underset{\text{(potassium carbonate)}}{(\text{or } K_2CO_3)} + 2\ H_2O$$

$$Na_2CO_3\ (\text{or } K_2CO_3) + \underset{\text{(calcium hydroxide)}}{Ca\,(OH)_2} \rightarrow \underset{\text{(calcium carbonate)}}{CaCO_3}\quad \underset{\text{regenerated to react again}}{\underset{\downarrow}{2\ NaOH\ (\text{or } 2KOH)}}$$

Chemical indicators are added to some brands of soda-lime so that a colour change occurs when the soda-lime becomes exhausted. Examples are Clayton yellow which changes from pink to yellow and ethyl violet which changes from colourless to violet when the soda-lime loses its efficiency. Too much reliance should not, however, be put on these chemical indicators; it is better to note the period during which the soda-lime has been in use. As a rough guide for this purpose, 1 kg soda-lime should last an anaesthetised adult of average weight for about eight hours.

When soda-lime canisters lie on their sides there is a tendency for the granules to fall away from the upper part of the canister so that the gases may be preferentialy channelled through this area without giving up their CO_2. For this reason, soda-lime canisters should be mounted vertically whenever possible.

Soda-lime and trichloroethylene. Soda-lime should never be used in the presence of trichloroethylene as the combination of heat and alkali may result in the breakdown of trichloroethylene into two toxic gases—dichloracetylene and phosgene. These produce cranial nerve palsies or even death.

Waters canister

This system has lost much of its popularity. Figure 9.7 shows this apparatus where the fresh gases are led in near the face mask or endotracheal tube and the patient breathes to-and-fro through the soda-lime canister which is placed between the patient and

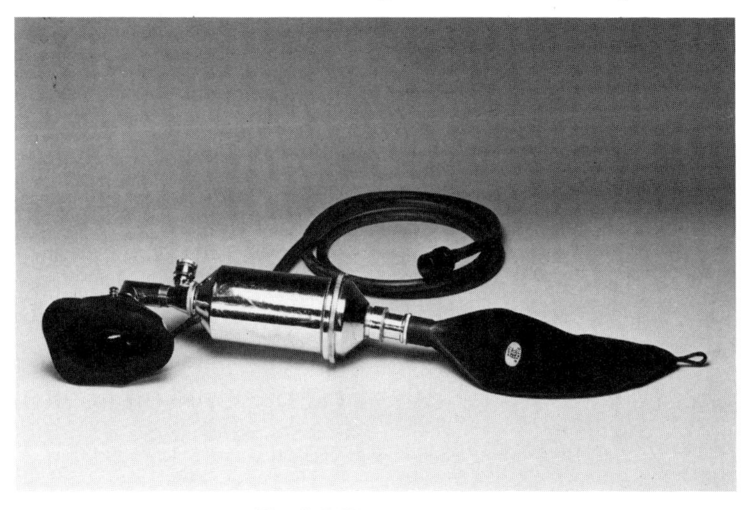

Fig. 9.7 Waters canister

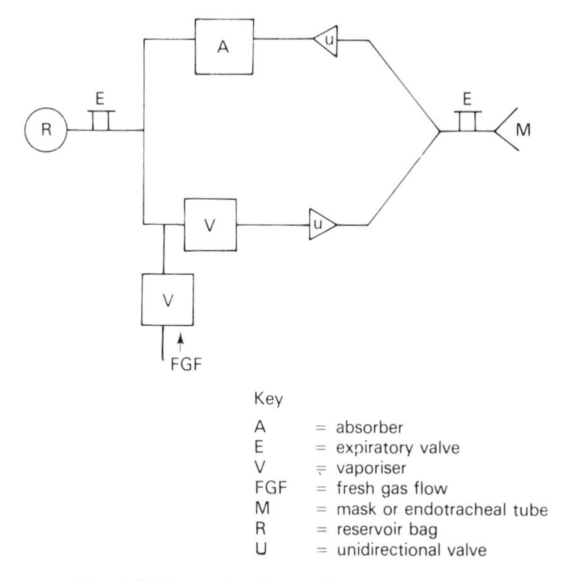

Fig. 9.8 Example of a circle arrangement

the rebreathing bag. The main reason for its fall from favour was (1) the awkwardness of the canister so close to the patient's face, (2) difficulty in preventing 'channelling' with horizontal canister, (3) a tendency to inhale alkaline dust from the soda-lime, and (4) the steady increase in dead space as the soda-lime nearest the patient became exhausted first. More recently the beneficial effects of this circuit in conserving heat have been used in hypothermic patients.

Circle systems
It has been stated above that there are many combinations for the relative positioning of the main components of the circle system. These components are two unidirectional valves, two T-piece connections to be placed next to the patient and at the fresh gas inflow point, a soda-lime canister, a reservoir bag and an overflow valve.

One possible arrangement of the components is shown in Figure 9.8. Without discussing the other possibilities in detail, it would, for instance, be pointless to have the overflow valve between the fresh gas inflow and the patient so that fresh gases were vented from the system without ever passing to the patient.

As indicated above, the circle systems may be used without

soda-lime for spontaneous or controlled respiration with fresh gas flows down to as low as the patient's alveolar ventilation without any build-up of carbon dioxide. For the average adult this means a fresh gas flow of about 4 litres/min.

When the fresh gas flow is reduced below the alveolar ventilation it is essential to have a soda-lime canister in the circuit to prevent build-up of CO_2.

Theoretically it is possible to use a circle system as a totally closed system. Once anaesthesia is established only the patient's basal requirement of 200–250 ml oxygen need be added to the system, the carbon dioxide being absorbed by the soda-lime and the patient losing no volatile anaesthetic to the atmosphere because of the closed system. In practice, this perfect balance is never attained for various reasons, such as the continued uptake of anaesthetic from the system by the patient, and imperfect absorption of CO_2. Concentrations of oxygen and anaesthetic in the circuit may vary considerably and this type of circuit is only safe in the hands of those very experienced in its use.

Position of vaporiser in the circuit. In circle systems the vaporiser may be outside the circuit (VOC) or inside the circle (VIC). In the case of VOC, the fresh gas passes through the vaporiser before joining the circuit where the concentration of anaesthetic will always be lower than the vaporiser setting as long as uptake by the patient is taking place. Eventually, as equilibrium is reached and the patient ceases to take anaesthetic from the circle, the concentration in the circle will rise towards the vaporiser setting.

The exception to this rule occurs when controlled respiration is used. This applies to any of the circuits where compression of the reservoir bag may cause a backflow into the vaporising chamber of gases which have already picked up the volatile anaesthetic. This 'pumping' action may produce concentrations of volatile anaesthetic higher than the vaporiser setting; to prevent this phenomenon some vaporisers or anaesthetic machines are now provided with a non-return valve to eliminate the backflow in the system.

In the case of VIC, the gases may pass through the vaporiser many times. In spontaneous respiration the resulting deep anaesthesia and respiratory depression slows the uptake of anaesthetic by the patient so that there is a certain built-in safety factor with this arrangement. However, if controlled respiration is used, this inherent safety is lost and high and potentially lethal concentrations of anaesthetic may be inspired.

10 Vaporisers and Inhalers

Vaporisation. Vaporisers and inhalers. The EMO inhaler.

VAPORISATION

Molecules in a liquid are constantly moving, the liquid not disintegrating because of the strong, mutual attraction of the closely packed molecules. Some of the molecules near the surface of the liquid move vertically with sufficient speed to overcome the attraction of the other molecules of the liquid. They become free in the atmosphere above the liquid where they are referred to as the vapour of the liquid. The rate of escape of the molecules is determined by the velocity of their movement, which depends on the temperature of the liquid. As the temperature rises the number of molecules that escape from the surface of liquid increases, so that the concentration of vapour above the liquid increases. Conversely, as the temperature of the liquid falls, the speed of movement of the molecules is reduced and the concentration of the vapour also falls.

Latent Heat of Vaporisation

This is a most important physical principle when discussing the vaporisation of volatile anaesthetic agents. Vaporisation requires the use of energy, as the natural tendency for the molecules of the liquid to adhere together has to be overcome. The energy is provided as heat, and this is called the latent heat of vaporisation of the liquid.

The latent heat varies from liquid to liquid, but is surprisingly high. For instance, while only 1 calorie of heat is required to raise the temperature of 1 ml water by 1 °C, it requires 580 calories to convert 1 ml water into water vapour (steam) without change of temperature (i.e. the latent heat of vaporisation of water is 580).

The heat required for vaporisation may be supplied from an external source, or may be taken from the liquid itself. In the latter case the temperature of the liquid falls, and this is what happens when a volatile anaesthetic liquid is vaporised. As we have seen above, a fall in temperature results in the volatile liquid vaporising less readily so that the amount of liquid converted into vapour falls. This means that as a stream of gases passes over a volatile anaesthetic liquid in a vaporiser, the concentration of vapour picked up will steadily fall due to the liquid cooling unless it is heated or some form of temperature-compensating mechanism is introduced.

The concept of latent heat also explains other phenomena seen in anaesthesia, e.g. the ice that tends to form on the power part of nitrous oxide cylinders as the gas is run off. The explanation here is that the lower part of the cylinder contains liquid nitrous oxide which has to be vaporised to replace the gaseous nitrous oxide being run off through the valve in the upper part of the cylinder. This vaporisation needs heat, which is taken first from the liquid nitrous oxide itself so that its temperature falls. Heat is taken next from the steel walls of the cylinder which become so cold that the water vapour in the atmosphere condenses on the outer surface of the cylinder and immediately freezes.

VAPORISERS AND INHALERS

Vaporisers and inhalers are pieces of equipment designed for vaporising volatile anaesthetic liquids. Vaporisers are usually described as having either plenum or draw-over characteristics. A plenum vaporiser is designed for use in a plenum anaesthetic system, i.e. a system where the vaporising gases arise from a high-pressure source such as a pipeline or cylinders. In this type of system no effort is required on the patient's part to draw the gases through the vaporiser, so it is not necessary that the

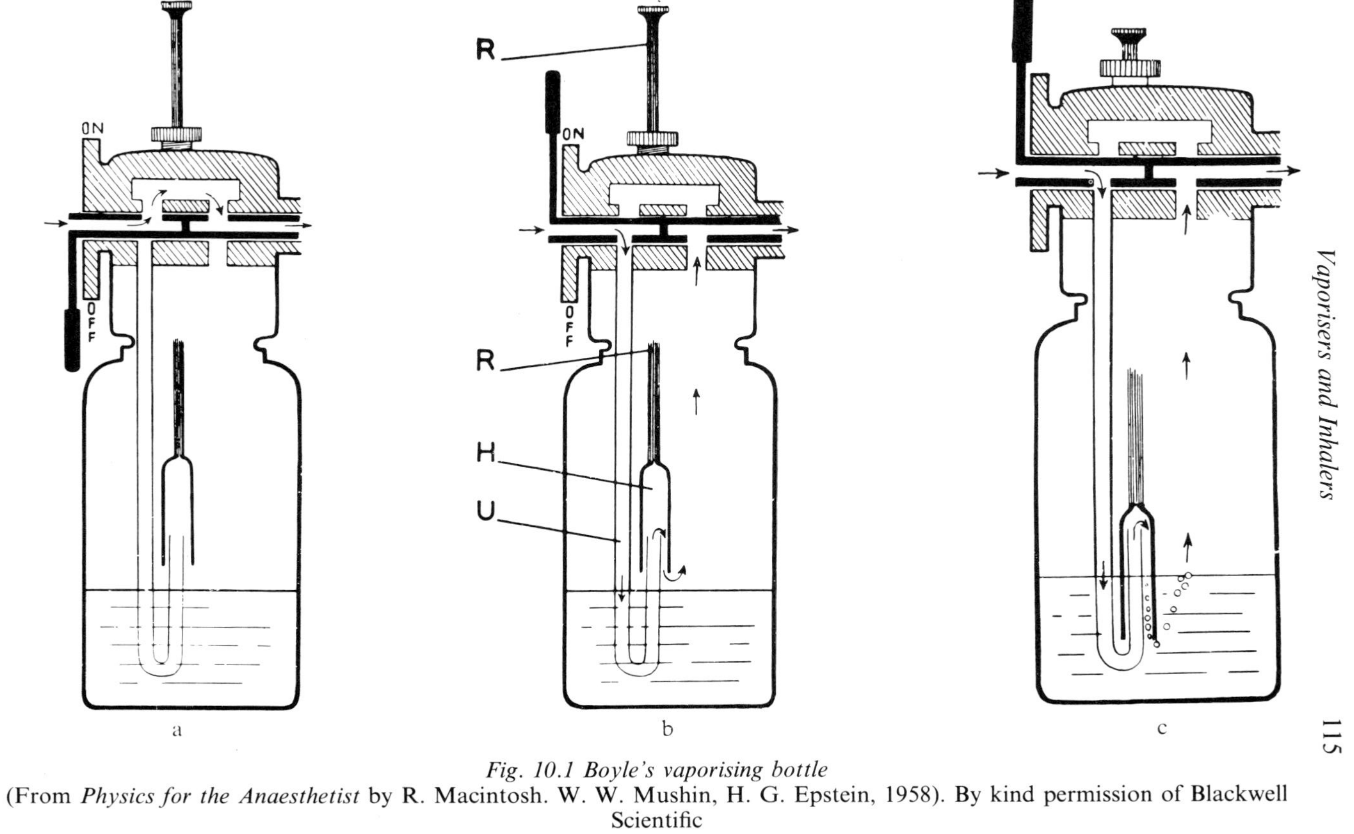

Fig. 10.1 Boyle's vaporising bottle
(From *Physics for the Anaesthetist* by R. Macintosh. W. W. Mushin, H. G. Epstein, 1958). By kind permission of Blackwell Scientific

resistance to flow of gases through the vaporiser be particularly low. Examples of this type of vaporiser are the Fluotec and Abingdon vaporisers.

In draw-over vaporisers (the inhalers all belong to this group) the vaporising vehicle (usually air) is drawn through the vaporiser by the patient's own respiratory effort. This means that the resistance of the vaporiser must be low so that the patient does not have to make too great an effort. Examples of this type of vaporiser are the EMO (Epstein–Macintosh–Oxford) inhaler and the OMV (Oxford Miniature Vaporiser). While plenum vaporisers cannot be used in draw-over systems, there is no reason why draw-over vaporisers cannot be used in plenum systems.

The basic arrangement of most modern vaporisers is similar to that of the bottles formerly supplied with the Boyle's anaesthetic apparatus. The construction is shown in Figures 10.1 a–c.

These vaporisers are essentially bottles with an on-off control lever. In Figure 10.1a the lever is in the 'off' position so that the entire flow of gases bypasses the vaporising bottle. In Figure 10.1b the lever is in the 'on' position so that the entire flow of gases passes into the vaporising bottle. The control lever may be placed in any intermediate position, thus varying the proportion of gas-flow diverted over the volatile liquid. Some Boyle's bottles had a further method of controlling the vapour concentration. This consisted of the rod R which could be used to lower the hood down over the open end of the tube U. As the hood was lowered the flow of gases escaping from the open end of the tube U were diverted closer and closer to the surface of the volatile liquid. Finally, as shown in Figure 10.1c, the hood could be lowered so that the gases were bubbled through the volatile agent, thus producing the maximum concentration of vapour achievable with this apparatus. Unfortunately the concentration of vapour steadily fell as vaporisation produced cooling of the liquid. With a volatile agent like ether the temperature, and therefore the concentration of ether vapour produced, fell so low that it might be inadequate for adequate anaesthesia. For this reason it was not uncommon to put two Boyle's bottles in series, or to surround the Boyle's bottle with a vessel containing warm water in an effort to maintain the ether temperature and therefore the concentration.

Temperature Compensating Devices

Many modern vaporisers conform to this basic configuration of a bottle with a main control knob or lever which divides the gas stream into two parts, one bypassing the vaporising chamber, and the other passing through it. In addition, many vaporisers now contain some temperature-compensating device, so that for any setting of the main control lever, the concentration of vapour leaving the vaporiser is constant. These temperature-compensating mechanisms are usually in the form of a bimetallic strip or a thermosensitive capsule.

Bimetallic strip

The bimetallic strip mechanism depends on the fact that different metals expand to different amounts when heated. A bimetallic strip consists of two bars of different metals riveted together, so that when the whole strip is warmed it bends as the metal with the greater coefficient of expansion lengthens relative to the

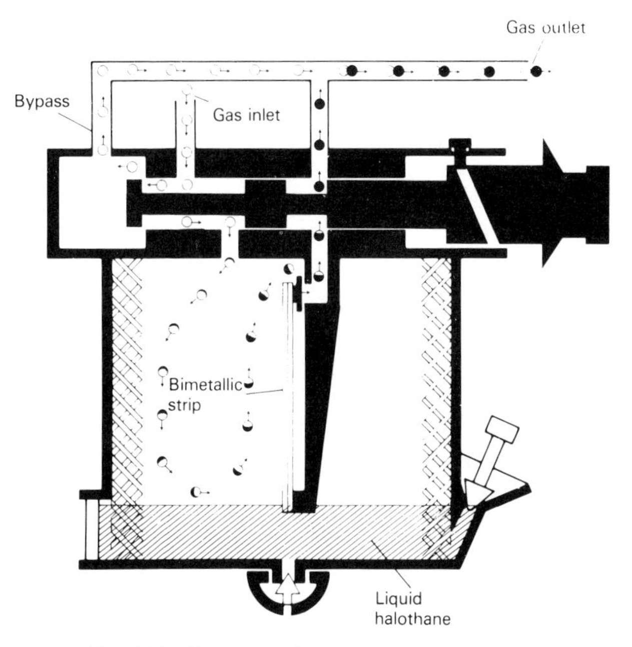

Fig. 10.2 Fluotec mark 2 vaporiser in 'on' position
(By kind permission of Cyprane Ltd, Keighley, Yorks)

other bar. The bimetallic strip is made to operate a valve regulating the proportion of the gas stream which bypasses the vaporising chamber. This can be seen in Figure 10.2 which shows a Fluotec mark 2 vaporiser. As the halothane in the vaporising chamber cools, the bimetallic bar tends to open the valve so that a higher proportion of the gas stream is diverted over the surface of the halothane. Conversely, if the halothane warms up, the bimetallic strip-operated valve tends to close and a higher proportion of the gas stream bypasses the vaporising chamber. In this way, the concentration of halothane emitting from the vaporiser remains constant despite alterations in temperature of the liquid halothane produced either by vaporisation or by changes in the ambient temperature.

Thermosensitive capsule
An example of a thermosensitive capsule is shown in the diagram of the EMO vaporiser (Fig. 10.3). In this case the capsule consists of a metal bellows which operates a plunger which opens and closes a valve. The bellows is surrounded by ether vapour in a closed container. In this case the valve alters the proportion of the gas stream which passes through the vaporising chamber. The capsule sits within the vaporising chamber so that a fall in the temperature of the ether in that chamber is accompanied by a fall in temperature of the ether vapour within the closed container. This causes an opening of the valve so that a higher proportion of the gas stream passes through the vaporising chamber. The converse applies if the temperature of the ether in

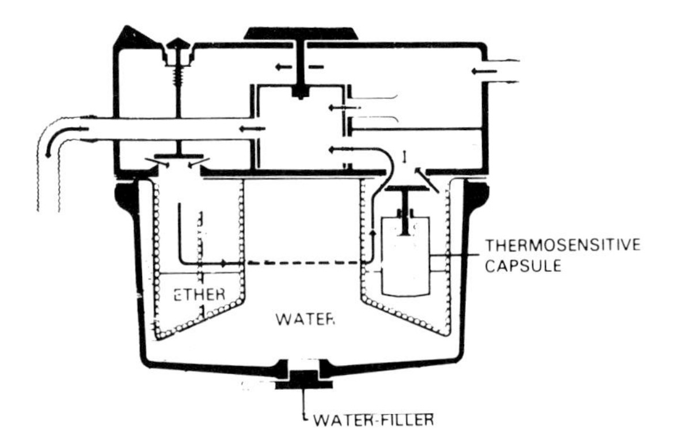

Fig. 10.3 Cross-section of EMO vaporiser

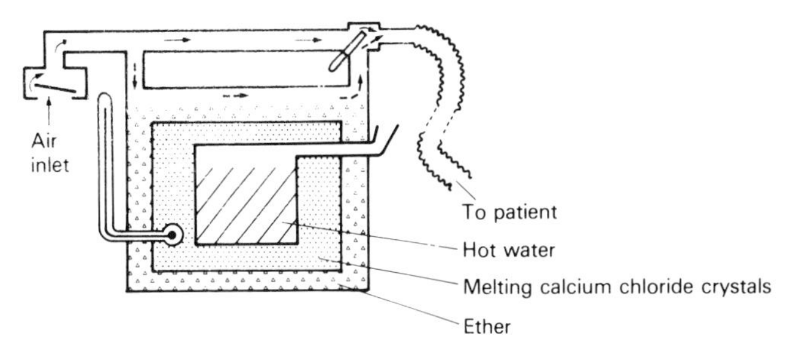

Fig. 10.4 Oxford vaporiser mark 1

the vaporising chamber rises. A similar method of temperature compensation is found in the Abingdon vaporiser.

Some vaporisers, e.g. the EMO and OMV, have a water-jacket or container surrounding the vaporising chamber. This is not a temperature-compensating device, but acts as a heat reservoir so that the temperature of the volatile agent does not tend to fall as quickly as if the vaporising chamber was surrounded simply by air.

Two other methods of dealing with the problem presented by the changes in vapour concentration associated with changes of temperature will be mentioned.

The first was the ingenious principle of the mark 1 Oxford vaporiser for ether (Fig. 10.4).

In this apparatus the vaporising chamber was surrounded by a vessel containing melting calcium chloride crystals. These have a constant temperature while in the melting state, and maintain the ether at a constant temperature. The other method is the 'copper kettle' apparatus which gained considerable popularity in the USA. This vaporiser consisted of a vaporising chamber made of copper, which has a high thermal conductivity, and was attached to an anesthetic table top of the same material. This arrangement ensured that the contents of the vaporising chamber remained at room temperature. The vaporiser is supplied with its own relatively low flow of oxygen which is divided into fine bubbles as it passes through the volatile agent. In this way, the oxygen flowing through the vaporiser is always completely saturated with anaesthetic vapour; this stream then joins the main stream of anaesthetic gases. Provided that the flow rates of the two streams and the temperature of the liquid (which stays constant) are known, the final concentration of the vapour in the emerging gas stream may be read off from tables. This

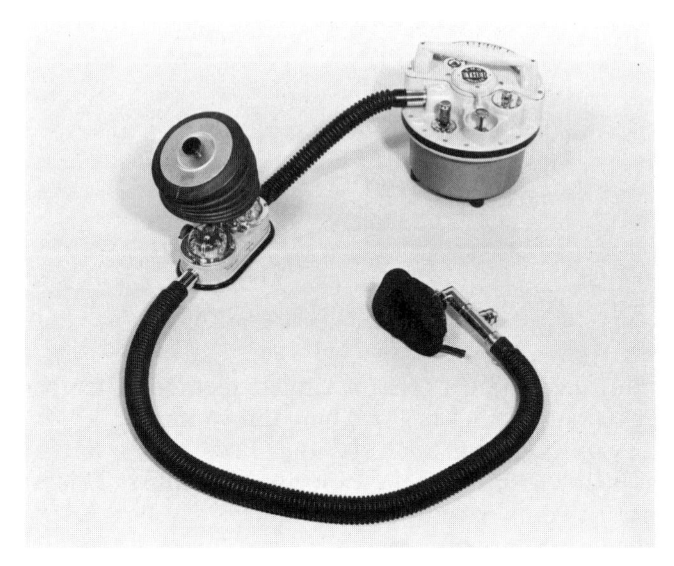

Fig. 10.5 EMO inhaler

relatively complicated system has never gained popularity in the UK.

THE EMO INHALER

The EMO ether inhaler (Fig. 10.5) is a temperature-compensated, draw-over ether vaporiser introduced in 1956. It is used with the OIB (Oxford Inflating Bellows) which consists of two unidirectional flap valves and a spring-loaded bellows. There is also a stopcock for adding oxygen directly to the bellows.

Ether concentrations of up to 20 % can be obtained by moving the lever on top of the vaporiser, these concentrations being kept accurate over a wide range of temperatures by the temperature-compensating device already mentioned which is located inside the casing of the vaporisor. The apparatus also has a water-jacket with a capacity of about 1200 ml.

This apparatus may be used simply with air as the vaporising vehicle with either spontaneous or controlled respiration. For the former a Heidbrink or non-return valve may be used. Controlled respiration may be performed with the OIB and a closed

Heidbrink valve by intermittently raising the face mask, or a thumb placed over the suction port of a Portex connection if the patient is intubated. More conveniently, an inflating valve such as the Ambu-E may be used, but in this case the magnet supplied with the OIB must be placed over the flap valve on the patient side of the OIB. If this is not done, the valve will not cycle into the expiratory (open from patient to atmosphere) position and the patient will become progressively overinflated with each breath.

The one situation in which the magnet must not be left in place over the flap valve is when the patient is breathing spontaneously with a Heidbrink valve. This will result in the patient rebreathing back into the bellows instead of out through the Heidbrink valve, which is very dangerous.

Oxygen may be added to the EMO system either by a T-piece system plugged into the inlet port of the EMO or via the stopcock on the OIB. The former is preferable (except when the OIB is being used simply for resuscitation) as oxygen added at the OIB will dilute the concentration of ether emitting from the EMO. It is important to remember that while ether and air are for practical purposes non-detonable, the addition of oxygen produces a most explosive mixture.

Further refinements of the EMO system are the addition of OMVs for halothane or trichloroethylene (which should be placed between the EMO and OIB) or its conversion into a plenum system for use with nitrous oxide and oxygen. The prior administration of about 2% halothane for 2–3 minutes has a powerful depressant effect on the coughing evoked by ether so that induction with the latter may be greatly facilitated.

Another important modification of the EMO system is the so-called Tri-Service (abbreviation for Army, Air Force and Navy) system. This involves the substitution of halothane and trichloroethylene OMVs for the EMO inhaler. This can be used for spontaneous or controlled respiration anaesthesia and its portability and efficiency was recently proved in the Falklands campaign.

Almost any operation can be carried out with the EMO system using air and ether alone. This fact, plus the robustness, reliability and portability of the EMO, makes it a most important piece of anaesthetic equipment worldwide, especially in underdeveloped countries where compressed gases may be either unobtainable or prohibitively expensive.

11 Volatile Anaesthetic Agents

Chloroform. Ether. Halothane. Trichloroethylene. Enflurane. Isoflurane.

Volatile anaesthetic agents depend on uptake by the lungs and subsequent diffusion across the alveolar capillary membrane into the bloodstream. Apart from using this method of administration, however, the volatile anaesthetic agents exert their effects like any other drug dissolved in blood, and therefore in terms of anaesthesia, possess the important properties of hypnosis, analgesia and relaxation in varying degrees.

Uptake by the lungs (Chapter 6) depends on the physical properties of the agent concerned as well as on variations in minute volume and alveolar ventilation. The importance of saturated vapour pressure in terms of the maximum vapour concentration of any particular agent, together with the importance of blood/gas solubility coefficients, have both already been emphasised. The values of these, for the volatile agents considered in this chapter, are listed in Table 11.1.

Although volatile agents are generally used for maintaining anaesthesia it is perfectly feasible to use them for induction, particularly in children; for this purpose some agents are much better than others. In general, however, we must consider the agents in terms of their contribution towards a balanced anaesthetic technique and therefore their relative properties in terms of hypnosis, analgesia and relaxation. These are summarised in Table 11.2 and it can be seen that the only agent that possesses

Table 11.1 Physical properties of volatile anaesthetics

	Boiling point °C	Saturated vapour pressure at 20 °C	Blood/gas solubility coefficient	Oil/H_2O solubility coefficient	MAC %
Halothane	50	243	2·36	330	0·77
Ether	35	442	12·1	3·2	1·92
Trichloroethylene	87·5	60	9·5	400	0·17
Enflurane	56·5	174·5	1·9	120	1·68
Isoflurane	49	250	1·4	174	1·15

all three properties is ether, which at the same time is explosive when used with N_2O or O_2 and therefore little used today. The volatile agents are broadly divided into ethers and hydrocarbons. The addition of halogen radicals (e.g. fluoride, chloride, bromide) to molecules of increasing size tends to increase their potency.

In addition to their pharmacological contribution to general anaesthesia, the volatile anaesthetic agents must be considered in terms of their effects on blood pressure, cardiac output, respiration, peripheral circulation and intracranial pressure; in many instances their routes of metabolism and excretion are also important.

Table 11.2 Pharmacological properties of volatile anaesthetics

	Hypnosis	Analgesia	Relaxation
Halothane	++		++
Ether	+	+	+
Trichloroethylene	+	++	(+)
Enflurane	++	?(+)	++
Isoflurane	++	?(+)	++

CHLOROFORM

Although chloroform possesses both hypnotic, analgesic and relaxant properties, its use in modern practice has been almost completely stopped. It produces a dose-related depression of blood pressure and respiration, by both an effect on the central nervous system and a direct depressant effect on the myocardium. Chloroform also produces severe dysrhythmias and, in particular, ventricular fibrillation that may lead to sudden death. Possibly this is caused by chloroform sensitising the myocardium to the circulating effects of adrenaline: for this reason adrenaline should not be used with chloroform. This agent also produces a delayed form of poisoning caused by toxic metabolites leading to centrilobular hepatic necrosis and death.

ETHER

Ether possesses hypnotic, analgesic and relaxant properties. However, it is a relatively soluble anaesthetic agent and therefore takes a long time to induce anaesthesia if used for an inhalational induction (Chapter 6), but ether is relatively cheap and is widely used in underdeveloped countries. It tends to produce raised levels of adrenaline and therefore an increased pulse rate and a relatively steady blood pressure. Hyperglycaemia, bronchial and coronary artery dilation, an increase in respiratory rate and dilation of the pupils are also results of catecholamine release. The relatively high blood solubility of ether means that recovery from this agent may be prolonged although it is excreted entirely unchanged.

HALOTHANE

Halothane is now widely used in a great many different anaesthetic techniques. It is an excellent hypnotic and, being relatively insoluble in blood, produces rapid induction of anaesthesia. It is also a good relaxant though not sufficient alone to allow abdominal surgery except in infants. Even so, halothane possesses no analgesic properties and therefore requires supplementary analgesia, either in the form of premedication or intra-operatively. It produces significant effects on blood pressure by depressing both the myocardium itself and the conductive tissue of the heart. Halothane also causes an overall reduction in peripheral resistance by producing vasodilation in skin which is partially balanced by vasoconstriction in skeletal muscle. Vagal stimulation results in a decreased pulse rate and aggravates the hypotension produced. Like other agents it produces dose-related respiratory depression. About 18 % of the inhaled halothane is metabolised by the liver, the remainder being excreted unchanged, but halothane has been shown to cause alterations in hepatic function, particularly after repeated exposure to the drug. Hepatitis following repeat halothane anaesthesia has been demonstrated unequivocally, but in only very few cases. Possibly this is due to a hypersensitivity reaction to a metabolite of halothane, but as the histological picture is identical to viral hepatitis it is possible that an exacerbation of such a disease may be the cause of the hepatitis. Other agents such as methoxyflurane have also been shown to produce hepatitis. Halothane relaxes the pregnant uterus and should not be used, except in very low concentrations, in pregnant patients.

TRICHLOROETHYLENE

Trichloroethylene (Trilene) is an excellent analgesic and weak hypnotic though its high blood solubility produces prolonged induction and recovery. It has relatively little effect on either blood pressure or pulse rate although it may produce cardiac dysrhythmias of all kinds, leading to hypotension. It has also been used in obstetrics for inhalation analgesia and is extremely cheap. Trichloroethylene should not be used with soda-lime in a closed circuit because toxic metabolites (Chapter 9) may be produced which cause cranial nerve damage. Trichloroethylene is excreted by the lungs almost entirely unchanged.

ENFLURANE

This comparatively new agent possesses many properties similar to halothane and is a good hypnotic and relaxant, though its analgesic properties are in some doubt. Its effects on the cardiovascular and respiratory system are similar to halothane, producing an overall reduction in blood pressure and heart rate. The main advantage of enflurane seems to be that it is metabolised to a far lesser extent than halothane and has not yet been implicated in postoperative hepatitis (enflurane metabolism is less than 3 %; halothane 18 %). Enflurane does not cause catecholamine release or associated problems and appears to be acceptable for inhalational induction of anaesthesia.

ISOFLURANE

Isoflurane is a halogenated ether and an optical isomer of enflurane. Unlike both halothane and enflurane, however, it does not depress myocardial contractility or conduction. Isoflurane produces hypotension by peripheral vasodilation and increasing doses of the agent will lower blood pressure and simultaneously increase the depth of anaesthesia. This tends to prevent the reflex tachycardia which results from other techniques of induced hypotension. Isoflurane is metabolised less than 0·3 % making it a suitable agent for use in patients with liver disease. For this reason, it is highly unlikely to be associated with the production of hepatitis.

12 Neuromuscular Transmission and Muscle Relaxant Drugs

History. Neuromuscular transmission. Types of neuromuscular block. Individual drugs. Nerve stimulators. Antibiotics and muscle relaxant drugs. Postoperative apnoea.

HISTORY

The early explorers of South America brought back reports of a mysterious arrow poison used by the South American Indians. Small quantities of this poison—curare—probably reached Europe, but it was not until 1851 that Sir Benjamin Brodie published a book describing some experiments with the substance. These included a description of how an ass treated with curare was kept alive by artificial respiration (happily not by mouth-to-mouth respiration, but by a bellows inserted in a tracheostomy!).

In 1850 Claude Bernard, the great physiologist, showed how the site of action of curare is neither on the nerve nor on the muscle, but on the neuromuscular junction.

Crude curare was made from various sources, but in 1935 King isolated one of the active constituents—the alkaloid d-tubocurarine which came from the roots of a small plant, *Chondrodendron tomentosum*.

In 1940 Bennet described the use of d-tubocurarine to soften the convulsions produced by electroconvulsive therapy. In 1942 Griffith and Johnson of Montreal described the first use of d-tubocurarine to provide muscle relaxation for surgery; this paper marked one of the milestones of modern anaesthesia.

Suxamethonium was introduced into clinical practice in 1951 at the Karolinska Institute in Stockholm.

NEUROMUSCULAR TRANSMISSION

The passage of an impulse down a nerve fibre is believed to be an electrical phenomenon. Similarly, the spread of an impulse across a muscle fibre causing it to contract is believed to be electrical. However, the transmission of the impulse from the nerve fibre to the muscle fibre is believed to be carried out by the chemical substance acetylcholine, and this occurs at special junctional areas between the nerve fibre and muscle fibre usually referred to as the neuromuscular or myoneural junction (Fig. 12.1).

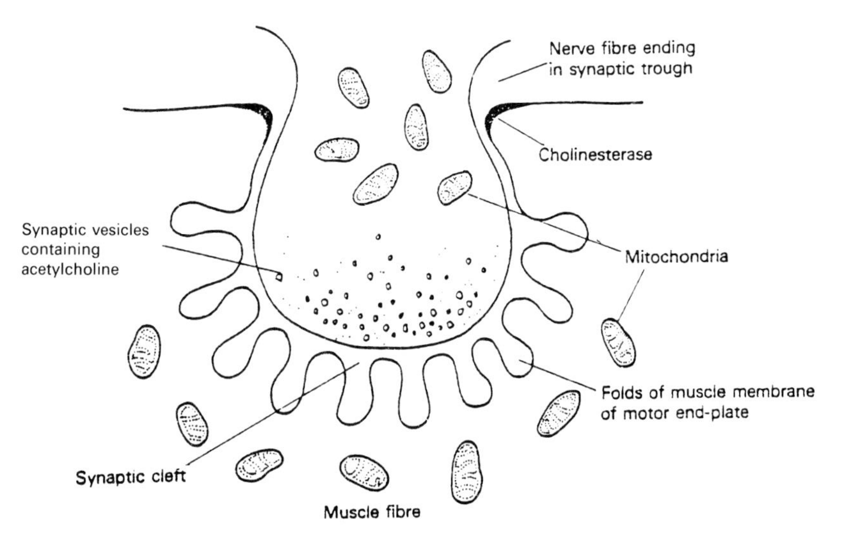

Fig. 12.1 Neuromuscular junction

The nerve-ending part of the neuromuscular junction is called the presynaptic or prejunctional area. The acetylcholine is manufactured in, stored in and, when a nerve impulse arrives, released from this area of the nerve ending.

The acetylcholine then crosses the extremely narrow gap to arrive at the muscle side of the neuromuscular junction. This is called the postsynaptic area or motor end-plate. The motor end-plate contains special acetylcholine receptor sites. On the arrival of sufficient acetylcholine the muscle membrane of the postsynaptic area becomes permeable to sodium ions, which pass into the muscle cell and produce sudden electrical depolarisation. If this current of depolarisation (also called the motor end-plate potential) reaches a certain magnitude the depolarisation spreads to the adjacent part of the muscle fibre (when it is called the muscle action potential) and is propagated across the surface of the muscle fibre, causing the contraction of the fibre in its wake.

In the meantime the acetylcholine is broken down in a fraction of a second by an enzyme called acetylcholinesterase, which is present at the motor end-plate. The neuromuscular junction is then ready to receive and transmit the next nerve impulse.

TYPES OF NEUROMUSCULAR BLOCK

Depolarising Block

Neuromuscular blocking agents of this group produce depolarisation at the postsynaptic membrane in the same way that acetylcholine does. However, once depolarisation has occurred it is maintained, so that when acetylcholine is released by the nerve stimulus it can produce no further depolarisation and paralysis occurs. The relaxation produced by depolarising block is preceded by a short period of muscle fasciculation as the agent produces depolarisation.

Non-depolarising Block

The non-depolarising blocking agents (also formerly called competitive inhibitory blocking agents) are believed to attach themselves to the receptor sites on the postsynaptic membrane to which the acetylcholine molecules normally become attached. The acetylcholine is prevented from reaching the end-plate receptor site in sufficient quantity to produce depolarisation, thus explaining the name given to this type of block.

If acetylcholine is present in sufficient concentration it is capable of removing the non-depolarising blocker from the receptor sites so that the neuromuscular junction can function again. This is achieved clinically by administering an anticholinesterase drug which inhibits the enzyme cholinesterase, whose normal function is to break down the acetylcholine at the neuromuscular junction. Thus the concentration of acetylcholine builds up and the block is overcome.

The anticholinesterase most frequently used in anaesthesia is neostigmine. Besides its action in reversing a non-depolarising block, however, neostigmine also has unwanted muscarinic effects (Chapter 14), the most important of which are bradycardia (or even cardiac arrest) and stimulation of bronchial and salivary secretion. These muscarinic actions of neostigmine are antagonised by atropine, so it is customary to give this with (or immediately before) the neostigmine in the usual adult dose of atropine 1·2–1·8 mg with neostigmine 2·5–5·0 mg. Nevertheless, the neostigmine usually just 'wins' in these proportions and few patients in the recovery room after this combination of drugs have a faster pulse than normal. This is not necessarily an indication of the patient's well-being, of course, but merely an indication that he has recently been given neostigmine.

As anticholinesterase drugs increase the concentration of acetylcholine at the neuromuscular junction, and as acetylcholine causes depolarisation, these drugs tend to have a depolarising blocking action of their own and to potentiate the effect of any depolarising agents that may be circulating. It is therefore unwise to give a short-acting depolarising agent in an attempt to reintroduce neuromuscular blockade after a non-depolarising block has been reversed by neostigmine. If neuromuscular block does occur it is likely to be prolonged.

Phase II Block (Dual Block)

If depolarising blocking agents are given repeatedly to produce a prolonged period of relaxation, the depolarising block eventually changes its nature. The block increasingly shows the properties of a non-depolarising block, in particular it being possible to at least partially reverse the block by an anticholines terase. The readiness with which this type of block becomes of clinical significance with intermittent suxamethonium varies from patient to patient but is seldom important with a dose of under 500 mg in a fit adult. A marked degree of dual block is best avoided—if intermittent suxamethonium or a suxamethonium drip is being used—by ensuring every now and again that the patient is adequately 'coming out' of the incremental doses of the drug.

INDIVIDUAL DRUGS

Depolarising Agents

Suxamethonium

Suxamethonium (Scoline), the only depolarising agent still in common clinical use, was introduced in 1951. Usually 75–100 mg are given to intubate a male adult, the effect coming on in a circulation time and lasting 3–5 minutes. The muscle fasciculations which it causes before paralysis may be violent. 'Suxamethonium pains' are skeletal muscle pains that occur in some patients after having suxamethonium. They are thought to be related in some way to the fasciculations, although their severity is not directly related to the degree of visible fasciculation. They occur most commonly and most severely in patients who are quickly ambulant after their anaesthetic and their incidence has been reported as being as high as 80 %. On the other hand, an incidence as low as 2 % has been reported after major thoracic surgery. They are also uncommon in children under nine and in the elderly. Their frequency and severity can be reduced by giving a small dose of a non-depolarising agent, e.g. 3 mg d-tubocurarine or 0·8 mg pancuronium at least two minutes before the suxamethonium. Unfortunately this technique slightly reduces the efficacy of the suxamethonium, which may be a disadvantage if intubation is urgent or difficult.

Other side-effects of suxamethonium associated with the muscle fasciculations are increased intraocular pressure due to contraction of the intraocular muscles and an increase in serum potassium due to muscle fibre rupture. The former complication may be dangerous in certain eye procedures (e.g. where there is a perforating injury to the eye or in cataract operations). The rise in serum potassium due to muscle damage is not usually serious unless the potassium concentration is already raised. In both these events it is probably better to avoid depolarising muscle relaxants or, if they are considered essential, to precede them with a small dose of a non-depolarising agent as described above.

The only other significant side-effect of suxamethonium is its tendency to produce bradycardia, especially after the injection of a second dose. This effect is blocked by atropine and many anaesthetists recommend that this drug be given intravenously —if not before the first, at least before the second dose of suxamethonium

While the commonest use of suxamethonium is to provide good intubating conditions, it may be used to provide relaxation for longer operations by giving incremental doses (of about 25 mg in an adult) or by using a suxamethonium infusion, e.g. suxamethonium 500 mg in normal saline 500 ml. Two problems make this less universally popular for prolonged muscle relaxation than the non-depolarising agents. The first of these is the possibility of dual block developing; the second is the relative difficulty of providing as smooth a level of muscular relaxation as with the longer-acting agents.

Suxamethonium (Scoline) apnoea. Suxamethonium is usually rapidly broken down in the plasma by a naturally occurring enzyme called plasma (or pseudo) cholinesterase. This usually gives suxamethonium an action of only 3–5 minutes. However, a few people possess an atypical pseudocholinesterase enzyme which has very little ability to break down suxamethonium. This abnormal enzyme is transmitted hereditarily by an abnormal gene and about one in 3000 people is affected. In these patients suxamethonium has a more prolonged action, often in the 2–4 hour range, the suxamethonium being broken down by alkaline hydrolysis, a process which does not play an important role in normal patients. Essentially the treatment consists of ventilating the patient, preferably with a mixture of nitrous oxide and oxygen until adequate respiration returns. Confirmation that the apnoea is due to this cause may be obtained by testing the patient's serum for atypical pseudocholinesterase. If the test is positive it is important to test close relatives in the same way to anticipate their extreme sensitivity to suxamethonium. Every effort should be made to avoid giving suxamethonium to those affected.

Non-depolarising Agents

The remaining agents discussed in this chapter all belong to this group. They are all slower in onset than suxamethonium, adequate conditions for intubation not usually occurring in under 2–3 minutes. As they do not produce depolarisation these agents do not produce muscle fasciculations or any of the complications associated with them. They are relatively long-acting, but their action is reversed by neostigmine. Probably the 'ideal' muscle relaxant would be a non-depolarising agent with an onset as rapid as that of suxamethonium and a very short action. Claims that various new agents almost fulfil these criteria have not been substantiated.

d-Tubocurarine chloride (Tubarine)

This purified alkaloid is the only naturally occurring substance at present in use as a neuromuscular blocking agent. It is relatively slow in onset (about 3 minutes) and lasts 30–45 minutes, although none of the non-depolarising agents has an abrupt end-point. For endotracheal intubation a dose of 40–45 mg is required in a 70 kg man, this being reduced by one-third for abdominal muscle relaxation if intubation has previously been carried out under suxamethonium. As with other non-depolarising agents, incremental doses are about one-fifth of the intubation dose. In the presence of halothane and ether the dosage requirements for d-tubocurarine are reduced, but it is unlikely that these agents act in precisely the same way as d-tubocurarine.

One of the main side effects of d-tubocurarine is its tendency to produce hypotension. It probably does this mainly by myocardial depression, but animal experiments suggest that it may have some blocking effect on the sympathetic ganglia and also some histamine-releasing action. As histamine may cause bronchospasm, theoretically this is not the relaxant of choice for asthmatics. The tendency to reduce blood pressure is made use of, especially in conjuction with halothane, as a method of producing controlled hypotension to reduce surgical bleeding. The local release of histamine after injection of d-tubocurarine is sometimes seen as an erythema and wealing up the line of the vein. These reactions are not serious and usually fade in a few minutes.

d-Tubocurarine is excreted unchanged by the kidneys, the biliary system providing an alternative route which may be particularly valuable when renal function is impaired.

In ill patients the effect of d-tubocurarine may be difficult to reverse completely with neostigmine, the respiration in particular remaining inadequate with 'see-sawing' movements of the abdomen and chest, and a 'tracheal tug', the larynx jerking downwards towards the chest with each inspiration. The mechanism of this resistance to neostigmine is unknown, but it seems to be commoner in the presence of a metabolic acidosis. This problem may arise with any of the non-depolarising drugs, as well as with d-tubocurarine.

Gallamine triethiodide (Flaxedil)

This was one of the earliest of the synthetic non-depolarisers. It is a little quicker in onset than d-tubocurarine, but has a slightly shorter duration of action—about 20–30 minutes. About 140 mg are required for intubation in a 70 kg man.

One of its main side-effects is that it blocks the cardiac vagus nerve, thus producing a tachycardia which tends to cause brisk oozing at the surgical incision. On the other hand, it tends to have a supportive effect on the blood pressure which makes it more popular for ill patients than d-tubocurarine.

It is excreted unchanged by the kidneys, which means that it may have a prolonged action in patients with renal failure. Its other undesirable property is that of all the non-depolarising relaxants gallamine is the one considered most likely to cross the placenta to the fetus in appreciable concentrations. With alternative agents available it is probably wise to avoid it in obstetrics. Gallamine has little or no histamine-releasing effect in man.

Pancuronium bromide (Pavulon)
This is one of the newer synthetic non-depolarising drugs, and is unusual in that it has a steroid ring configuration. Its rapid onset makes it a popular choice where a non-depolariser is to be used for endotracheal intubation, and its duration of action probably lies between that of gallamine and d-tubocurarine. A 70 kg man would require 8–10 mg for good intubating conditions and a woman 6–8 mg. Incremental doses of about one-fifth these amounts are required.

The effects of pancuronium on the cardiovascular system are to produce a tachycardia (usually mild or moderate) and sometimes a slight increase in blood pressure. It is not believed to release histamine or cross the placenta in significant amounts.

Pancuronium is excreted largely unchanged by the kidneys, but metabolism in the liver and excretion in the bile are a valuable alternative excretory mechanism.

Alcuronium chloride (Alloferin)
This is another synthetic agent with a rate of onset almost as fast as pancuronium and a similar duration of action. About 20 mg is required for good intubating conditions in a male adult. It has little or no effect on the pulse rate or blood pressure, the tendency being to produce a slight fall in the latter. It has only a mild histamine-releasing action.

Like d-tubocurarine and pancuronium it is excreted mainly by the kidneys, but may also be excreted in the bile.

Vecuronium bromide (Norcuron)
This is one of the newer drugs with a speed of onset similar to pancuronium and a medium duration of action (20–30 minutes). The dose is the same, or slightly larger than that for pancuronium. It has the least effect on the cardiovascular system of any of the relaxants, causing neither tachycardia nor hypotension, and it does not release histamine. It is excreted mostly in the bile and only to a small extent through the kidneys, making it a useful drug in cases of renal failure.

Atracurium besylate (Tracrium)
Another relatively new non-depolarising drug, atracurium has a speed of onset and duration of action similar to that of vecuronium. About 40 mg is recommended to intubate a 70 kg

patient. Atracurium is unique in that it is broken down in the plasma mainly by a process known as 'Hofmann elimination' which occurs at plasma pH and body temperature. The termination of action of this drug is not dependent on metabolism or excretion by either the liver or the kidneys, so it is useful in hepatic or renal failure (Chapter 32). Under normal circumstances its action is reversed using atropine/neostigmine.

Atracurium has minimal effects on the heart and blood pressure, and has a weak histamine-releasing action.

It should be noted that anaesthetic agents (e.g. halothane) or surgical manoeuvres (e.g. peritoneal traction) which cause vagal stimulation are more likely to produce a bradycardia when cardiovascularly inactive drugs like vecuronium or atracurium are being used rather than tachycardia-inducing agents like pancuronium or gallamine.

ANTIBIOTICS AND MUSCLE RELAXANT DRUGS

Several antibiotics, including streptomycin, neomycin, kanamycin, polymyxin, bacitracin, colomycin and viomycin, have neuromuscular blocking properties. They tend to potentiate non-depolarising block and deaths have been reported when large doses of some of these antibiotics have been given to patients under anaesthesia. Particularly high doses may be given intraperitoneally. The block produced is partly reversed by neostigmine but calcium appears to be more effective.

NERVE STIMULATORS

Portable, battery-powered nerve stimulators are becoming increasingly popular (Fig. 12.2). By means of two electrodes placed over a peripheral nerve (commonly the ulnar nerve at the wrist) they can apply a variety of different types of stimulation the effect of which is seen by contraction of a muscle supplied by that nerve (usually the adductor muscle of the thumb). These types of

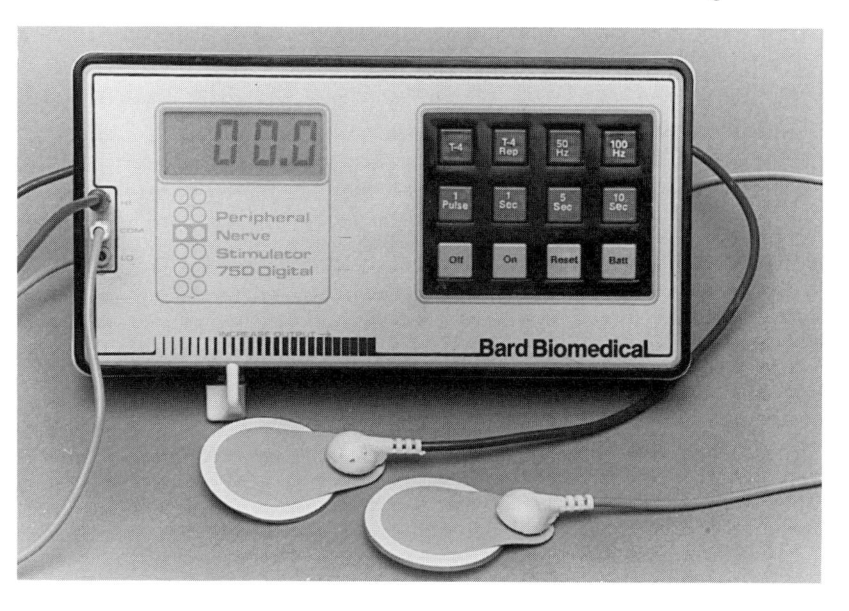

Fig. 12.2 A typical battery-powered nerve stimulator

stimulation are usually single stimuli eliciting a twitch response as tetanic bursts at rates of 50 or 100 cycles/second or as bursts of four stimuli at a rate of 2/second—the well-known 'train of four' stimulation.

By studying the effects of these different stimuli on the response by the adductor pollicis it is possible to estimate the degree of neuromuscular blockade. This is useful not only in adjusting increments or infusions of muscle relaxants, but also in deciding whether residual neuromuscular blockade is responsible in cases of postoperative apnoea. The nerve stimulator is less useful in deciding between depolarising and non-depolarising blocks as nearly all prolonged blocks are non-depolarising in nature.

POSTOPERATIVE APNOEA

There are many reasons why a patient may not breathe (or may breathe inadequately) at the end of an anaesthetic. In some cases remedial treatment may be possible; in others, given time, normal spontaneous respiration will return of its own accord. Whatever the cause, it is fundamental that the patient be ventilated until normal respiration returns.

Some of the many causes of prolonged apnoea are given below. Often, in any one case, more than one of these factors may be involved.

Depression of the Respiratory Centre

Depression of the respiratory centre in the brain occurs by residual effect of a narcotic premedication or residual traces of induction or maintenance agents—e.g. thiopentone or halothane.

Hypocapnia

This commonly plays at least a part in the apnoea often seen at the end of a controlled respiration anaesthetic. There is no stimulus to the medullary respiratory centre to recommence breathing until the arterial PCO_2 returns to its normal level.

Hypercapnia

This is a less common cause of apnoea, being usually due to a fault in the anaesthetic circuit.

General State of the Patient

The gravely ill patient, e.g. one with severe hypotension, is less likely to breathe at the end of the operation. In addition, some new illness, such as a myocardial infarction or cerebrovascular accident, may have occurred during the anaesthetic.

Atypical Plasma (Pseudo) Cholinesterase

The apnoea which occurs in patients with this abnormal enzyme when they are given suxamethonium is described on p. 132.

Low Normal Plasma (Pseudo) Cholinesterase

This most commonly occurs in the presence of liver disease, in patients who have been contaminated with certain organic phosphorus insecticides and in patients given ecothiopate iodide eye drops.

Phase II Block

This type of block is mentioned on p. 130 and usually follows the administration of an excessive amount of suxamethonium.

Acid–Base and Electrolyte Disturbances

The difficulty in reversing the effects of d-tubocurarine in the presence of a metabolic acidosis has also been mentioned. A similar position may arise in the presence of a low serum potassium.

13 Analgesics and Anti-emetics

Opiate analgesics. Neuroleptanaesthesia. Opiate antagonists. Opiate-like analgesics. Anti-emetics.

OPIATE ANALGESICS

Analgesia is one of the fundamental requirements of a balanced anaesthetic and, apart from certain volatile or gaseous anaesthetic agents which possess analgesic properties, modern anaesthetists employ many opiate or related substances to produce intra-operative analgesia. As such, these drugs may be given either as premedicants or, equally commonly nowadays, during anaesthesia. More recently there has been a tendency for increasingly large doses of, in particular, the synthetic opiate fentanyl to be used intra-operatively to abolish many of the potentially harmful effects of anaesthetic and surgical 'stress'.

There are several pharmacological effects common to all the opiate analgesics and their derivatives:

Analgesia	Gastrointestinal sphincteric spasm
Sedation	Histamine release
Respiratory depression	Addiction
Depression of the cough reflex	Cardiovascular depression
Nausea and vomiting	Constipation and bowel atony

Although it has been possible with some of the newer synthetic opiate analgesics to produce drugs with fewer side effects than morphine or pethidine, it has so far been impossible to obtain a drug free from either addiction or respiratory depression, while at the same time maintaining satisfactory analgesia. However, the wider therapeutic ratio (i.e. the ratio between the effective dose and the toxic dose of the drug) of fentanyl and phenoperidine have made it possible to give far larger doses of these drugs for intra-operative analgesia and stress. In addition to the side-effects of opiate analgesics given above, it is important to consider the various drugs available in terms of their duration of action because this is one of the factors governing the wide range available.

Morphine

As one of the oldest and most effective of the analgesic agents, morphine is used as the standard with which the newer analgesics are compared. Morphine is a potent analgesic and also possesses a distinct euphoric action. The important side-effects are:

Respiratory depression
This tends to limit to 10–15 mg intramuscularly, the dose that may be given in a spontaneously breathing patient but the therapeutic ratio is sufficient to allow up to 100 mg to be given in one hour without toxic effects if the patient is ventilated. Morphine may also be used as a respiratory depressant in intensive care to control patients on artificial ventilation.

Depression of the cough reflex

Nausea and vomiting
It is a good idea to give an anti-emetic with morphine.

Smooth muscle constriction
Constriction of the smooth muscle of the large bowel produces constipation and may also produce breakdown of bowel anastomoses. Morphine may produce bronchospasm which, together with histamine release, makes its use undesirable in asthmatics.

Addiction
Although addiction may be a problem with long-term administration of morphine, this is uncommon if the drug is used only to treat acute pain; it is cruel to withhold morphine from a patient in pain for fear that they may become addicted.

Hypotension
Moderate cardiovascular depression and hypotension occur with normal doses of morphine. When given intramuscularly morphine lasts 3–4 hours and intravenously $1\frac{1}{2}$–3 hours.

Pethidine

Pethidine is a synthetic analgesic similar to morphine, producing analgesia together with respiratory depression, suppression of the cough reflex, nausea and vomiting, hypotension and is a drug of addiction. Pethidine does not produce as much euphoria and sedation as morphine nor does it release histamine. Some patients are sensitive to pethidine and sweat, vomit, have vertigo and may become confused. Pethidine relaxes smooth muscle and it may be useful for renal and biliary colic after large-bowel surgery. Given intramuscularly, 50–100 mg last about 180 min and intravenously 20–30 mg last 60–120 min.

Diamorphine (Heroin)

A powerful analgesic, sedative and respiratory depressant, diamorphine is about twice as potent as morphine and useful in patients undergoing postoperative ventilation and in left ventricular failure, where it helps by decreasing anxiety and by producing mild respiratory depression and sedation. The main problem of diamorphine is addiction and for this reason it is not available in the USA. The normal dose is 5–7·5 mg intramuscularly.

Papaveretum (Omnopon)

This drug is a mixture of purified opium alkaloids containing

50 % morphine and 50 % other opium alkaloids, e.g. codeine, thebaine and papaverine. Clinically 20 mg of papaveretum are equal to about 10 mg morphine. The actions and side-effects of papaveretum are similar to morphine.

Fentanyl (Sublimaze)

This synthetic analgesic drug is derived from pethidine and is similar to phenoperidine. Like phenoperidine it has virtually no effect on the cardiovascular system. Fentanyl has an extremely wide therapeutic ratio and is now used in varying doses from 2 to 20 μg/kg for intra-operative analgesia. To a certain extent the size of the dose influences its duration of action. With the smaller doses, analgesia and respiratory depression last about 30 min after an intravenous injection, while with larger doses this may be prolonged for up to 2–3 hours. Fentanyl is a powerful respiratory depressant but has relatively few other side-effects, and its use is restricted to intra-operative analgesia. In some countries a combination of fentanyl and droperidol (Thalamonal) is commonly used both intramuscularly and intravenously

Fentanyl is also used in very large doses (20–50 μg/kg) during cardiac surgery to produce profound analgesia and obtund all reflex responses. This is particularly advantageous in patients with a compromised coronary circulation in whom any increase in cardiac work due to tachycardia or hypertension might precipitate relative myocardial ischaemia and angina.

Alfentanil (Rapifen)

Alfentanil is a short-acting version of fentanyl, particularly suitable for use in day-case anaesthesia or for administration by intravenous infusion. Like fentanyl, it is a powerful analgesic, but the respiratory depressant effect is relatively shortlived and less profound, making it suitable for administration in limited doses to spontaneously breathing patients (6–8 μg/kg). It is cardiovascularly stable and provides good reversible analgesia and sedation when administered as an infusion to ventilated patients in intensive care.

Phenoperidine

Like fentanyl, phenoperidine is a synthetic pethidine derivative causing respiratory depression but with relatively little effect on the cardiovascular system. Its longer duration of action, about two hours after intramuscular injection and one hour after intravenous injection, makes it more useful than fentanyl for intensive care when both analgesia and respiratory depression are required in patients on artificial ventilation. In some patients phenoperidine also has an emetic action.

Levorphanol (Dromoran)

This potent analgesic is of longer duration than morphine. It is a good sedative and one of the best postoperative analgesics available, rarely producing nausea and vomiting. It may also be given intravenously, a dose of 1–4 mg producing 2–3 hours of analgesia.

Methadone (Physeptone)

A synthetic analgesic this is similar to morphine with similar side-effects. The chief difference between the two drugs is that the duration of methadone, two hours, is half that for the analgesia following intramuscular morphine. Methadone also produces less euphoria and is used to treat opiate addiction and drug withdrawal.

NEUROLEPTANAESTHESIA

Neuroleptanaesthesia is a dissociative anaesthetic state, similar to ketamine anaesthesia, produced by administering fentanyl and droperidol. Since only small doses of fentanyl are used the patients breathe spontaneously and, although sedated and analgesic, are able to move to command. Although this technique is advantageous in some conditions—for example, neuroradiological procedures—where complete analgesia is not needed, supplementary agents are required to produce surgical anaesthesia. Neuroleptanaesthetic induction of anaesthesia is also used, particularly in poor-risk patients for vascular surgery, because this technique results in minimal disturbance of cardiovascular haemodynamics.

OPIATE ANTAGONISTS

Until recently all the available opiate antagonists were opiate drugs producing analgesia in their own right and only producing antagonism of the opiate side-effects such as respiratory depression when given in conjunction with another drug such as morphine.

Naloxone (Narcan)

Naloxone is a synthetic opiate antagonist derived from oxymorphone and does not possess any opiate activity of its own. In a dose of 0·1–0·4 mg it will antagonise any of the opiate analgesics, although analgesia and respiratory depression are antagonised equally. Its duration of action is between 45 and 90 min; naloxone may therefore need to be given in repeated doses when morphine or another long-acting drug has just been administered.

Nalorphine (Lethidrone)

This acts as a competitive inhibitor of morphine to antagonise the respiratory depressant effects, but it is not possible to antagonise these without also removing the benefit of analgesia. Mixtures of opiates and nalorphine have been unsuccessful in producing selective analgesia without respiratory depression. Repeated doses of nalorphine may cause hypertension and may exacerbate symptoms in drug addiction. Nalorphine has also been used to reverse opiate-induced neonatal respiratory depression.

Levallorphan (Lorphan)

This synthetic opiate antagonist has a longer effect than nalorphine or morphine and has been used in obstetrics in particular. It was combined with pethidine as Pethilorfan but this was unsuccessful.

OPIATE-LIKE ANALGESICS

The search for an analgesic as powerful as morphine but without the additive or respiratory depressant side-effects has been intensive and several drugs have been produced. However, all of these have proved to be addictive to a certain degree and also tend to produce nausea and vomiting and in some patients—particularly the elderly—confusion or disorientation. They also possess properties of opiate antagonism for which some, e.g. pentazocine, were initially developed. They may be used to reverse respiratory depression caused by other opiates.

Pentazocine (Fortral)

This analgesic is derived from nalorphine, with mild respiratory depression. It has now been shown to be addictive and may cause disorientation and hallucinations. It raises pulmonary artery blood pressure so should not be used in patients with myocardial infarction, and it also produces moderate falls in systemic blood pressure; 30 mg pentazocine are equivalent to 10 mg morphine given intramuscularly.

Phenazocine (Narphen)

A more potent synthetic analgesic than pentazocine, 3 mg being equivalent to 10 mg morphine, phenazocine may be given by mouth or sublingually but in other ways is similar to pentazocine.

Buprenorphine (Temgesic)

This long-acting member of the group produces good cardiovascular stability and moderate respiratory depression. It may also produce nausea and vomiting in some patients. So far, reports of its use in premedication or intra-operatively are somewhat disappointing although its long duration of action may make it useful in the treatment of postoperative pain.

Meptazinol (Meptid), Nalbuphine (Nubain)

These partial opiate agonist drugs, like pentazocine, will reverse opiate-induced respiratory depression. They are potent analgesics but do not possess the euphoric properties of the opiates. They may also cause nausea, vomiting and confusion, particularly in elderly patients.

ANTI-EMETICS

Several drugs used in anaesthesia, particularly the opiate analgesics, produce nausea and vomiting. This is usually produced by stimulation of the vomiting centre which lies close to the respiratory centre in the medulla of the brain. The chemoreceptor trigger zone, another area stimulated by emetic drugs, lies superficial to the true vomiting centre. Vomiting may be initiated not only centrally but also by peripheral effects such as food or other irritants in the stomach. The drugs used to prevent vomiting are commonly phenothiazines. This group of drugs, the chief of which is chlorpromazine, has many actions (e.g. sedative, hypotensive, anti-emetic, antihistaminic, atropine-like and vasodilatory). Various members of the group each have one predominant effect (e.g. anti-emetic) and possess many of the other actions (e.g. sedation) as secondary effects.

Perphenazine (Fentazin)

Perphenazine is a phenothiazine with a marked anti-emetic

action. It also has sedative properties. The other common side-effect is hypotension due to α-adrenergic blockade and peripheral vasodilation. Its action lasts 6–12 hours. After perphenazine some patients may develop extrapyramidal signs such as tremor and rolling of the eyes together with confusion. Patients look frightened and alarmed but this oculogyric crisis may be treated with intravenous atropine, promethazine or benztropine (Cogentin).

Prochlorperazine (Stemetil)

Another phenothiazine drug used as an anti-emetic and in the treatment of nausea and vomiting due to motion sickness, migraine and Ménière's disease. Unlike perphenazine this does not cause noticeable sedation and has fewer other side-effects.

Metoclopramide (Maxolon)

This drug is not a phenothiazine but acts as an anti-emetic, both centrally by depressing the vomiting centre and peripherally by stimulating gastrointestinal emptying and therefore removing the peripheral stimulus to vomiting. Metoclopramide has few side-effects and is a useful anti-emetic drug but, like perphenazine, may cause extrapyramidal reactions.

Anticholinergic Agents

Both atropine and more particularly hyoscine (scopolamine, Kwells) possess an anti-emetic action but also tend to cause central nervous system depression. This is why it is recommended not to drive a car after taking anti-emetics for sea sickness.

Droperidol, Haloperidol

These butyrephenone drugs also possess significant anti-emetic action by depressing the chemoreceptor trigger zone. They are probably the most powerful anti-emetics available but cause sedation and, in some patients, confusion and hallucinations. They are really suitable only for prolonged anti-emesis in patients who require appreciable sedation, or, for example, in faciomaxillary surgery when the jaw is being wired together and when postoperative nausea and vomiting may produce serious problems.

Domperidone (Motilium)

This long-acting anti-emetic acts as a dopamine antagonist on the vomiting centre in the brain. Its prolonged effect makes it particularly suitable for oncology patients receiving cytotoxic drugs and it does not appear to produce excessive sedation.

14 Autonomic Pharmacology

Cholinergic agents. Anticholinergic drugs. Anticholinesterases. Sympathomimetic amines. Adrenergic blocking drugs. α-adrenergic blocking drugs. β-adrenergic blocking drugs. Combined α- and β-adrenergic blocking drugs. Angiotensin-converting enzyme (ACE) inhibitors. Calcium channel blockers.

This chapter deals with the more detailed pharmacology of the individual drugs already mentioned in Chapter 2.

CHOLINERGIC AGENTS

These are drugs with an acetylcholine-like action.

Carbachol

This drug mimics the actions of acetylcholine and is more resistant to destruction by cholinesterase. It possesses both muscarinic (parasympathetic) and nicotinic actions, although unless atropine is given concurrently to block the muscarinic actions these will tend to predominate. Carbachol therefore mainly stimulates the parasympathetic system dilating peripheral blood vessels, reducing heart rate and lowering the blood pressure. It is used to increase bladder tone in postoperative retention and to promote gut movement in intestinal atony. It may cause increased salivation.

Methacholine

This cholinergic agent also possesses predominantly muscarinic effects and is used in a similar way to carbachol, though relatively rarely nowadays. The side-effects are similar to carbachol.

ANTICHOLINERGIC DRUGS

Atropine

Atropine blocks the action of acetylcholine on the parasympathetic nervous system and by producing parasympathetic blockade causes (1) tachycardia, (2) drying of the secretions of the mouth, gut and tracheobronchial tree, (3) relaxation of the smooth muscle of the gut, and (4) dilation of the pupil (in large doses only).

Main uses of atropine
To abolish bradycardia induced by vagal stimulation. It is not effective in bradycardia due to heart block or digitalis overdose.

As premedication to reduce secretions in the tracheobronchial tree and to reduce the effects of vagal stimulation during intubation and surgery.

To counteract the parasympathetic effects of neostigmine, which is used to reverse muscle relaxants and in the treatment of myasthenia gravis.

As eyedrops in the form of homatropine to dilate the pupil for long periods.

Hyoscine (Scopolamine)

Hyoscine resembles atropine and produces similar effects as a result of parasympathetic blockade. Hyoscine also possesses a central effect which is different from atropine. While atropine stimulates the central nervous system, hyoscine tends to depress the cortex and produce sedation. Hyoscine also affects other parts of the brain causing amnesia and reducing motion sickness. For this reason, hyoscine is used to treat travel sickness. The cardiac effects of hyoscine are less marked than those of atropine when the drugs are given in comparable dose.

Glycopyrrolate (Robinul)

Glycopyrrolate is a recently introduced anticholinergic drug, which blocks the action of acetylcholine on the parasympathetic nervous system. Its main use is in combination with anticholinesterase drugs such as neostigmine for the reversal of neuromuscular blockade and a combined preparation of the two drugs has recently been introduced. Glycopyrrolate produces less cardiovascular stimulation than atropine and since it does not cross the blood–brain barrier, excitatory side-effects do not occur.

ANTICHOLINESTERASES

Neostigmine (Prostigmine)

Acetylcholine is normally broken down by cholinesterase into choline and acetic acid. Neostigmine is an anticholinesterase which increases the concentration of acetylcholine by preventing its breakdown. The acetylcholine produced possesses both muscarinic and nicotinic effects, the muscarinic stimulating the parasympathetic nervous system causing increased salivation, gut activity and bradycardia. These effects are antagonised by atropine. The nicotinic effects of acetylcholine are exerted at the skeletal neuromuscular junction and therefore antagonise the effect of non-depolarising neuromuscular blocking drugs—for example, curare. Neostigmine, therefore, is used to antagonise the effects of these relaxants and is given in combination with atropine to prevent the muscarinic side-effects which would otherwise occur. Neostigmine is also used in the same way to treat the muscle weakness of myasthenia gravis. Too much neostigmine may produce depolarisation of the muscle end-plate, also causing muscle paralysis—the cholinergic crisis of myasthenia gravis. This is in contrast to the normal weakness which occurs in this condition due to a relative lack of acetylcholine.

Pyridostigmine (Mestinon)

This is another anticholinesterase drug which possesses less activity than neostigmine. However, as its muscarinic actions are weaker and its duration of action is longer it is more useful than neostigmine in treating myasthenia gravis. It may also be given by mouth which is an advantage in this condition.

Physostigmine

This agent is a more potent anticholinesterase than neostigmine, with a greater effect on the cardiovascular system, the eye and the salivary secretions. Unlike both neostigmine and pyridostigmine, physostigmine crosses the blood–brain barrier, increasing the central nervous concentration of acetylcholine as well as the peripheral levels. This has been used to great effect in counteracting excessive central depression resulting from some drugs—e.g. phenothiazine, hyoscine and the tricyclic antidepressants, which are thought to act by reducing the central nervous concentrations of acetylcholine.

Edrophonium (Tensilon)

This short-acting anticholinesterase is mainly used as a diagnostic test in cases of muscle weakness, thought to be due to myasthenia-like acetylcholine deficiency.

SYMPATHOMIMETIC AMINES

Adrenaline

The actions of adrenaline may be divided into alpha (α) and beta (β) (Table 14.1). The beta effects of adrenaline are further subdivided into β_1, the effects on the heart, and β_2, the effects on the bronchi. Adrenaline stimulates the α-receptors of the sympathetic nervous system, producing peripheral vasoconstriction,

Table 14.1 The α- and β-actions of adrenaline

α Actions	β_1 Actions	β_2 Actions
Dilation of pupil Peripheral vaso-constriction Coronary vaso-constriction Intestinal sphincter contraction Piloerection in skin Sweat production	Increased heart rate Increased myocardial contractility Coronary vasodilation	Bronchodilation

and the β_1 receptors producing an increase in pulse rate and myocardial contractility. It is used to treat cardiac arrest, stimulating the heart without causing peripheral vasodilation which might cause a fall in blood pressure and decreased coronary perfusion. Adrenaline also relaxes the smooth muscle of the bronchi by its β_2 effect and hence is useful in treating bronchospasm. It is also used with local analgesics for its vasoconstrictor properties to decrease the rate of absorption of the local analgesic. Adrenaline may be used in the treatment of angioneurotic oedema and other hypersensitivity reactions.

Table 14.2 The α- and β-agonists and blockers

Adrenaline effect	Stimulated by	Blocked by
α	Adrenaline Noradrenaline (Ephedrine) (Amphetamine)	Phentolamine Phenoxybenzamine
β (non-specific)	Isoprenaline (Dopamine) Ephedrine Amphetamine	Propranolol Labetalol
β_1 (specific)	Dobutamine	Practolol Oxprenolol Sotalol Atenolol
β_2 (specific)	Salbutamol	—

Noradrenaline (Levophed) (Table 14.2)

Noradrenaline is a naturally occurring catecholamine which causes a pronounced increase in blood pressure by peripheral vasoconstriction and, to a lesser extent, by stimulating myocardial contractility. Noradrenaline, therefore, is predominantly an α-adrenergic stimulator, and because of its pronounced alpha effects, causes a reflex slowing of the pulse rate. The vasoconstriction causes poor tissue perfusion and reduces renal blood flow; noradrenaline is therefore hardly ever used alone except in extreme circumstances. Noradrenaline does possess a mild β-adrenergic stimulatory effect which is apparent only when the drug is given in combination with an α-adrenergic blocker (e.g. phentolamine). This has been used to some effect in cardiac surgery.

Isoprenaline (Suscardia)

In contrast to noradrenaline, isoprenaline exhibits mainly the beta actions of adrenaline. It is a powerful cardiac stimulant, increasing both the pulse rate (chronotropic effect) and the force of contraction (inotropic effect). It also causes peripheral vasodilation by relaxing smooth muscle and so may cause a fall in blood pressure. Isoprenaline may also be used in treating bronchospasm, when it may be given either by inhalation using an inhaler or a Bird ventilator, subcutaneously or sublingually. Overdose of isoprenaline results in atrial tachycardia and arrhythmias, especially ventricular ectopics, ventricular tachycardia and even ventricular fibrillation.

Dopamine (Intropin)

Dopamine acts in a similar way to isoprenaline, producing predominantly β-adrenergic stimulation, although it has been suggested that this drug is more effective on the peripheral blood vessels than on the heart itself because it does not cause such a severe tachycardia when given systemically. Dopamine in low doses acts on specific dopaminergic receptors within the kidney producing selective renal vasodilation and simultaneously increasing the blood pressure to a satisfactory level, while larger doses of dopamine are used for their direct myocardial stimulant action, increasing the force of contraction and the cardiac output and therefore the blood pressure. Hence dopamine infusions are used widely in intensive care to treat such conditions. High doses of dopamine may produce peripheral vasoconstriction as a result of a small α-adrenergic effect. Dopamine exerts only a mild effect on bronchial smooth muscle.

Ephedrine

Ephedrine is a synthetic drug related chemically to adrenaline. It raises the blood pressure mainly by increasing heart rate and myocardial contractility although it also causes some peripheral vasoconstriction. As well as being used as a vasopressor, ephedrine is useful as a bronchodilator in patients with bronchospasm. It has been used in the treatment of myasthenia gravis, as it improves neuromuscular conduction.

Amphetamine

In general, the actions of amphetamine resemble those of ephedrine but tend to be more apparent as central nervous stimulants. Amphetamine has both α- and β-adrenergic stimulatory effects, producing an increase in blood pressure and heart rate. However, because of its pronounced central stimulation and abuse by drug addicts amphetamine has now been withdrawn.

Salbutamol (Ventolin)

Salbutamol is a β-adrenergic stimulant with a highly selective action on bronchial muscle receptors (β_2 action). Used predominantly for the relief of bronchospasm, it may be administered by inhalation, orally or intravenously. When used by the latter route, salbutamol also produces mild cardiac stimulation and a degree of peripheral vasodilation which has been employed with some success when treating cardiogenic shock.

Dobutamine (Dobutrex)

Dobutamine is a β_1-adrenergic stimulant, producing an increase in myocardial contractility. It does not cause noradrenaline release, so peripheral vasoconstriction and hypertension are not common. It is claimed to be a more specific cardiac stimulant than dopamine.

ADRENERGIC BLOCKING DRUGS

Drugs have now been specifically developed to block the different effects of adrenergic stimulation (Table 14.2). The beta effects of adrenaline can be subdivided into β_1, which are the cardiac effects, and β_2, which are the effects on the bronchi. α-Adrenergic blocking drugs therefore block the alpha effects of adrenaline, β_1 blockers the cardiac effects of isoprenaline, and β_2 blockers, the bronchial effects (Table 14.2).

α-ADRENERGIC BLOCKING DRUGS

Phentolamine (Rogitine)

Phentolamine is an α-adrenergic blocking drug which is also a direct myocardial stimulant. It blocks the actions of adrenaline, noradrenaline and related compounds on peripheral blood vessels, thus producing vasodilation. This will cause a fall in blood pressure and central venous pressure and therefore extra fluid will be required to maintain the circulation.

Phentolamine is used:

1. To promote vasodilation, for example during cardiopulmonary bypass.
2. To antagonise vasoconstriction, for example due to Gram-negative septicaemia.
3. As a direct myocardial stimulant, the vasodilation being antagonised by noradrenaline.
4. To antagonise the vasoconstrictive effects of noradrenaline.

5. To control the acute hypertensive attacks in patients with phaeochromocytoma.

Phentolamine is relatively short-acting drug, its effect lasting between 15 and 30 min after intravenous injection.

Phenoxybenzamine

This α-adrenergic blocking drug exerts its effect only slowly but produces a prolonged action, decreasing slowly over 3–4 days. Phenoxybenzamine is usually used in the treatment of abnormal peripheral vasoconstriction and in the long-term control of phaeochromocytoma, particularly in the pre-operative preparation of such patients. Phenoxybenzamine therapy requires careful intravenous fluid management to counteract the gradual fall in central venous pressure as a result of increase in the intravascular space. It may produce postural hypotension and a reflex tachycardia if the fluid volume is not accurately corrected.

β-ADRENERGIC BLOCKING DRUGS

Propranolol (Inderal)

Propranolol is a β-adrenergic blocker antagonising both the β_1 and β_2 effects of isoprenaline on the heart and bronchi. It causes a fall in heart rate and cardiac output and a decrease in myocardial oxygen consumption. It may, however, cause bronchoconstriction and should not be used in asthmatics. Propranolol is used:

1. To control ectopic beats. It is more effective in the control of atrial ectopics than ventricular. It is useful in the treatment of arrhythmias due to digitalis overdose.
2. To control supraventricular tachycardia.
3. To control the tachycardia which may develop when hypotensive drugs (e.g. pentolinium) are used.
4. To control tachycardia or ventricular arrhythmias due to excess adrenaline.

5. To reduce myocardial oxygen consumption and thereby the frequency of angina.

Practolol (Eraldin)

Practolol is a β_1-adrenergic blocker and by being cardiospecific does not cause bronchoconstriction and may be used in asthmatics. It does not depress the myocardium as much as propranolol as it has certain sympathomimetic properties of its own. It has a better anti-arrhythmic action than propranolol but is not so good for treating angina. The duration of action of practolol is longer, 10 hours compared with two hours for propranolol. It is now available only in hospitals for intravenous use due to several cases of retroperitoneal fibrosis and uraemia. It may also rarely cause conjunctivitis and keratitis.

Oxprenolol (Trasicor), Sotalol (Beta-Cardone), Atenolol (Tenormin)

These are β_1-selective adrenergic blocking drugs, the principal effects of which are slowing of the heart rate with a consequent reduction in myocardial oxygen consumption. Oxprenolol also has some sympathomimetic action of its own and is used in treating angina and dysrhythmias.

COMBINED α- AND β-ADRENERGIC BLOCKING DRUGS

Labetalol (Trandate)

This agent possesses both α- and β-adrenergic blocking effects and has been advocated for hypertension, as not only does it reduce myocardial oxygen consumption, but it also acts as a peripheral vasodilator. However, its α-blocking effects are much milder than its beta effects and are also much shorter in duration, and for this reason the predominant effects of labetalol are similar to other β_1-adrenergic blocking drugs.

Labetalol is now widely used to produce moderate reduction in blood pressure during elective surgery. By inducing vasodilation and minimising any reflex tachycardia, the fall in blood pressure is posturally dependent and controllable.

ANGIOTENSIN-CONVERTING ENZYME (ACE) INHIBITORS

Captopril (Capoten), Enalapril (Innovace)

This new group of drugs is used in the treatment of hypertension, chiefly in patients with hypertension secondary to renal causes. Like other agents used to control blood pressure, their use should be continued during surgery. Their action is not sufficiently acute to make them suitable for elective hypotension during anaesthesia.

CALCIUM CHANNEL BLOCKERS

Nifedipine (Adalat), Verapamil (Cordilox), Diltiazem (Tildiem)

These drugs, introduced for the control of cardiac dysrhythmias, are being increasingly used for the control of blood pressure and for the reduction of myocardial oxygen consumption in patients with ischaemic heart disease and angina. Like patients receiving β-adrenoceptor blocking drugs, treatment with calcium channel blockers should continue during surgery, although their effect may enhance the hypotensive effect of halothane and enflurane. Their speed of onset of action makes them unsuitable for intraoperative induced hypotension.

15 Hypotensive Anaesthesia and Hypothermia

Hypotensive anaesthesia. Controlling vascular tone. Reduction of cardiac output. Background anaesthetic technique for elective hypotension. Ganglion-blocking drugs. α-Adrenergic blocking drugs. β-Adrenergic blocking drugs. Direct-acting peripheral vasodilator drugs. Extradural and spinal anaesthesia. Hypothermia.

HYPOTENSIVE ANAESTHESIA

Operative blood loss occurs as a result of either arterial bleeding, venous bleeding or capillary oozing, and the control of these three forms of blood loss is achieved in different ways. A reduction in systemic arterial blood pressure by using hypotensive drugs will reduce but not abolish arterial bleeding, because cut vessels will always bleed. Venous bleeding is worsened by venous congestion and a high venous tone and therefore techniques such as intermittent positive pressure ventilation (IPPV) and posture will help to reduce venous congestion while regional anaesthetic techniques (e.g. epidurals) abolish venous tone. Capillary ooze depends on arterial blood pressure and venous congestion, but can also be abolished by localised vasoconstriction using dilute solutions of a vasoconstrictor (e.g. adrenaline).

The reduction of systemic arterial blood pressure by a hypotensive anaesthetic technique is used in two distinct situations. Firstly, to make possible operations that would otherwise be impossible (e.g. neurosurgery and cardiac surgery) and, secondly, to reduce operative blood loss and make surgery easier (e.g. plastic, maxillo-facial, orthopaedic, ENT and eye surgery). Hypotensive anaesthetic techniques vary widely, the main distinction being between drugs that can produce an extremely rapid reduction in blood pressure (e.g. sodium nitroprusside) and those which produce a relatively gradual falling blood pressure (e.g. ganglion-blocking drugs and epidurals). As mentioned, hypotensive anaesthesia should be employed as an extension of the concept of balanced anaesthesia, using specific drugs to produce arteriolar vasodilation. The supplementation of hypotensive techniques with a good anaesthetic, together with IPPV and posture, is also essential.

CONTROLLING VASCULAR TONE

The pharmacology behind hypotensive anaesthesia lies in controlling vascular smooth muscle tone, because vasodilation without expansion of the fluid volume results in hypotension. Blood vessel size is controlled by sympathetic nervous system activity (Chapter 2) and increase in sympathetic activity produces vasoconstriction, while abolition of sympathetic activity produces vasodilation. With the exception of those drugs which act directly on the smooth muscle of the blood vessel walls, hypotensive techniques interrupt the sympathetic outflow at various sites.

The preganglionic sympathic nerves leave the spinal cord to synapse within the sympathetic ganglia. Acetylcholine is the transmitter substance of these synaptic sites, this being a nicotinic action. Remember that acetylcholine is also the transmitter at the parasympathetic ganglia. Noradrenaline, however, is the transmitter substance between the post-ganglionic sympathetic neurone and the smooth muscle of the blood vessels. Sympathetic outflow may therefore be interrupted in the following ways:

1. *Central sedation* produced by general anaesthesia causing a degree of vasodilation.

2. *Ganglion blockade* and competitive inhibition of acetylcholine (e.g. hexamethonium, pentolinium, trimetaphan).

3. *Direct competition* with the effects of noradrenaline (α-adrenergic blocking drugs—e.g. phentolamine).

In addition, hypotensive anaesthesia may also be achieved by direct-acting smooth muscle vasodilators (sodium nitroprusside, glyceryl trinitrate) and by reducing the cardiac output, thus inevitably reducing blood pressure.

REDUCTION OF CARDIAC OUTPUT

Cardiac output depends on venous return to the heart, which itself depends on both a negative intrathoracic pressure and on the pumping action of muscles surrounding blood vessels. Muscular relaxation together with IPPV (instead of the negative pressure created during spontaneous ventilation) will tend to reduce venous return to the heart and hence reduce cardiac output. Halothane, usually in combination with IPPV, also produces hypotension. In addition to vasodilation, halothane also directly reduces cardiac output. This it does by (1) direct myocardial depression, (2) slowing the heart rate as a result of vagal stimulation, (3) decreasing the rate of conduction of impulses through the heart, and (4) inhibiting the baroceptor reflex, thereby preventing the reflex rise in heart rate resulting from hypotension. The cardiovascular effects of enflurane are similar to those of halothane. Isoflurane, however, does not produce significant myocardial depression making it now the best volatile agent for producing moderate hypotensive anaesthesia.

BACKGROUND ANAESTHETIC TECHNIQUE FOR ELECTIVE HYPOTENSION

A small dose of isoflurane combined with IPPV provides a good background anaesthetic for elective hypotension. This is best augmented by muscle relaxation using curare, as this drug also possesses ganglion-blocking effects which tend to interrupt sympathetic activity.

This combines with both the effects of isoflurane and the mechanical effects of ventilation to produce a moderate fall in blood pressure which can be enhanced with various pharmacological agents.

GANGLION-BLOCKING DRUGS

These drugs (hexamethonium, pentolinium, trimetaphan) block preganglionic to postganglionic neuronal transmission by competitive inhibition of acetylcholine, the transmitting substance released in all autonomic ganglia, both sympathetic and parasympathetic. As these drugs act on both parts of the autonomic nervous system, they produce effects resulting from both sympathetic and parasympathetic blockade.

Main Actions of Sympathetic Blockade

Sympathetic nervous activity maintains peripheral vascular tone and interruption of this by sympathetic blockade will produce vasodilation and therefore hypotension. This fall in blood pressure will be posturally sensitive, being made worse if the patient is in the foot down position. Hypotension resulting from sympathetic blockade is augmented by the effects of (1) gravity, (2) venous pooling, and (3) a decreased cardiac output, resulting from the decreased venous return, as more blood is retained in the periphery.

Main Actions of Parasympathetic Blockade

Although the desirable effects of ganglion blockade are essentially to produce hypotension as a result of vasodilation, the effects of these drugs are also seen at the parasympathetic ganglia. Interruption of parasympathetic activity produces (1) mydriasis (due to blockade of the ciliary ganglion), (2) decreased intra-ocular pressure, (3) decreased gastric secretion, (4) decreased intestinal tone, (5) difficulty in micturition, and (6) tachycardia.

This tachycardia may be due either to parasympathetic blockade or possibly to a baroceptor reflex resulting from the hypotension produced. In clinical practice the increased heart rate produced by ganglion-blocking drugs presents the greatest problem, the effects being most marked with hexamethonium and trimetaphan, and least with pentolinium. Trimetaphan also exhibits tachyphylaxis, i.e. increasing doses of the drug are required to maintain the same effect. This tachycardia is often adequately controlled with a β-adrenergic blocking drug (e.g. propranolol).

The ganglion-blocking agents are generally used to produce a relatively slow fall and rise in blood pressure most suited to plastic surgery and similar procedures. The duration of the hypotensive effect varies from one agent to another, being about 15–20 min with hexamethonium and trimetaphan and 45 min with pentolinium.

α-ADRENERGIC BLOCKING DRUGS

The transmitting substance released from the postganglionic sympathetic nerve (*see* Fig. 2.5) is noradrenaline, the site of action being an α-adrenergic one. α-Adrenergic blocking agents all produce vasodilation by competitive inhibition at the alpha site. The drugs used may conveniently be divided into those producing a relatively permanent effect lasting several days which is irreversible (phenoxybenzamine), and those producing acute α-blockade lasting 10–30 min (phentolamine). α-Adrenergic blockade not only produces peripheral vasodilation which may result in compensatory tachycardia, but also produces congestion of mucous membranes and constriction of the pupil. These drugs do not block the positive chronotropic or positive inotropic effects of adrenaline on the heart. Details about the pharmacology of phenoxybenzamine and phentolamine are given in Chapter 14. Several other drugs (e.g. droperidol and some phenothiazines such as chlorpromazine) also possess mild α-adrenergic blocking activity. The ergot alkaloids, with the exception of ergometrine, also produce peripheral vasodilation and this is used for treating migraine.

The combined α and β blocking effects of labetalol are particularly useful in the production of elective hypotension. The vasodilation resulting from α-blockade wears off considerably more quickly than the β-blocking effect.

β-ADRENERGIC BLOCKING DRUGS

The main contribution of these agents to hypotensive anaesthesia results from the bradycardia and the consequent reduction in cardiac output. There is no doubt that a tachycardia greatly increases intra-operative blood loss and that, conversely, a dry and satisfactory operating field is often achieved with normal blood pressure but a slow heart rate. For this reason many anaesthetists use intravenous propranolol in fit patients to reduce the heart rate and therefore reduce bleeding. The individual β-blocking agents are discussed in more detail in Chapter 14.

DIRECT-ACTING PERIPHERAL VASODILATOR DRUGS

Although some direct-acting vasodilators (e.g. hydralazine and diazoxide) are used in the long-term control of hypertension, the prolonged action of these agents makes them unsuitable for the acute intra-operative control of blood pressure. For many years the nitrites (e.g. amyl nitrite and glyceryl trinitrate in tablet form) have been used to produce coronary vasodilation in the relief of angina and, more recently, sodium nitroprusside, a drug with a nitrite-like action, has been available as an intravenous preparation to produce hypotension. Glyceryl trinitrate is now also available in intravenous form for intra-operative use.

Sodium Nitroprusside (SNP)

This drug, which is administered as an intravenous infusion, produces an extremely rapid fall in arterial blood pressure which is dose-dependent and which is brought about by peripheral vasodilation. Sodium nitroprusside dilates arteries and veins equally and, for this reason, maintains blood flow to vital organs at lower blood pressures than most other hypotensive techniques. It is widely used for elective hypotension in operations where fine and rapid control of blood pressure is essential (e.g. neurosurgery, cardiac surgery and vascular surgery). It is also used as a vasodilating agent in intensive care and to treat acute hypertensive emergencies. The action of nitroprusside is short-lived, wearing off within two minutes of discontinuation, and for this reason it is best given as an intravenous infusion using a drip controller to maintain regular administration. The normal dose used should not exceed 1·5 mg/kg as a total dose or 10 μg/kg per min.

Glyceryl Trinitrate (GTN)

Also prepared in the form of an intravenous infusion for intra-operative hypotension, this drug produces a slower fall and rise in blood pressure than nitroprusside, but this may sometimes be beneficial. Glyceryl trinitrate is also used in intensive care in similar situations to sodium nitroprusside. The solution is relatively unstable and has to be made up fresh before each administration. Nevertheless, the drug provides accurate and fine control of blood pressure by peripheral vasodilation. Both sodium nitroprusside and glyceryl trinitrate are made up as 0·01% solutions for slow intravenous infusion.

EXTRADURAL AND SPINAL ANAESTHESIA

These are discussed in detail in Chapter 42.

HYPOTHERMIA

When the human body is cooled, its metabolic rate is reduced and therefore the oxygen consumption of various organs is correspondingly reduced. As an adjunct to general anaesthesia hypothermia is most commonly used during surgical procedures on the heart and brain. By lowering the temperature and hence reducing the oxygen consumption of the organ concerned it is possible to prolong the period of circulatory arrest to that organ while surgery is performed. It is still used in the treatment of congenital cardiac abnormalities and, in some centres, during cerebral aneurysm surgery, although in the latter case hypotensive techniques have largely superseded hypothermia.

Methods of Hypothermia

These are divided into two main methods.

Surface hypothermia
This may be achieved in three ways: (1) by immersion in a bath of iced water after the patient has been anaesthetised and is relatively vasodilated; (2) by evaporation; the patient first being given a drug such as chlorpromazine to prevent shivering and then being exposed to a cold air fan, the evaporation produced resulting in the body surface cooling, and (3) by using a cooling blanket which is usually wrapped round the patient rather than laid under his back.

Blood cooling
This includes cardiopulmonary bypass, and moderate hypothermia is still employed while patients are on bypass for valvular surgery.

Possible Problems of Hypothermia

Reduction in cerebral blood flow
Reduction in cerebral flow does occur, but this is matched by a corresponding fall in cerebral oxygen consumption and is not serious in normal circumstances.

Cardiac dysrhythmias
At core temperatures of 28°C and lower, abnormal cardiac contraction occurs, particularly in the form of ventricular extrasystoles which may lead to ventricular fibrillation if left untreated.

Renal and hepatic blood flow

Both these are decreased during hypothermia, resulting in reduced urine output and distal tubular function. However, proximal tubular function within the kidney remains normal even at low body temperatures so that the coarse control of the fluid and electrolyte concentration of the urine is maintained.

Blood coagulation

As body temperature falls the clotting time of whole blood is increased.

Oxygen carriage

At low temperatures the oxygen dissociation curve shifts to the left, resulting in less oxygen being carried by a given quantity of haemoglobin. This, however, is balanced by the reduction in oxygen demand of the tissues.

16 Pre-Anaesthetic Visit and Assessment

Perusal of notes. Interview and examination of patient. Intercurrent drug therapy. Lung function tests. The anaesthetic out-patient clinic.

Only in cases of dire emergency should an anaesthetist meet his patient for the first time in the anaesthetic room. This is a good working rule which at times, unfortunately, has to be broken, e.g. when patients are admitted for surgery on the same day.

The pre-operative visit benefits both the anaesthetist and the patient. It gives the anaesthetist the opportunity to check the patient's pre-operative preparation, to assess his psychological and physical state, to request any further investigations he may consider essential to decide what anaesthetic technique he will use and perhaps even to begin to consider what sort of post-operative analgesia may suit the patient. It gives the patient the opportunity to ask questions about the anaesthetic (and frequently about surgery). In addition, especially with modern operating theatre clothes-changing disciplines, fewer ward nurses accompany the patient as far as the anaesthetic room, so that the anaesthetist's may be the only familiar face that he sees there.

PERUSAL OF NOTES

The patient's notes should provide the anaesthetist with most of the important information he needs. They should contain not only the patient's history and clinical examination but also the results of any haematological, biochemical or radiological examinations. The investigations will vary widely depending on the patient's physical status and the operation intended, but for patients of African origin and from countries bordering the Mediterranean they should include testing for sickle-cell disease (Chapter 17).

INTERVIEW AND EXAMINATION OF PATIENT

Interview

Although the anaesthetist may have gathered all the information he requires from the notes, it is still important for him to speak to and possibly examine the patient. Not only does it give him the chance to repeat some of the questions and ask some of his own, but it also gives him the opportunity to form some degree of rapport with the patient. Questioning and examination along the following lines is the minimum that is necessary for a patient who has not already been 'clerked', but will not be wasted even if he has. The reason for some of the questions will be discussed in detail later in this chapter.

Is your general health good? Many patients, especially younger ones, will reply in the affirmative. This encourages the anaesthetist to think that nothing particularly adverse will be disclosed by further questions.

Have you ever had any serious illnesses? This may be taken to mean anything that necessitated admission to hospital, although some quite serious illnesses (e.g. myocardial infarction and pneumonia) are sometimes treated at home. However, the patient usually considers these serious enough to mention. A history of rheumatic fever is also usually elicited by this question, although it may be wise to ask about it specifically.

Have you ever had any operations or anaesthetics? By putting the question in this way dental-chair anaesthetics, which many patients do not regard as operations, will not be missed. The operations, their dates and whereabouts should be listed as it may be possible to obtain the anaesthetic notes if necessary.

Were you told of any problems associated with any of your anaesthetics? This may reveal a history of avoidable complications (e.g. suxamethonium pains or even the occasional suxamethonium apnoea). More commonly the patient may give a history of distressing nausea or vomiting after the operation and it may be possible to identify some causative agent.

Do you know of any family history of problems with anaesthetics, or operations? While this question seldom produces an affirmative answer, if it is not asked routinely the anaesthetist may miss the possibility of the patient having one of the hereditarily transmitted conditions such as abnormal pseudocholinesterase or malignant hyperpyrexia.

Do you have any pain in your legs or chest on taking exercise? This question is asked to elicit a history of claudication or angina. It is the first question in evaluating cardiorespiratory function and, like many of the later questions, if answered in the affirmative it is followed by further questioning to find out how long the patient has had the symptom, how readily it comes on, if the patient knows anything that will get rid of it, etc.

How easily do you get short of breath? Can you walk up a flight of stairs or a hill reasonably briskly without having to stop for breath, or are you out of breath at the top? Can you sleep lying down or do you need several pillows to avoid feeling breathless?

Do your ankles swell?

Do you have a cough? If the answer is in the affirmative it is important to inquire about the colour, quantity and consistency of the sputum.

Do you smoke? A patient who smokes may show signs of an irritable respiratory tract under the anaesthetic but, more important, he is much more likely to suffer respiratory complications postoperatively.

Do you suffer from indigestion? An affirmative answer should be followed by more detailed questioning about the presence and nature of abdominal pain and history of acid regurgitation. The latter may be caused by a hiatus hernia—of considerable potential danger to the patient during anaesthesia.

Do you have hay fever? While not itself a life-endangering disease, hay fever indicates that the patient has an allergic tendency.

Do you have asthma? This disease covers all ranges of severity and the patient will often be on medication either in tablet form or by inhaler. The treatment may have to be prescribed for the period of the operation, and the premedication and anaesthetic agents used can be chosen to some extent to try to avoid bronchospasm if general anaesthesia is to be given.

Do you have any allergies? The commonest allergies are probably to antibiotics, but many drugs, as well as other stimuli, may be incriminated (e.g. dogs, cats and horses). It is most important to inquire carefully about the drug allergies and determine their nature. Many will be genuine allergic reactions, but others, especially reactions to local anaesthetics in the dental chair, are simply vasovagal attacks.

Are you on pills or tablets? These commonly include digoxin or other cardiac glycosides, diuretics, antihypertensive drugs, tricyclic antidepressants, monoamine oxidase inhibitors, tranquillisers, sleeping tablets, oral antidiabetic drugs, insulin (by injection) or steroids. Notes on the importance of some of the drugs are given below.

Do you drink wine or spirits? Patients who drink alcohol regularly and excessively often have an alarming resistance to general anaesthetic agents.

Do you have any false teeth? Enquiries should also be made about crowns or elaborate dental work. It is wise to ascertain whether there is anything else artificial about the patient (e.g. a false eye, wig, or a false limb). The patient is unlikely to come to the operating theatre wearing a false limb, but may wear a wig or false eye without mentioning it. These latter objects may prove disconcerting during anaesthesia, especially if the false eye is relied on to provide information about the depth of anaesthesia!

This list of questions needs much modification from patient to patient; questions about angina and claudication would be inappropriate for a young child.

Examination of Patient

The two main systems of interest to the anaesthetist are the cardiovascular and the respiratory systems. These should be examined quickly but carefully. While examining the patient's pulse and taking his blood pressure it is good practice for the anaesthetist to look for likely sites for intravenous needles or cannulae.

It is also important for the anaesthetist to check the upper respiratory tract. He should not only ask about the patient's teeth but he should also ask the patient to open his mouth as widely as possible. Not all patients can open their jaws wide and a very few have congenital trismus, which may lead to extreme difficulty with intubation. Other factors that may lead to difficulty in maintaining an airway with a face mask or in visualising the larynx include protruding teeth, a receding lower jaw and a somewhat immobile cervical spine.

After the history-taking and examination the anaesthetist should complete his pre-operative visit by discussing with the patient points relating to the anaesthesia and surgery. Night sedation is first discussed and if necessary prescribed, and then the patient told what, if anything, he will be allowed to eat or drink on the day of the operation. The anaesthetist should then describe in what way he will induce anaesthesia in the anaesthetic room, where the patient is likely to waken up, what pain he is likely to feel from the operation and what methods will be available to relieve the pain. It is also as well to tell the patient if an intravenous infusion will be running when he wakes because this routine piece of equipment to the anaesthetist may be frightening to the patient if it is unexpected. Also worth mentioning is the possibility of muscle pains if suxamethonium is to be given and the possibility of some degree of sore throat if endotracheal anaesthesia is to be used.

Patients undergoing abdominal and thoracic surgery are particularly liable to underventilate and retain sputum because of the pain associated with deep breathing and coughing: they should be told pre-operatively the importance of these actions and of the help they may obtain from nursing staff and physiotherapists. All patients should be told of the value of early leg movements (or even simple foot-waggling). These help to prevent venous stasis and deep venous thrombosis.

The patient should then be asked if there is any other point upon which he wishes clarificaton. Quite a few patients will take this opportunity to ask for more information about the operation. It is remarkable how poorly informed many patients are so soon before surgery.

With young children the pre-anaesthetic visit tends to be simpler but is, if anything, even more important than in an adult. It is best to give children an honest but simple description of what will happen, because they may feel cheated if they are told one thing, only to find something different taking place.

In summary, the pre-anaesthetic visit is a most important part of the whole ‘anaesthetic incident’. From it the anaesthetist can gain a great deal of information, and the patient, it is to be hoped, a little confidence.

INTERCURRENT DRUG THERAPY

Many patients who present for anaesthesia are already on some form of medication. Apart from the significance of the condition that is being treated, many of the drugs may react adversely with agents during anaesthesia, or produce other disconcerting effects. However, it is now established as a good working principle with most drugs that patients should be maintained on their usual medication right up to the time of operation. Provided the anaesthetist is aware of the patient’s intercurrent drug therapy and any likely interaction with anaesthetic agents, it is considered in the patient’s best interests to have minimal interruption of their drug treatment. There are only a few firm exceptions to this rule; monoamine oxidase inhibitors (see below) and lithium (used in manic-depressive states) are two of these. A brief discussion of some of the groups of drugs patients may be taking when presenting for anaesthesia is given below.

Antihypertensive Agents

Although fashions for particular agents or groups of agents change, antihypertensive drugs of one kind or another represent one of the commonest groups of drugs being taken by patients coming for anaesthesia. Because of the risk of potentiation of agents used during anaesthesia which themselves may cause hypotension (e.g. halothane, d-tubocurarine) it was once thought that they should be stopped long enough before the anaesthetic for their effect to wear off. Very few anaesthetists now hold this view. Indeed, temporary discontinuation of treatment is now thought to be even more dangerous, with the risk of a cerebrovascular accident or myocardial infarction. During anaesthesia also, the untreated patient seems to be at increased risk, with wild swings of blood pressure, particularly high blood pressure occurring at laryngoscopy and intubation.

These patients' underlying cardiovascular status is of course poor, but provided that care is taken with anaesthetic agents which produce hypotension in their own right, and provided that a steep or sudden head-up tilt is avoided (because of the dramatic fall in blood pressure that it may cause), there seems little doubt that these patients are more safely anaesthetised if their antihypertensive therapy is continued throughout the operation.

It should be remembered that the summative hypotensive effects of anaesthesia and these drugs may continue into the postoperative period; it is therefore wise to sit these patients up or let them get out of bed more cautiously than is usual.

Steroid Therapy

The therapeutic use of adrenal cortical hormones (steroids) is common in many conditions, including collagen diseases such as rheumatoid arthritis and asthma. The effect of this treatment is to suppress the secretion of adrenocorticotrophic hormone (ACTH) from the patient's own pituitary gland and, without stimulatory effect, the patient's own adrenal cortex atrophies. If the patient is then exposed to some stress, such as anaesthesia and operation, the adrenal cortex may not be able to respond as normal, and acute adrenal insufficiency will occur. This may present as sudden hypotension and the patient may die unless intravenous steroids are given immediately.

The suppressant effect on the adrenal cortex of therapeutically administered steroids may continue long after the treatment has stopped. The suppression is probably related to the dosage and duration of the therapy but may be significant after treatment for as short a period as one week, and the adrenal cortex may not recover completely for weeks or months. Various regimens of steroid cover have been recommended, depending on the size and duration of steroid treatment, how long has elapsed since the course of steroids finished (assuming that the patient is not still on the course), and the severity of the expected stress from the anaesthetic and operation. Sometimes the administration of 100 mg hydrocortisone sodium succinate given intramuscularly with the premedication will be adequate, while at others the extra steroid cover, whether given parenterally, or orally, may have to be continued for several days. In any case, it is important that the patient be maintained on a shock chart for 24–48 hours post-operatively or until the administration of additional steroids has ended.

Monoamine Oxidase Inhibitors (MAOIs)

This group of drugs was used in the 1960s for angina and for depressive states. Fortunately their use for angina has ceased, and for depressive states it is much less common than before. Severe, sometimes fatal reactions were reported with two entirely different groups of drugs. Firstly, catastrophic rises in blood pressure, leading at times to acute subarachnoid haemorrhage, were seen when patients taking these drugs were given vaso-pressors. Secondly, pethidine in conjunction with MAOIs at times produced profound collapse, hypotension and death. While barbiturates, morphine and other narcotics are probably safer than pethidine, they should be treated with the utmost caution. It is also recommended that patients on MAOIs should avoid certain foods, including Bovril, Oxo and other meat extracts, cheese, Marmite, yoghurt, pickled herrings and red wine.

The residual effects of MAOIs linger for a considerable time and it is recommended that if possible they should be stopped for three weeks before anaesthesia.

Monoamine oxidase inhibitors

Approved name	*Proprietary name*
phenelzine	Nardil
iproniazid	Marsilid
isocarboxazid	Marplan
tranylcypromine	Parnate
tranylcypromine + trifluoperazine	Parstelin (Parnate + Stelazine)
pargyline	Eutonyl

Tricyclic Antidepressants

These antidepressants (e.g. amitriptyline, imipramine) are probably the commonest group of drugs in use at present. They may potentiate the cardiovascular effects of adrenaline and noradrenaline, causing hypertension and cardiac dysrhythmias and it is thought that this has been the cause of deaths in the dental chair, where 1:80 000 adrenaline is often used with a local analgesic.

Sedatives and Tranquillisers

Almost any of the drugs in this huge group (e.g. phenobarbitone, diazepam) may have some (although not usually dangerous) effects on anaesthesia. In summary, where patients are on a fairly acute course of one of these drugs there is a tendency for their sedative effects to summate with that of general anaesthesia, while if the treatment is long-term the patients tend to be resistant to the effects of general anaesthesia. This statement applies also to the tricyclic antidepressants and indeed to most psychotropic agents.

LUNG FUNCTION TESTS

In the vast majority of patients presenting for anaesthesia, lung function tests are unnecessary, and in any case add little to what can be learned from clinical examination, with careful assessment of the patient's degree of breathlessness. They are indicated more often in the respiratory cripple requiring major surgery, or in patients about to undergo lobectomy or pneumonectomy. They are also useful in evaluating various forms of treatment by comparing results before and after treatment, e.g. in assessing the efficacy of bronchodilators, or of epidural analgesia in the relief of postoperative pain. Examples of such tests are arterial blood gases, vital capacity (VC), forced expiratory volume in one second (FEV_1) and peak flow rate (PFR).

THE ANAESTHETIC OUT-PATIENT CLINIC

The concept of an anaesthetic out-patient clinic in which patients can be assessed and the above types of problem clarified before their admission to hospital is an excellent one. Investigations and treatment can be carried out where required as an out-patient so that the possibility of delaying the operation after admission can be reduced. It also gives the opportunity to summarise the findings on a pre-operative assessment form.

Unfortunately, few anaesthetic departments can cope with the work involved if all patients are referred to the clinic as soon as they are put on the surgical waiting list. The alternative is to be selective, e.g. to see only patients for major surgery, who have systemic disease or who are to have special types of anaesthesia, e.g. hypotensive techniques. Another problem of anaesthetic out-patient clinics is that they tend to become ineffectual if the waiting list is excessively long.

17 Anaesthesia and Intercurrent Diseases

Obesity. Neurological and muscular conditions. Epilepsy. Parkinson's disease. Malignant hyperpyrexia (malignant hyperthermia). Serum hepatitis (hepatitis B antigen; Australia antigen). AIDS (acquired immune deficiency syndrome). Sickle-cell haemoglobinopathies. Atypical pseudocholinesterases. Porphyrias. Rheumatoid arthritis.

With an ageing population the incidence of intercurrent illness in patients presenting for surgery is increasing. Most common are diseases of the cardiovascular and respiratory systems. These and endocrine disorders are discussed elsewhere. In this chapter a variety of diseases—some quite common, some quite rare—are collected. Many of these conditions are inherited; some are of unknown aetiology. The importance of some of them lies in the fact that in their presence the administration of an anaesthetic which would be perfectly reasonable in a normal person may have serious, or even fatal consequences.

OBESITY

Next to cardiovascular and respiratory disease, obesity is one of the commonest disorders occurring in patients presenting for anaesthesia. Usually it is an incidental finding, but occasionally the surgery (e.g. apronectomy, intestinal bypass) may be treatment of the obesity itself.

The anaesthestist's difficulties begin with technical ones. For example, lifting and positioning the patient may be difficult; veins may be hard to find; the airway may be awkward to maintain in patients with short, fat necks and large tongues, and endotracheal intubation may present a problem. Even the blood pressure may not be easy to take accurately because of difficulty in applying the sphygmomanometer cuff satisfactorily to an obese arm.

Obese people are susceptible to a great many other conditions. Among these are ischaemic heart disease, hypertension, bronchitis, diabetes mellitus, varicose veins, gallstones, abdominal and hiatus hernia, arthritis of the legs and increased susceptibility to industrial, household and street accidents. The cardiovascular and respiratory problems are likely to be of the greatest interest to the anaesthetist, obese patients in particular having a tendency to hypoxaemia due to splinting of the chest and abdominal walls by adipose tissue, to the increased amount of intra-abdominal fat and to alterations in the ventilation/perfusion ratio in the lungs.

Management

Most anaesthetic techniques, which would normally be appropriate for the surgery being performed, are acceptable but it is important to ensure that ventilation is adequate. The main underlying principles are to use a method which ensures that the patient rapidly regions consciousness and does not suffer from residual neuromuscular blockade. Not only do obese patients have difficulty in maintaining their airways and ventilation if still drowsy or suffering from residual curarisation, but, as respiratory and venous thrombotic complications are commoner in them, early active movements and ambulation are also important.

NEUROLOGICAL AND MUSCULAR CONDITIONS

Myasthenia Gravis

This disease is due to an abnormality of the neuromuscular junction and is characterised by weakness of skeletal muscle, this weakness being progressive with exercise. Myasthenia gravis varies widely in its severity, its rate of onset and the number of muscles involved. The muscle weakness recovers partially with rest and with anticholinesterase drugs and, although the theory that the disease is caused by the presence of a circulating curare-like drug has now been discounted, it may help clinically to think of the condition as being caused in this way. Thus, in addition to the improvement in muscle strength in response to anticholinesterase drugs, e.g. neostigmine or pyridostigmine, these patients are extremely sensitive to non-depolarising muscle relaxants and resistant to depolarising relaxants.

Anaesthetic management
Myasthenic patients are usually on long-term anticholinesterase drugs. Anaesthesia may be required for incidental surgical conditions or for thymectomy, removal of the thymus gland now being recommended as treatment in certain types of myasthenia.

If possible, it is wise to avoid the use of muscle relaxants in these patients. Anaesthesia may be induced with thiopentone, and if endotracheal intubation is required it can usually be carried out under nitrous oxide, oxygen and halothane, with or without topical analgesia of the larynx. If controlled respiration is needed it can usually be easily carried out with this same anaesthetic sequence. IPPR will certainly be required for thymectomy, where a sternum-splitting incision may be used. If respiratory function has been severely reduced pre-operatively, it may be necessary to ventilate these patients electively for several days postoperatively.

Myasthenic Syndrome (Eaton–Lambert Syndrome)

This is a condition of muscle weakness usually associated with bronchial carcinoma, although the latter may not have been clinically diagnosed. It differs from myasthenia gravis in that the muscle weakness tends to improve with exercise rather than deteriorate. In addition, patients tend to be sensitive both to depolarising and to non-depolarising relaxants.

Dystrophia Myotonica

This is an inherited disease with onset usually in the patient's early thirties. The weakness of the muscles which occurs is associated with difficulty in relaxing after contraction. This may be seen as difficulty in relaxing the grip after a handshake or after clenching the fist to facilitate venepuncture. Associated features are baldness, cataracts, testicular atrophy and cardiomyopathy. The myotonia or muscular contraction may be accentuated by suxamethonium, which should therefore be avoided. Non-depolarising agents may be used, but may not be effective in producing muscular relaxation. Thiopentone has been reported as causing profound respiratory depression and regional techniques or halothane-based inhalational anaesthesia seem the safest methods of anaesthesia.

Multiple Sclerosis

Although the effects of general anaesthesia on this neurological condition have not been carefully evaluated there is no anaesthetic technique which is known to have a definite, detrimental effect on this disease. Even central nerve-blocking techniques (e.g. epidural analgesia) have been performed without worsening the condition. However, in advanced cases there may be much muscle wasting, and it is likely that small doses of anaesthetic and analgesic drugs will go a long way. In addition, the autonomic nervous system may be involved in the condition so that the patient's blood pressure may drop in response to stresses (e.g. doses of drugs and changes in posture) which would have little or no effect on healthy individuals.

Lastly, as in any of these conditions associated with muscle weakness, patients may have difficulty in coughing up sputum after operation and are consequently prone to chest infections.

EPILEPSY

Patients on anti-epileptic drugs should be maintained on them until pre-anaesthetic starvation, and given them again as soon as possible postoperatively. Most general anaesthetics tend to have a sedative effect on the central nervous system, but several agents, especially methohexitone, ketamine and enflurane have been shown to produce convulsions and should not be used in epileptic patients. Thiopentone is the induction agent of choice. It should also be remembered that as hypoglycaemia is a stimulus to convulsions, when an epileptic patient is allowed no oral sustenance for a considerable time because of anaesthesia or surgery, it is worth setting up an intravenous dextrose infusion.

Status Epilepticus

The convulsions can usually be treated initially with a relatively low, careful intravenous injection of thiopentone or diazepam. If the convulsions return they may be treated with an intravenous infusion of diazepam, thiopentone, or phenytoin. The hypoxic and self-destructive physical effects of the convulsions may be controlled with suxamethonium and in the longer term by curare, but it must be remembered that the brain-storm continues and in addition to the muscle relaxant, anti-epileptic drugs must be used.

PARKINSON'S DISEASE

This condition is associated not only with involuntary tremor and a shuffling gait but also with an immobile face which may belie a still active brain.

Until recently treatment has consisted mostly of atropine-like drugs and antihistamines, but more recently levodopa has been introduced, this being converted to dopamine in the brain. Under general anaesthesia this drug tends to produce lability of the blood pressure and cardiac dyshythmias. For this reason, halothane should be avoided and, as the drug has a relatively short action, it should be stopped for 6–12 hours before anaesthesia.

MALIGNANT HYPERPYREXIA (MALIGNANT HYPERTHERMIA)

Although it must have existed before that date, this condition was first described in 1962 as a result of an investigation of the family of a patient who nearly died of hyperpyrexia under general anaesthesia. Findings showed that out of 37 relatives who had been given general anaesthesia, ten had died. Other similar cases and family histories were soon reported from around the world and it became clear that the condition was inherited. The apparent sudden appearance of the disease was no doubt due not only to the fact that the condition had not previously been recognised as a clinical entity, but also to the fact that two of the most powerful triggers to the condition, namely suxamethonium and halothane, were becoming increasingly popular in anaesthetic practice at about that time.

Malignant hyperpyrexia, which is believed to be due to an abnormality of the muscle-fibre membrane, may be triggered by various pharmacological agents including lignocaine, atropine, diazepam, pancuronium and the phenothiazines, or simply by stress, but easily the most powerful triggering agents are suxamethonium and halothane. Hence it is probably the prime example of an intercurrent condition where administering normally acceptable anaesthetic agents may do devastating harm.

The first sign of the condition may be a failure to relax after suxamethonium, or even increased muscle rigidity. The patient's temperature then rises rapidly, an increase of several degrees centigrade per hour being possible. The patient becomes hot and flushed with a tachycardia. As metabolism outstrips the oxygen supply, cyanosis appears, respiratory and metabolic acidosis produce a profound fall in pH and the serum potassium rises rapidly. Death is common in the severe, untreated case.

Treatment

Until recently the treatment has been largely symptomatic, with the infusion of cold sodium bicarbonate to combat metabolic acidosis, insulin and glucose to try to restore serum potassium and surface cooling, steroids and procaine in an attempt to relax muscle rigidity. While sometimes successful, procaine was occasionally required in doses likely to produce cardiovascular collapse. As malignant hyperpyrexia is to some extent dose-related, discontinuation of any possible trigger-agents may also help.

Recently, dantrolene sodium (Dantrium), a skeletal muscle relaxant, has been shown to be remarkably effective in preventing or treating malignant hyperpyrexia in pigs (some strains of which are extremely susceptible to the condition). Case reports are now appearing describing a similar life-saving effect in man. To be effective in severe cases dantrolene should be given within half-an-hour to an hour of the onset of the condition. It has recently become available in the UK, is expensive but now has a shelf-life of three years. It is hoped that it will be available in enough hospitals to be used effectively on any patient who needs it.

SERUM HEPATITIS (HEPATITIS B ANTIGEN; AUSTRALIA ANTIGEN)

The viral hepatitis referred to by the above names (see also Chapter 46) varies in severity from a subclinical infection to fatal liver failure. Its importance lies not in any particular difficulty in anaesthetising these patients, but in the risk of infecting theatre personnel. Spread is mainly blood borne, but may also be transmitted by body secretions or close physical contact. Serum testing can identify degrees of infectivity and, in the cases of highest risk, disposable gloves and gowns should be used when handling patients. For further details of how to deal with these cases, referral should be made to local hospital policy. For personnel inadvertently contaminated an antiserum is available.

AIDS (ACQUIRED IMMUNE DEFICIENCY SYNDROME)

While at the time of writing this is numerically a less serious problem than serum hepatitis in the UK, several factors have led to the government making energetic efforts to disseminate information about prevention of spread of this disease. These features include the high mortality rate (probably 100%) in those infected who develop symptoms, the absence (at present) of any cure or antiserum, and the fact that the virus is sexually transmitted (both homosexually and heterosexually), with a consequent explosive potential for its spread.

The virus can be isolated from blood, semen, tears, saliva and breast milk, but is transmitted principally by sexual intercourse, or transfusion or inoculation by infected blood or blood products. Vomit, sputum, urine, faeces and pus are possibly dangerous if contaminated with blood. The virus is not transmitted by ordinary physical contact, so the risk of infection of theatre personnel is less than with serum hepatitis, precautions being concentrated on the disposal or disinfection of articles, e.g. needles, syringes, theatre instruments and drapes contaminated by spilt blood.

SICKLE-CELL HAEMOGLOBINOPATHIES

This heading covers many genetically transmitted conditions where the patient has an abnormal haemoglobin. Normal haemoglobin is referred to as haemoglobin A. In sickle-cell disease the abnormal haemoglobin is referred to as haemoglobin S. In sickle-cell anaemia an abnormal gene is inherited from both parents (the homozygous state) so that nearly all the haemoglobin is abnormal, and the condition is also referred to as HbSS. In sickle-cell trait, the abnormal gene is inherited from only one parent (the heterozygous state), so there is a mixture of normal and abnormal haemoglobin. This condition is referred to as HbAS.

Under certain circumstances, which include hypoxia, hypercarbia, hypothermia and acidosis, the abnormal haemoglobin (HbS) may distort and rupture the red blood cells. The distorted cells (called 'sickle' cells) form aggregates in the smaller blood vessels causing infarction in many organs, or the rupture of the red blood cells leads to haemolytic anaemia. Sickling may occur under anaesthesia, especially if hypoxia, hypercarbia, hypothermia or hypotension are allowed to occur. This is much more likely in the case of sickle-cell anaemia than the trait, where lesser amounts of abnormal haemoglobin are present.

ATYPICAL PSEUDOCHOLINESTERASES

The apnoea which may result when suxamethonium is given to patients with inherited, abnormal pseudocholinesterases is discussed in Chapter 12. If a patient is found to have this abnormal enzyme it is important to test close relatives to discover whether they are similarly affected.

PORPHYRIAS

The porphyrins are pigments produced in the liver and bone marrow and involved in the synthesis of haem. Disorders in the metabolism of porphyrins are called 'porphyrias' and result in overproduction of some of the porphyrins or their precursors. There are several porphyrias, but only acute intermittent porphyria will be considered here.

Acute Intermittent Porphyria

This inherited condition often presents in young adults. There may be acute onset of abdominal pain; there is often a peripheral neuropathy with paraesthesiae and weakness of trunk and limb muscles, which may cause respiratory embarrassment. There may also be tachycardia and hypertension. During an attack the urine turns dark on standing due to a high concentration of porphobilinogen.

An acute attack of porphyra may be triggered by any of the barbiturates, which are *absolutely* contraindicated in this condition.

RHEUMATOID ARTHRITIS

This is a general systemic disease which in its acute phase may show tachycardia, fever and anaemia. Typically, the small joints of the fingers and toes are the first to become affected, but other joints are frequently involved and are of interest to the anaesthetist. Such joints include the temporomandibular joint and the joints of the cervical spine where stiffness may lead to difficulty in intubation, and the costovertebral joints where limitation of movement may lead to a reduction in vital capacity and a tendency to postoperative pneumonia. Lastly, patients with rheumatoid arthritis may be on, or have recently taken, a course of steroids.

18 Anaesthesia and Endocrine Disease

Thyroid gland. Adrenal gland. Pituitary gland. Parathyroid glands. Pancreas.

The endocrine glands consist of the pituitary, thyroid, parathyroids, adrenals, ovaries, testes and the endocrine portion of the pancreas. The pituitary gland synthesises several 'trophic' hormones that are responsible for controlling the output from the other endocrine glands. These glands produce several hormones which control many of the phsyiological and metabolic functions of the body. For this reason, reduced or excessive activity of any of them may produce severe metabolic disturbance as seen, for example, in thyrotoxicosis or diabetes. The endocrine glands present anaesthetic problems in two situations. Firstly, when a patient undergoing elective surgery is coincidentally suffering from an endocrine disorder and is receiving treatment; and, secondly, when the endocrine disorder itself is to be treated surgically by removal of part or all of the gland.

THYROID GLAND

Hyperthyroidism

Unless emergency surgery is indicated, it is wise to avoid anaesthetising a patient with thyrotoxicosis, either for thyroidectomy or a coincident conditional. Pre-operative restoration of normal thyroid function is obtained by using antithyroid drugs, e.g. carbimazole (Neo-Mercazole), and then iodine is given immediately pre-operatively to decrease the vascularity of the gland. Symptomatic treatment of hyperthyroidism is often by β-adrenergic blockade to reduce the tachycardia, and general sedation to reduce hyperexcitability and shaking. If the patient must be anaesthetised in a hyperthyroid state the anaesthetic should be a deep one with adequate pre-operative sedation and effective β-blockade.

Hypothyroidism

This is usually a chronic condition which either arises spontaneously or results from excessive treatment of hyperthyroidism by irradiation or surgery. As the thyroid gland controls metabolic activity, underactivity of the gland causes a patient to be sluggish and prone to hypothermia, hypoglycaemia, muscle weakness and coma. He may also suffer from respiratory depression and may only metabolise drugs slowly. Satisfactory treatment is obtained by chronic administration of thyroxine, but hypothyroidism may occur, for example, when the patient suffers coincidental intestinal obstruction and fails to absorb his thyroxine. In this case, the patient may appear tired or listless but it may only be when he fails to wake up from an anaesthetic that hypothyroidism is suspected. In this case it is essential to give T3 (tri-iodothyronine) to restore normal thyroid activity.

Thyroid crisis

After partial thyroidectomy a thyroid crisis occasionally occurs, this being a severe increase of the symptoms of hyperthyroidism. It is important to keep the patient cool and sedated and to control his hypertension and tachycardia, which is usually achieved with β-blockade and, if necessary, digoxin to prevent the development of congestive cardiac failure. The overactive remaining thyroid tissue is treated with intravenous iodine and carbimazole or thiouracil.

ADRENAL GLAND

The adrenal glands are divided into the cortex, which secretes cortisol and aldosterone, and the medulla, which is part of the sympathetic nervous system and responsible for secreting adrenaline and noradrenaline.

Hyperadrenalism—Primary Cortical (Conn's Syndrome)

This rare condition is associated with a high concentration of aldosterone and low serum potassium in the blood. The patients also suffer from hypertension and impaired renal function. Anaesthesia for removing what is usually a benign cortical adenoma must take account of the metabolic problems in a similar way to anaesthetising patients in renal failure. Pre-operative treatment with spironolactone may return the blood pressure and serum potassium to normal levels.

Hyperadrenalism—Secondary Cortical (Cushing's Disease)

Excess pituitary production of adrenocorticotrophic hormone (ACTH) leads to excessive activity of the adrenal cortex. This produces sodium retention, oedema and hypertension together with other changes which resemble the side-effects of steroid therapy, e.g. 'moon-face' and striae.

Hypoadrenalism—Primary Cortical (Addison's Disease)

In this condition atrophy of the adrenal cortex and medulla occurs and the patients become pigmented, weak, hypotensive and sometimes have considerable electrolyte disorders. Pre-operative treatment with hydrocortisone and fludrocortisone is necessary to restore their metabolic balance before surgery.

Hypoadrenalism—Secondary Cortical

This usually occurs in patients who are or have recently been on steroid therapy. The side-effects of steroid therapy are important, and include euphoria, a thrombotic tendency, delayed wound healing, mild glycosuria, sodium and water retention and osteoporosis. Anaesthesia itself is only a moderate stress unless accidental hypothermia occurs or the operation is prolonged. Normal steroid cover with hydrocortisone (Chapter 16) is satisfactory for patients who are receiving or who have recently received steroid therapy, mineralocorticoid (fludrocortisone) cover not usually being necessary.

Medullary Hyperadrenalism (Phaeochromocytoma)

Tumours of the medullary portion of the adrenal gland are rare but nevertheless present considerable anaesthetic problems. A phaeochromocytoma is a tumour of chromaffin tissue which may be either benign or malignant, single or multiple. It may occur anywhere along the sympathetic chain as well as in the adrenal gland itself. As sympathetic tissue is involved, there is excessive production of noradrenaline and adrenaline. The patients usually present with paroxysmal hypertension and sweating, together with headache and palpitations. Pre-operative control of wild fluctuations of blood pressure with both α- and β-adrenergic blockade is essential to provide a smooth anaesthetic. Failure to do this may produce such severe rises in blood pressure that a cerebrovascular accident may occur. Death may also result from ventricular arrhythmias.

Bilateral Adrenalectomy

This is usually carried out as a further operation in the treatment of disseminated breast cancer and, apart from needing to maintain the patient on steroid cover postoperatively, the main anaesthetic problems are that the patients are often frail with numerous bone secondaries, pleural effusions and electrolyte disorders.

PITUITARY GLAND

Hyperpituitarism

Although the pituitary gland produces several trophic hormones, it is disorders of the production of growth hormone which may present anaesthetic difficulties. Overproduction of growth hormone in adults leads to acromegaly with considerable overgrowth of the jaws, tongue, pharynx and larynx, and thickening of the vocal cords. The hands become spade-like and the skin may be extremely tough. It may be difficult to anaesthetise and intubate these patients and care must be taken not to precipitate respiratory obstruction only to find intubating the patient impossible. Once anaesthetised, patients with acromegaly do not present severe anaesthetic problems, but they are prone to obstruction and hypoxia in the recovery room and careful post-operative observation is essential.

Hypopituitarism

Reduced pituitary activity is associated with a reduction in the production of growth hormone together with other trophic hormones and the patients are generally lethargic with a low basal metabolic rate. These patients may be exceptionally sensitive to barbiturates and narcotic analgesics and general anaesthesia may precipitate coma in patients with severe metabolic disorders. Reduced levels of ACTH and thyroid stimulating hormone (TSH) may produce secondary effects due to failure of hormone production of these glands.

PARATHYROID GLANDS

Hyperparathyroidism

The parathyroid glands control the blood calcium concentration, which is essential for normal nerve and cardiac conduction. Parathormone, the hormone secreted by the parathyroids, increases the mobilisation of calcium from bone and in hyperparathyroidism a high serum calcium may be associated with metabolic disorders requiring treatment with diuretics and calcitonin. The cause is usually a parathyroid adenoma requiring surgical removal; this condition is particularly common in patients with renal failure on dialysis.

Hypoparathyroidism

Hypoparathyroidism is usually a complication of thyroidectomy, the glands being removed inadvertently with the thyroid. A reduced serum concentration of calcium may be accompanied by muscle spasms and tetany, the treatment being intravenous calcium gluconate. Anaesthesia in patients with parathyroid disorders does not usually present any additional difficulties to those encountered with the thyroidectomy except that many of the patients may be in renal failure, the cause of their parathyroid disorder.

PANCREAS

The endocrine portion of the pancreas secretes insulin and glucagon respectively from the beta and alpha cells of the islets of Langerhans. These two hormones are responsible for controlling blood sugar and diabetes mellitus is probably the commonest endocrine disorder likely to produce anaesthetic difficulties.

Management of Diabetic Patients during Anaesthesia and Surgery

In most cases, diabetes does not cause problems if the anaesthetist accepts that the patients are essentially normal people with impaired or absent insulin production. If their diabetes is well under control pre-operatively there is no reason why it should not remain so throughout the operation. Patients should arrive in the anaesthetic room not only with a normal or slightly raised blood sugar level but also with normal glycogen stores, glycogen being stored in the liver and used to maintain a normal blood sugar level. It is important, therefore, that they are starved for the minimum time pre-operatively and are operated on at the beginning of the list at a predetermined time.

Pre-operative knowledge of the stability of their diabetic regimen is essential and in many cases little or no additional treatment is required. Diet-controlled diabetics can simply be starved pre-operatively in the normal way, as the only problem likely to develop is hyperglycaemia. To err on the side of hyperglycaemia is a far safer way of conducting the anaesthetic. Patients on oral hypoglycaemic drugs should stop these 1–2 days before surgery and will therefore tend to become hyperglycaemic. Those on insulin should be controlled by whatever regimen is necessary, depending on the urgency of the operation, the degree of control of the diabetes and the expected postoperative course.

In general, patients who are undergoing a short operation may simply omit their morning dose of insulin and their breakfast, knowing that they will be eating later in the day. In major surgery, however, it is essential not only to maintain a normal blood sugar level but also to ensure that glucose passes into the cells where it can be used for metabolism; this can be achieved only by simultaneous administration of glucose and insulin. In this event a reduced morning dose of insulin together with a 5% dextrose infusion is usual. In more complicated cases, or when the diabetes is out of control, it is most satisfactory to change the patient on to a sliding scale of Actrapid insulin controlled on four-hourly blood or urine glucose estimations. Frequent measurements of blood sugar and intravenous administration of glucose and insulin are probably the best and most accurate way of controlling diabetes during anaesthesia.

More recently, slow intravenous insulin infusions have been successfully used to treat diabetic hyperglycaemia and these are likely to become widely used for intra-operative control of diabetics undergoing major surgery. In the Alberti regimen 10 units of Actrapid insulin and 10 mmol potassium chloride are added to 500 ml 10% dextrose which is then infused over four hours. This fail-safe system means that variations in infusion rate cannot produce an imbalance of either glucose and insulin or hypokalaemia.

19 Interpretation of Electrocardiogram

Pre-operative ECG interpretation. Intra-operative ECG interpretation. Common intra-operative dysrhythmias and their treatment.

Although electrocardiography (ECG) is a specialist subject in itself, the use of monitoring and the simple interpretation of dysrhythmias are extremely important in anaesthetic practice. There is little excuse for failing to monitor the electrocardiogram (ECG) during anaesthesia and although this is simply a record of the electrical activity of the heart and does not reflect peripheral blood flow, abnormalities may give an early indication of problems during anaesthesia.

When excitable tissue, either nerve or muscle, is activated to produce either contraction or impulse transmission, this is effected by a change in permeability of the cell membrane, allowing sodium ions to flow in and potassium ions to flow out of the cell. This depolarisation, as it is known, results in a change in electrical charge inside the cell, and is followed by a repolarisation process when the charge returns to normal. Resting cells are negatively charged with respect to the outside while depolarised cells become positive. If electrodes are placed in certain positions on the chest wall or the limbs, changes in electrical activity in the heart due to contraction are detected at the electrode as a change in charge. If this electrical activity is then demonstrated on the ECG, an upward deflection of the baseline reflects a positive change and a downward deflection a negative change, this being

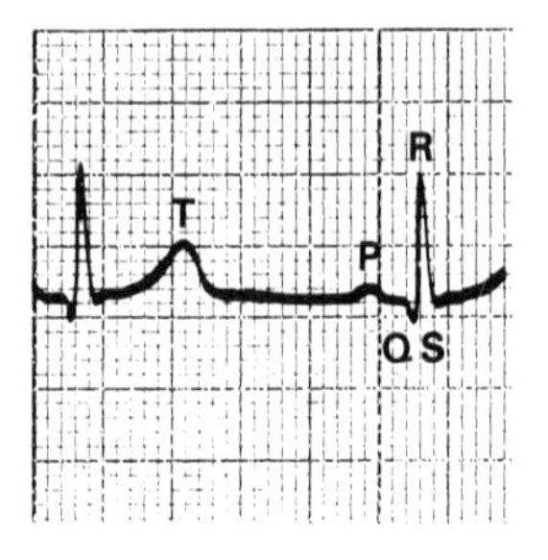

Fig. 19.1 Normal ECG waveform

the basis of the ECG recording. The ECG waveform (Fig. 19.1) reflects the changes in charge occurring at different points in the cardiac cycle.

The heart lies in a fixed position in the chest, so if these changes in charge are viewed from the right arm or the left arm for example, the appearance will differ. By using different leads it is possible to examine the different parts of the heart for abnormalities of contraction or conduction, reflecting, for example, myocardial ischaemia or heart block. The intra-operative use of ECG monitoring, however, is limited to a single lead that is designed to reflect major disturbances in rate and rhythm rather than to diagnose focal areas of ischaemia which requires a full 12-lead ECG.

PRE-OPERATIVE ECG INTERPRETATION

Pre-operative ECG records should be obtained routinely from patients with a history of cardiac disease and also those in the older age group undergoing major surgery. In patients in whom cardiac problems are expected, it is important to have a pre-operative baseline ECG with which to compare any post-operative change. Normal ECG assessment includes the following.

Rate

The paper speed of a normal ECG recording is 25 mm a second, and as the small squares on the ECG paper are 1 mm, this means that the paper travels at 25 small squares (five large squares) per second; 300 large squares are therefore covered every minute, and by dividing into 300 the number of large squares between the same point (usually the R wave) of two ECG complexes, the heart rate is derived (e.g. 300/5 = heart rate of 60). This is applicable only to patients with a regular heart beat (sinus rhythm).

Cardiac Rhythm

Normal sinus rhythm is diagnosed by the presence of a P wave, reflecting atrial contraction, before each QRS complex (Fig. 19.1). This results in a regular heartbeat which will vary only slightly with respiration (sinus arrhythmia).

The normal pacemaker of the heart (the sino-atrial node) initiates impulses at a regular rate, which travel across the atrium to the atrioventricular node and then down the bundle of His which divides to supply the right and left ventricles. Normal ECG complexes of the type shown in Figure 19.1 reflect contractions which are initiated from the atrium (supraventricularly).

The absence of P waves preceding some or all of the cardiac complexes, which are nevertheless of a supraventricular type, indicates that the normal pacemaker is not functioning. If the rate is regular, this implies that another area of the atrium has taken over the task of pacemaker, e.g. the A-V node or, if the rate is irregular without P waves and usually relatively fast, this is indicative of atrial fibrillation. A number of P waves regularly preceding each cardiac contraction indicates atrial flutter with a degree of heart block that allows only one in every three or four impulses to cross the atrioventricular septum and pass down the bundle of His.

In nodal rhythms, the impulse rises in or near the A-V node. In this case, normal, regular QRS complexes are seen. The P waves may either be present, but the P-R interval short, or lost within the QRS complex.

Ventricular ectopic beats (Fig. 19.2) are very different in appearance from supraventricular contractions. They appear broader and are irregular: they are not preceded by a P wave and may occur at any stage in the resting period or, occasionally, during cardiac contraction. Regular runs of ventricular beats

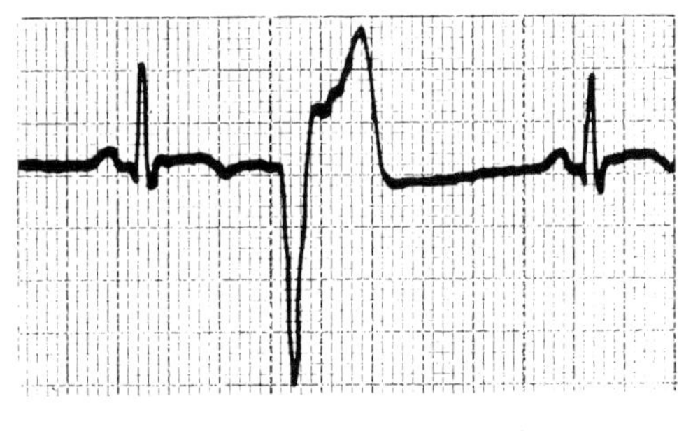

Fig. 19.2 Ventricular ectopic beats

(ventricular tachycardia) or coupled beats (one supraventricular, one ventricular) are both indicative of conduction disturbances or myocardial ischaemia.

Conduction Defects

The interpretation of conduction defects on the ECG is a specialised procedure, but irregular rhythms or broad, biphasic R waves are often indicative of conduction abnormalities in the ventricles.

Myocardial Ischaemia

Recent myocardial ischaemia is reflected by ST-segment elevation (Fig. 19.3) particularly in the chest leads, often accompanied by flattening or inversion of the T wave. Large Q waves in the chest leads are indicative of old myocardial ischaemia.

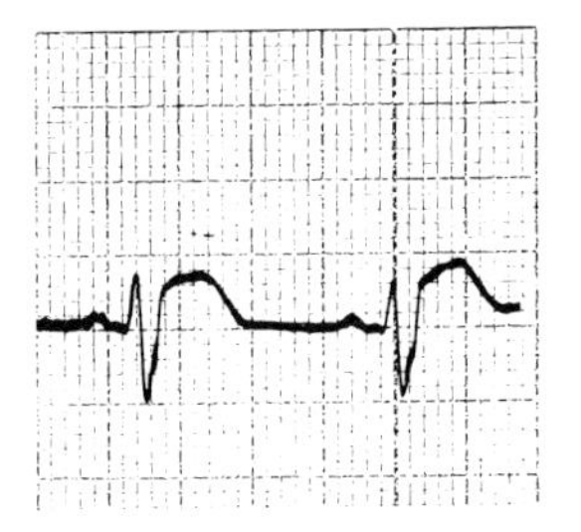

Fig. 19.3 ST-segment elevation—myocardial ischaemia

Metabolic Disturbances

Hyperkalaemia is the most important metabolic disturbance detectable on the ECG. High-peaked T waves indicate severe hyperkalaemia requiring emergency treatment with either calcium or glucose and insulin.

INTRA-OPERATIVE ECG INTERPRETATION

In this situation the ECG is used mainly as a rate and rhythm monitor, although severe changes in the appearance of the ECG complex with the leads remaining in the same position may be interpreted as myocardial ischaemia if they follow some important clinical event. It is then wise to repeat a 12-lead ECG in the immediate postoperative period. Apart from the detection of dysrhythmias, use of the intra-operative ECG is important because it gives an early indication of inadequate anaesthesia. A tachycardia is produced as an early response to almost every intra-operative problem. Hypoxia or hypercarbia, due either to inadequate ventilation, circuit faults, or ventilator disconnection, inadequate analgesia or sedation and excessive blood loss all lead to a tachycardia, which is easily detectable on the ECG.

COMMON INTRA-OPERATIVE DYSRHYTHMIAS AND THEIR TREATMENT

Disorders of Sinus Rhythm

Sinus tachycardia

An increase in heart rate is produced as an early response to many anaesthetic problems although it will not occur in patients on β-adrenergic blockade. The anaesthetic technique should be examined for inadequate gas flow or oxygenation, inadequate analgesia or sedation, and also the presence of excessive blood loss requiring transfusion.

Sinus bradycardia
This is a common dysrhythmia, often produced by anaesthetic agents, particularly halothane and suxamethonium, which stimulate the vagus nerve, producing a bradycardia. It is important to remember that normal, fit patients' heart rates are far slower when they are asleep, sometimes being as slow as 40 beats per min. Although a full vagal blocking dose of intravenous atropine is 2 mg, it is often possible to increase the heart rate to an acceptable level with a very small dose of atropine (0·2–0·3 mg). Excessively slow heart rates may also produce other dysrhythmias (see below).

Supraventricular Dysrhythmias

Wandering pacemaker and nodal rhythm
It is not infrequent during anaesthesia for the pacemaker in the atrium to shift from the normal sino-atrial node to another area of the atrium or to the A-V node itself. If the atrial impulses are coming from varying sites in runs of three or four beats, which then change to a slightly different supraventricular complex, this is known as a wandering pacemaker. Nodal tachycardia has already been mentioned. Supraventricular dysrhythmias may occur as a result of sinus bradycardia, presumably because the normal rate is insufficient to prevent additional beats occurring. For this reason they often respond well to atropine, producing a slight increase in heart rate.

Atrial fibrillation
It is relatively uncommon for atrial fibrillation to occur during anaesthesia in a patient who is in sinus rhythm pre-operatively, unless the pericardium is disturbed during thoracic surgery. If atrial flutter or fibrillation do arise, however, it may be necessary to digitalise the patient urgently to prevent a fall in cardiac output resulting from lack of atrial contraction. Intravenous ouabain or lanatoside C is often useful instead of digoxin in such an emergency.

Supraventricular tachycardia
This dysrhythmia is again relatively rare during anaesthesia, but it may occur particularly if the patient is inadequately anaes-

thetised. Like a severe sinus tachycardia, it is sometimes controllable with additional analgesia or sedation but may require β-adrenergic blockade or verapamil (p. 160) to reduce the heart rate.

Ventricular Dysrhythmias

Ventricular ectopic beats may occur in any patient, particularly if he is anxious or inadequately anaesthetised, and are frequently seen during induction when this period is monitored on the ECG. The occurrence of the occasional ventricular ectopic is probably of no importance, particularly if it is present on the pre-operative ECG, but regular ectopics occurring either in groups of three or four or coupled with a supraventricular beat, are more serious. As a general rule, an incidence of more than one ventricular ectopic in five beats requires treatment and this rule may be extended if cardiac output is impaired. Ventricular ectopics may also reflect myocardial ischaemia and should be carefully evaluated. Intravenous lignocaine (50–100 mg) is usually sufficient to treat intra-operative ventricular ectopics, although, as in the case of supraventricular dysrhythmias, a change in anaesthetic technique may be required. Occasionally a lignocaine drip is necessary to abate the ventricular dysrhythmia permanently. Intravenous disopyramide may also be useful. However, both these drugs cause myocardial depression and may therefore aggravate the hypotension that frequent ectopics tend to produce, and treatment should be given only when absolutely necessary. Care should also be taken to ensure that patients are metabolically normal since hypokalaemia, in particular, may predispose to ventricular dysrhythmias. Occasionally, ventricular ectopic beats are produced in response to a sinus bradycardia, again presumably because the inherent excitability of the ventricle takes over. Intravenous atropine in small doses may again be useful.

20 Intravenous Techniques: Central Venous Pressure

Technique and equipment. Complications. Central venous pressure.

The hypodermic syringe is usually believed to have been invented in 1853 by Pravaz of Lyons. A year later a syringe and a needle were introduced by Alexander Wood, a Scotsman and, over subsequent years, various anaesthetic agents were injected intravenously including chloral hydrate, chloroform, and ether. In 1924 the first barbiturate was given intravenously, and in 1935 the most famous intravenous anaesthetic agent of them all, thiopentone, was introduced in the USA. Reusable metal intravenous cannulae began to be replaced by the disposable plastic variety in the middle 1950s. Improvements in their quality, changes in the versatility of their design and the variety of substances of which they are made have been continuing ever since. As regards hypodermic needles, the old reusable type which had to be sharpened periodically has been almost completely replaced by disposable needles.

The common uses of intravenous techniques are for taking venous samples, for administering drugs (in particular for inducing and maintaining anaesthesia), for the transfusion of blood or infusion of other fluids, for various radiological procedures, for central venous pressure measurement and for catheterisation of the right side of the heart. For long-term intravenous feeding a central venous line is almost essential.

TECHNIQUE AND EQUIPMENT

The commonest sites for venepuncture are the superficial veins of the dorsum of the hand or of the forearm. The veins on the back of the hand are often the easiest to use, but for cannulation for intravenous infusion a straighter vein on the forearm tends to be less temperamental. It is essential that the lighting be good and preferably oblique as it tends to make the veins more obvious. The venous outflow from the arm should be occluded by a tourniquet or by an assistant squeezing the arm. The nearer the venepuncture is performed to the venous obstruction, the more distended and easier to see and palpate will the vein be.

Having occluded the venous outflow, various techniques may be used to make the vein more obvious. These include lightly tapping the vein with the fingers (firm slapping may be painful), actively or passively clenching the patient's fingers, allowing the arm to hang below the level of the heart, or occasionally by applying warmth over the intended venepuncture site. The junction of two veins, if convenient, is the best site for venepuncture because the vein is less likely to escape from the probing needle. It is also wise to pierce the skin and vein in two separate movements because the vein is less likely to be transfixed by the jerking movement which tends to accompany the passage of the needle or cannula through the skin. Needles should always be advanced at least several millimetres up the lumen of the vein to ensure that the entire needle bevel remains within the vein during injection. Blood should always be aspirated before injection. Similarly, cannulae should be advanced a few millimetres before removing the needle as it is possible for the latter to be within the vein and blood to be aspirated while the shoulder of the cannula has not yet passed through the vein wall into the lumen.

Other veins useful, especially in emergencies, are the external jugular vein which tends to fill when the patient is placed head-down, and the veins in the antecubital fossa. The veins on the medial side of the latter site should not be used routinely because there is an appreciable risk of injection into an artery or of damaging the median nerve. However, it may be a useful site for rapid infusion in a hypovolaemic patient until other more convenient veins appear as the circulating blood volume is restored.

Other useful injection sites, especially in babies, are the scalp, the front of the wrist and the saphenous vein in front of the medial malleolus at the ankle. The legs should be avoided if possible for infusions in adults because of the risk of unpleasant thrombophlebitis.

Types of Equipment

Winged needles
These needles have two flexible plastic wings attached to the shank of the needle and a length of flexible tubing which ends in either a female Luer adapter or a rubber bung. The wings serve as a needle-holder and as an aid to secure taping of the needle after venepuncture. These needles are deservedly popular for induction and intermittent injections during anaesthesia, but even if securely fixed in position they retain the disadvantage of a needle compared with a cannula, namely that they are more likely to cut out of the vein. Other types of non-disposable needles used for intermittent injections, e.g. Gordh and Mitchell needles, have declined in popularity since the introduction of disposable winged needles.

Cannulas and catheters
These are made of various substances including polyvinyl chloride (PVC), nylon, silastic, polyethylene, polypropylene and Teflon, or other materials may be Teflon-coated. The difference between a cannula and a catheter is simply one of length, anything under about 12 cm being considered a cannula.

The cannula is a 'needle-inside' device. Catheters may also be manufactured in this way, but have the disadvantage that the longer the catheter, the longer and more unwieldy the needle it contains. In addition, it cannot be supplied with a stilette to aid insertion, as the needle is already inside the catheter.

Another common type of catheter is the 'catheter-inside-needle' design. This is more convenient to insert, and is usually advanced still containing a stilette. The serious disadvantage of this design is that should the catheter ever be withdrawn relative to the needle, it is possible to shear off the distal part of the catheter against the bevel of the needle and the fragment may migrate centrally in the vein as an embolus.

A third type of catheter is inserted through a cannula. The cannula is inserted over a needle in the usual way, and after withdrawing the needle the catheter is inserted through the cannula.

The final type of catheter is supplied alone and is intended for insertion by surgical cut-down.

Seldinger Technique

This technique was originally devised for the insertion of catheters into veins or arteries for radiological investigations. A needle or cannula is used to insert a flexible guide-wire into the chosen vein. The needle is then removed and a tapered dilator threaded over the guide-wire to enlarge the hole in the vein. The dilator is then removed and a large cannula threaded over the guide-wire which in turn is then removed. This cannula can then be used to pass a variety of catheters, e.g. triple lumen, Swan-Ganz, for anaesthetic or intensive care purposes.

COMPLICATIONS

Complications of intravenous techniques range from trivial to life-endangering. Minor problems include haematoma formation at the injection site and temporary erythema or wealing along the line of the vein due to a localised allergic reaction to the substance injected.

A more unpleasant complication of venepuncture is inflammation of the vein (phlebitis). Sooner or later this occurs with any prolonged venous cannulation and is caused by a combination of the irritating effect of infused fluids on the vein wall and bacterial action caused by bacteria entering through the puncture site in the skin. Fluids administered into a central venous catheter are rapidly diluted by the large volume of blood, so that their irritant action is greatly reduced, and if care is taken to maintain the puncture site sterile, these central venous lines may remain in situ for weeks.

When phlebitis occurs, apart from the redness and tenderness of the overlying skin the vein rapidly becomes blocked by thrombus (thrombophlebitis). Fortunately, these thrombi are firmly attached to the vein wall by the inflammation, so seldom give rise to emboli. However, if the blockage occurs in a large enough vein (e.g. the femoral vein) this alone may lead to disability owing to the oedema produced in the limb.

Embolism of catheter fragments caused by faulty technique has already been mentioned. Catheter embolism may also occur if the shaft of a cannula or catheter separates from the hub due to faulty bonding of the two parts—a much less likely occurrence with improved methods of manufacture.

Air embolism may occur when entry is made into a vein where the pressure is subatmospheric. For this reason patients should be placed head-down to raise the pressure in the neck veins before performing venous cannulation. Air may also gain entry to the venous system with some methods of forced transfusion (e.g. Martin's pump) but not with the methods whereby the infusion bag is squeezed from outside (Fenwal, Tycos pressure infusers) because infusion automatically stops when the bag is empty.

CENTRAL VENOUS PRESSURE

In recent years the measurement of central venous pressure has become an important aid in managing seriously ill and especially hypovolaemic patients. The veins concerned are the large intra-thoracic veins leading to the right side of the heart, i.e. the superior and inferior venae cavae.

To understand central venous pressure it helps to consider the circulation as being divided into three parts: (1) the venous system, which returns the blood down a gradient from the periphery to (2) the heart, which pumps the blood out into (3) the arterial system, which provides a varying peripheral resistance. It also makes it easier to consider the left ventricle as being the heart's pump and the right side of the heart and pulmonary circulation simply as part of the venous system leading to it.

The normal central venous pressure is 0–12 cm H_2O measured where the mid-axillary line crosses the 4th intercostal space with the patient supine. In the presence of hypovolaemia the venous return and the central venous pressure fall. The body attempts to maintain the blood pressure by venoconstriction to reduce venous pooling and improve venous turn, and by vasoconstriction on the arterial side to increase peripheral resistance. Only after these compensatory mechanisms have failed does the blood pressure fall. Thus the central venous pressure is a more sensitive index of reduced blood volume than blood pressure. It is safe to infuse fluids quickly provided that the central venous pressure does not rise above normal limits.

Conversely, the central venous pressure tends to rise above normal in overtransfusion. It also rises when the pump, i.e. the heart, fails. Common examples of this condition are a heart

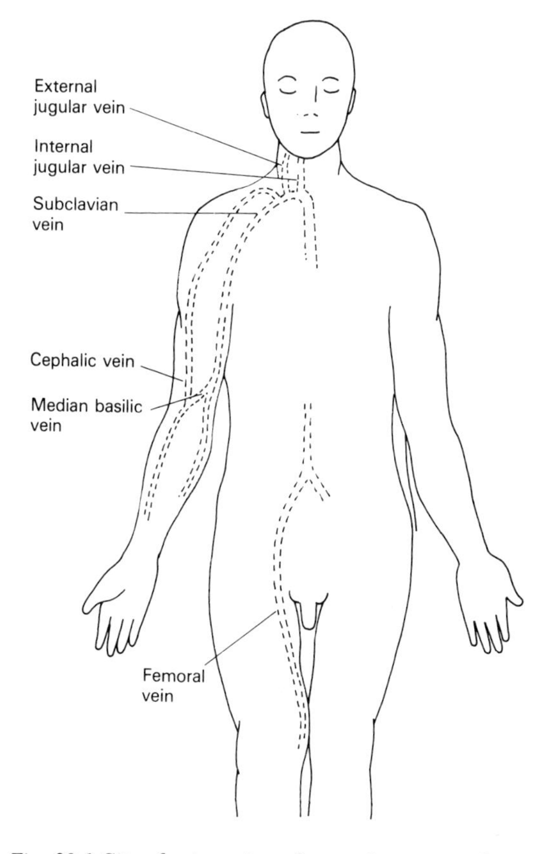

Fig. 20.1 Sites for insertion of central venous catheters

weakened by acute or chronic myocardial ischaemia, or 'poisoned' by depressant anaesthetic agents such as thiopentone or halothane. Clearly, these two groups of factors causing a rise in central venous pressure may be interrelated, it being much easier to overtransfuse a weak heart.

Central Venous Pressure Catheter Techniques

The various routes by which catheters may be inserted into the central veins are shown in Figure 20.1 and summarised below with some of the advantages and disadvantages of the various approaches. The complications described above for catheters apply, of course, catheter embolisation being a real danger with some types of equipment. Care must be taken to avoid infection, it being wise to insert the catheter with a full aseptic technique, to apply an antibiotic locally to the injection site and to apply an occlusive dressing, which should be changed regularly.

The ideal position for the catheter tip is in the superior vena cava. A catheter which has stopped too peripherally will give an incorrect reading, while a catheter which has been inserted too far may perforate the wall of the right atrium. If the catheter is advanced even further it may enter the right ventricle, which has a much higher pressure. A rough guide to the length of catheter to be inserted may be gained by holding another catheter (or the catheter's stilette) against the patient's skin along the line of the vein that has been used. Even so, accurate confirmation of the position of the catheter tip (provided that it is radio-opaque) can be made only by x-ray examination of the chest.

Methods of Central Venous Catheterisation

Veins in the arm

The large vein on the radial side of the wrist or the veins in the antecubital fossa may be used. In the latter site the approach through the median basilic vein on the medial aspect of the elbow is more likely to prove successful than the cephalic vein on the outer aspect of the antecubital fossa. All the arm veins require long catheters which makes them less likely to be successful than a more central approach, but, as they are free from some of the serious complications of the direct approaches to the neck veins (e.g. pneumothorax), they should usually be the first choice.

External jugular vein
With the patient slightly head-down venepuncture of this vein may be easy. However, for an approach so close to the central veins, this method is unfortunately accompanied by a rather high failure rate in accurate placement of the catheter.

Subclavian vein
The patient should be placed head-down to distend the vein and to prevent air embolism. Supraclavicular and infraclavicular techniques are used. They have the highest success rates, but also the highest incidence of pneumothorax.

Internal jugular vein
The patient is placed head-down and the skin pierced about 3 cm above the clavicle. This approach also has a high success rate and pneumothorax is less likely. However, there is some risk of producing a haematoma if the neighbouring carotid artery is pierced, and on the left side damage to the thoracic duct may result in a chylothorax.

Femoral vein
The femoral vein should be avoided if possible for central venous catheterisation because the incidence of thrombophlebitis and oedema of the leg is high when this site is used.

21 Endotracheal Intubation

History. Indications. Equipment. Techniques. Complications. Difficult intubation ('Difficult Intubation Box').

HISTORY

The first uses of endotracheal intubation were in the treatment of asphyxia neonatorum and in cases of drowning. For these purposes, in 1754, Benjamin Pugh, a Chelmsford surgeon, designed a tube made from a coiled wire covered with soft leather, and in 1788, Charles Kite, a surgeon of Gravesend, designed a curved metal cannula which he used in several cases of apparent drowning in the River Thames. These earlier tubes were introduced blindly into the larynx, usually with the help of the operator's finger.

In 1880 anaesthesia was administered for the first time through an endotracheal tube.

The next main advance in endotracheal intubation was the invention of the first laryngoscope by Kirstein in 1895, but the instrument was somewhat primitive and did not gain widespread popularity. Not until an improved laryngoscope was designed by Chevalier Jackson in 1920 did intubation under direct vision become a more widespread technique. Added impetus to the popular use of endotracheal intubation occurred in the 1914–18 war, which resulted in a great many casualties requiring surgery to the head and neck. During this period Magill introduced the orotracheal tube with an inflatable cuff.

Many different designs of laryngoscope were used, but the

Macintosh laryngoscope, today almost the standard laryngoscope for adult intubation worldwide, was introduced in 1943.

INDICATIONS FOR ENDOTRACHEAL INTUBATION

There is some variation among individual anaesthetists as to exactly which patient they consider requires intubation, but the following are typical indications.

For Head and Neck Operations or Remoteness from Patient

For most operations on the head and neck, and especially for those on the upper respiratory tract, endotracheal intubation is desirable or even essential.

On other occasions it may be desirable that the anaesthetist keeps some distance away from the patient. This might happen, for instance, in anaesthesia for x-ray procedures where, to avoid excessive irradiation, it is essential that the anaesthetist be remote from the patient.

To Prevent Aspiration of Gastric Contents into the Lungs

Under general anaesthesia the respiratory tract is completely safe from contamination by gastric contents only when an endotracheal tube has been passed and its cuff inflated. For this reason endotracheal intubation is indicated in most emergency anaesthesia.

When Intermittent Positive-pressure Ventilation is to be Used

It is difficult and dangerous to ventilate a patient with a face mask for any length of time, there always being the possibility of regurgitation, especially if the stomach is inadvertently inflated. This also means that endotracheal intubation is routine for thoracic anaesthesia, where IPPV is necessary to prevent collapse of the lung once the pleural cavity has been opened.

When the Airway is Difficult

In some patients it may be difficult or impossible to maintain an airway for any length of time with a face mask. The degree of difficulty varies in different patients and also depends on the strength of the anaesthetist's fingers. The patient's position may also make using a face mask difficult, e.g. the prone position.

For Ill Patients, or with Complicated Anaesthetic Techniques

Where perfect control of the airway is essential at all times it is better to use endotracheal intubation. Examples of this include the very frail or ill patient, or when some special technique is being used, e.g. hypotensive anaesthesia.

For Resuscitation

The apnoeic patient is most effectively and safely ventilated through an endotracheal tube, although simpler methods, such as mouth-to-mouth respiration or ventilation with a face mask are usually effective if equipment for intubation is not to hand. In conditions of upper respiratory tract obstruction (e.g. due to inflammation), endotracheal intubation may be necessary to provide adequate respiration.

In longer-term intensive care, nasotracheal or orotracheal intubation may be continued for several days while the problem as to whether the patient requires a tracheostomy is resolved.

EQUIPMENT

Familiarity with the equipment required for endotracheal intubation is best learned in the anaesthetic room. The following is intended as a general introduction.

Laryngoscopes

Traditional laryngoscopes are divided into two groups: the

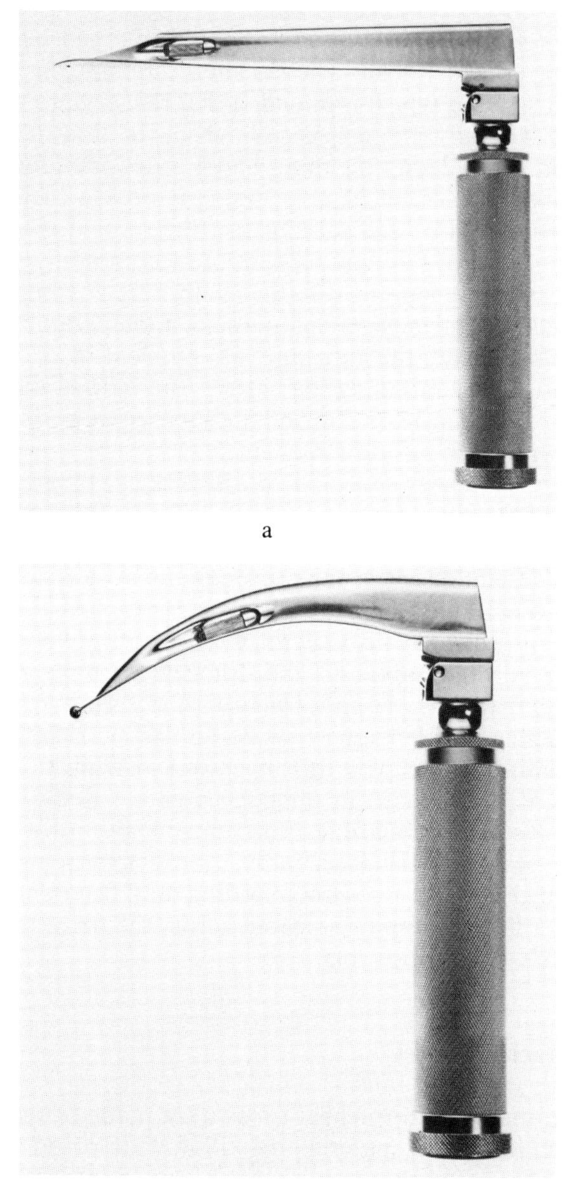

Fig. 21.1 (a) Straight-bladed laryngoscope (Soper pattern). (b) Macintosh laryngoscope

straight-bladed type (Fig. 21.1a) and the curved-blade type (Fig. 21.1b), the Macintosh. The essential difference is that with the straight-bladed type it is intended that the laryngoscope blade be passed behind the epiglottis, which it lifts forwards. The Macintosh blade, on the other hand, is designed for passing into the vallecula—i.e. in front of the epiglottis, which is indirectly lifted forwards by pressure against the root of the tongue.

Both types of laryngoscope are now commonly supplied with batteries in the handle. The tiny bulb, screwed into a socket on the blade, has always tended to make a temperamental electrical connection, and the introduction by Penlon of a Macintosh laryngoscope containing the battery and bulb in the handle with the light carried to the tip of the laryngoscope blade by fibre-optics has been an improvement.

The most recent development in laryngoscopes is a fibre-optic instrument where both light and vision are carried down the same flexible rod, the intention being to pass the instrument within an endotracheal tube through the nose or mouth (usually the former) and when the pharynx is reached to visualise the vocal cords directly through the flexible optical system. When the flexible laryngoscope and endotracheal tube have been passed through the cords, the endotracheal tube is slid further down into the trachea and held there while the laryngoscope is removed. Two main reasons why this ingenious instrument has not been more frequently used in difficult cases are firstly, because it is expensive and there are few instruments about for anaesthetists to gain skill with them; secondly, even if a vasoconstrictor spray is applied to the nose, some bleeding may occur, and any blood or other fluid becoming smeared across the tip of the instrument renders vision impossible.

Endotracheal Tubes

Traditionally, endotracheal tubes were made of red rubber and tubes made of this material are still in widespread use. The next material used was latex rubber, which is reinforced with a wire (or now more commonly a nylon) spiral to prevent it from kinking. More recently, endotracheal and tracheostomy tubes have been made of PVC.

Advantages claimed for tubes made in this material include disposability, reduced irritant effect on the tracheal mucosa in long-term use and the provision of 'low-pressure' cuffs, which exert less pressure on the tracheal mucosa and are therefore less likely to cause mucosal sloughing. These last benefits, which depend on the properties of PVC, tend to be lost when economies dictate that the tubes be re-used, any form of heat sterilisation producing changes in the nature of the plastic. At present, red rubber tubes are still the most popular in everyday clinical practice.

The commonest patterns of tube are the Magill (*see* Fig. 21.2), the Oxford (*see* Fig. 21.3) and the armoured latex tubes mentioned above. These are numbered in millimetres according to their internal diameter.

The Magill endotracheal tube

These tubes (Fig. 21.2) have a continuous curve and are invariably supplied by the manufacturers cut to an excessive length, as required by the British Standards Institution. The anaesthetist must then cut the tube to the length which he thinks is correct for the patient. A tube that is too short may slip out of the larynx, while one which is too long tends to intubate the right main bronchus because it is more in a straight line with the

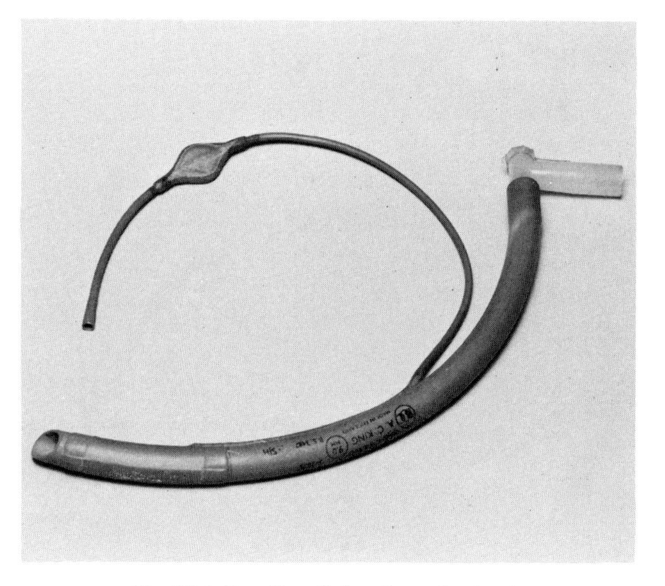

Fig. 21.2 Magill cuffed endotracheal tube

trachea than is the left main bronchus. If this happens, ventilation of the left lung will be diminished or absent, especially if the inflated cuff occludes the left main bronchus. The other disadvantage of the Magill tubes is that, of the three patterns described, they are the most easily kinked. The Magill tubes are designed for either nasotracheal or orotracheal intubation, those for the former being rather thinner-walled so that they take up less space in the nose. The smaller size of Magill tubes are not supplied with inflatable cuffs because in small patients these would take up too large a proportion of the available airway. The larger sizes of tubes are available with (and are usually used with) inflatable cuffs. Nasotracheal tubes are not usually supplied with inflatable cuffs, but there is now available a nasotracheal tube with a flush-fitting cuff which is inflated by a tube running within the wall of the tube itself. Thus the inflating mechanism makes little difference to the external dimensions of the tube, and this is a useful piece of equipment when a cuffed nasotracheal tube is required.

The Oxford endotracheal tube

This tube (Fig. 21.3) is L-shaped, which conforms better with the anatomy of the upper respiratory tract. The internal diameter of

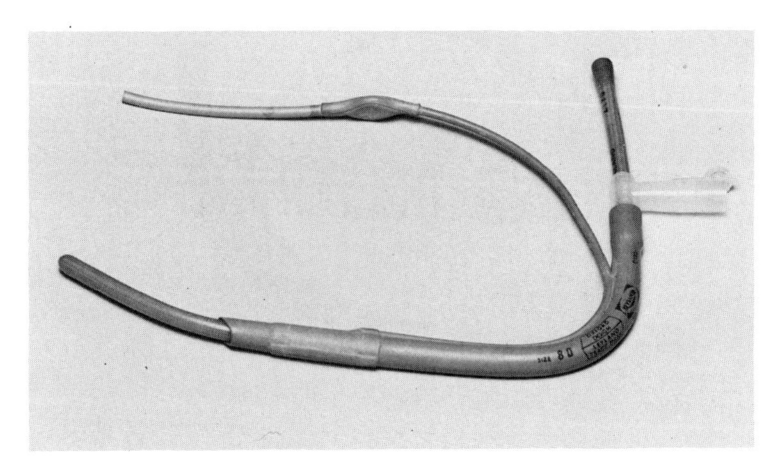

Fig. 21.3 Oxford cuffed endotracheal tube with introducing bougie

these tubes is constant, but the proximal part of the tube which lies in the mouth and pharynx is thicker than the distal part; hence this tube is virtually unkinkable. The other main advantage of the Oxford tubes is that they are supplied by the manufacturers in lengths which increase with the diameter. These lengths have been carefully calculated so that, provided the anaesthetist chooses the diameter of the tube that is correct for the patient, the length is almost invariably correct without further trimming. The smaller sizes of Oxford tube are only supplied uncuffed, but the variable thickness of the rubber means that the tubes are tapered and more likely to make an airtight fit than the smaller sizes of Magill tube. Oxford tubes are difficult to pass unless a malleable bougie or stilette is passed through and beyond the tube and given a further curve anteriorly. Attempts to pass Oxford tubes without this aid probably explain the relative lack of popularity of these excellent tubes. Because the bevel of the Oxford tubes faces posteriorly it is possible to obstruct the end of the tube in situations where the neck is acutely flexed forward, e.g. in certain neurosurgical procedures. This problem may be avoided by cutting a small hole in the anterior wall of the tube opposite the bevel. Obstruction can similarly occur with Magill tubes, but as their bevel faces laterally, this obstruction is likely to occur with lateral deviations of the trachea, as might be caused by a thyroid tumour.

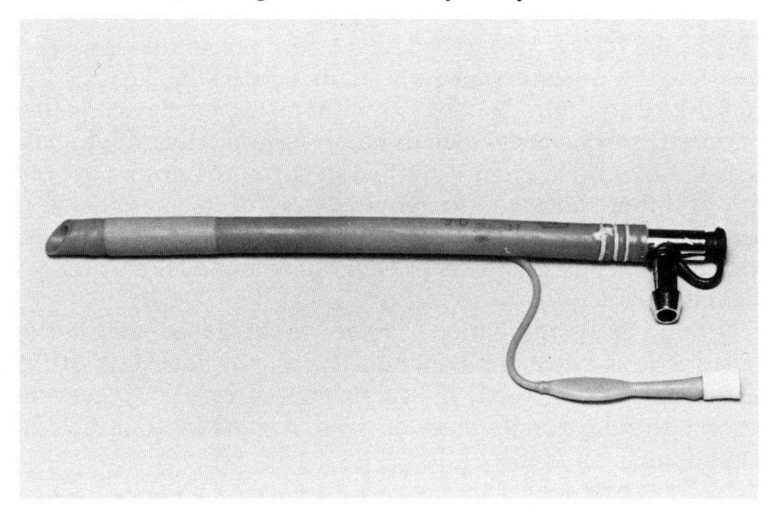

Fig. 21.4 Latex armoured cuffed endotracheal tube

Latex armoured endotracheal tube

The earlier tubes of this type (Fig. 21.4) were also called 'flexo-metallic', being made by repeatedly dipping a wire spiral in latex rubber. The spiral is now usually made of nylon; the reinforced part is virtually unkinkable but, as they are relatively expensive and difficult to insert without an introducer, they tend to be reserved for procedures where kinking of an endotracheal tube is more likely (e.g. neurosurgical anaesthesia). It is most important that the endotracheal connector be pushed right in as far as the beginning of the nylon spiral, and preferably tied in that position with thread. Otherwise, any part of the latex tube left unsupported between the connector and nylon spiral is liable to kinking.

TECHNIQUES OF ENDOTRACHEAL INTUBATION

Endotracheal intubation can be carried out by three methods: under deep general anaesthesia; with the help of a muscle relaxant; or under local analgesia.

Intubation under Deep General Anaesthesia

This is the 'classical' method of performing intubation. Very deep levels of anaesthesia have to be induced so that larynoscopy and intubation may be effected without the patient coughing. Formerly, single agents such as chloroform or ether might have been used, or these agent vaporised in nitrous oxide and oxygen. It was often quicker and required less deep anaesthesia to perform nasotracheal intubation blind without a laryngoscope, with the patient's spontaneous respiration stimulated by carbon dioxide.

Endotracheal intubation under spontaneous respiration anaesthesia is much less commonly practised nowadays except occasionally in children, in whom nitrous oxide, oxygen and halothane quite rapidly produce good, if short-lived, intubating conditions.

Intubation under Muscle Relaxant Anaesthesia

Neuromuscular blocking agents have transformed the ease with which excellent intubating conditions can be provided. The agent providing the best conditions is suxamethonium which, if given in adequate doses, produces profound relaxation within a few seconds. The main disadvantage of this muscle relaxant is its propensity for producing a high incidence of muscle pains in those patients ambulant soon after surgery.

The non-depolarising muscle relaxants can produce almost as good conditions, but take 2–5 minutes to do so. They have the advantage of not causing muscle pains.

Intubation under Local Analgesia

This method is much less commonly employed, being both time-consuming and less pleasant for the patient. Various techniques are possible, e.g. the administration of a local analgesic lozenge to the patient followed by spraying of the upper part of the larynx with local analgesic from a spray placed in the pharynx. The larynx below the vocal cords can be made analgesic by passing the spray through the cords from above or by injection of local analgesic solution by a needle passed through the crico-thyroid membrane. It is important to keep the total dose of local analgesic solution below the toxic level.

COMPLICATIONS OF ENDOTRACHEAL INTUBATION

It is clear from the list of indications given earlier in the chapter that in some circumstances endotracheal anaesthesia is considered mandatory. There are other circumstances where the indications are more equivocal and certainly some anaesthetists sometimes intubate for convenience rather than necessity. In this context it is important to remember that the passage of an endotracheal tube does not guarantee trouble-free anaesthesia. There is a formidable list of minor and major sequelae and, while serious complications are rare, they can lead to the death of the patient. The following are some of the sequelae of endotracheal anaesthesia.

Complications Arising during Intubation

Potentially, the most serious complication which can arise is that the endotracheal tube is not introduced into the larynx at all, but is passed behind the larynx into the pharynx and oesophagus. It is a good rule for the anaesthetist that 'if in doubt, take it out' and ensure that the patient is adequately oxygenated before the next attempt at intubation.

Trauma arising during laryngoscopy
Damage may occur to lips, teeth, other parts of the mouth, pharynx or larynx. These injuries may cause discomfort, or may be frankly dangerous—for example, in the case of teeth passing into the bronchi, or oedema or haematoma of the larynx causing respiratory obstruction.

Trauma arising during insertion of endotracheal tube
Injury may be caused by the endotracheal tube, or by a protruding introducer (especially a metal one) used to aid its insertion. A nasotracheal tube may perforate the nasopharyngeal mucosa causing a false passage which may ultimately lead to retropharyngeal abscess or mediastinitis. Trauma to the larynx may lead to surgical emphysema of the neck or mediastinum or even to pneumothorax.

Cardiac dysrhythmias
Disturbances of cardiac rhythm at intubation are probably due to afferent impulses travelling up the vagus nerve and producing reflex excitation of the vagus or sympathetic system. Thus a wide variety of dysrhythmias is seen, ranging from sinus bradycardia and atrial or ventricular extrasystoles to asystole or ventricular fibrillation. These disturbances are usually transient but may be serious, especially if associated with other adverse factors such as hypoxia, hypercarbia or hyperkalaemia. Intravenous atropine will block the vagal excitatory effects, but may accentuate the sympathetic effects.

Complications during Endotracheal Anaesthesia

These are usually caused by mechanical faults or failures and include foreign bodies within the lumen of tubes or connectors, kinking tubes, or obstruction caused by cuff defects. An overinflated endotracheal tube cuff may herniate downwards over the end of the tube and cause respiratory obstruction. Bubbling has occurred between the layers of latex rubber in armoured tubes, again causing obstruction. Many of these faults have been almost eliminated by improved manufacturing techniques.

Complications Occurring during Extubation

Cardiac dysrhythmias may again occur at extubation or during tracheal suction. Laryngeal spasm of varying degree is not uncommon at extubation.

Complications Occurring after Extubation

Sore throat is the commonest complication of endotracheal intubation and occurs to some extent in about half the patients intubated. Laryngitis is much less common and pronounced laryngeal oedema is rare, except in children where the use of too large a tube may lead to enough oedema to cause obstruction in these small airways. Even more rarely, a granuloma of the vocal cords may follow endotracheal intubation.

This list should serve as a reminder that although with better training of anaesthetists and more refined manufacturing of equipment the incidence of severe complications of endotracheal anaesthesia is low, the risk of minor complications is appreciable even in the best hands. These factors should always be borne in mind before deciding to perform endotracheal intubation.

DIFFICULT INTUBATION ('DIFFICULT INTUBATION BOX')

Endotracheal intubation can present varying degrees of difficulty usually as a result of congenital or acquired anatomical abnormalities of neck mobility, jaw shape or limitation of mouth opening (trismus), or of dentition. A variety of techniques and gadgets ranging from the simple to the complicated have been described to overcome this problem. Each anaesthetist will have his favourites among these, but it is important that there should be in or near each anaesthetic room a choice of these special items of equipment in a clearly labelled 'Difficult Intubation Box'. The following is by no means a comprehensive list of possible contents, but gives an idea of some useful items: Magill endotracheal intubation forceps (to lift the tube forwards into the larynx); right-handed Macintosh laryngoscope blade (to avoid unilaterally difficult problems, e.g. dentition); straight-bladed laryngoscope; rubber-covered flexible wire introducer (Macintosh-Leatherdale); long gum-elastic endotracheal introducer (Eschmann—long enough to be introduced on its own into the larynx and the endotracheal tube then passed over it); 12 G intravenous cannula and connector to connect cannula to oxygen supply (this is meant for passing through the cricothyroid membrane, i.e. below the vocal cords, so that oxygen can be fed directly into the trachea when ventilation by a face-mask is impossible); tracheostomy tubes; epidural catheter and Tuohy needle (this is also for passing through the cricothyroid membrane, but under local analgesia, the catheter being passed up into the mouth or oropharynx. The catheter is then retrieved through the nose or mouth and an endotracheal tube then threaded over it down into the larynx. When it reaches the cricothyroid membrane the catheter is cut short at the skin over the membrane and the endotracheal tube passed further into the trachea).

22 Principles of Ventilators

Requirements of ventilation. Ventilator types. Gas flow during inspiration. Inspiratory time. Effect of leaks or obstruction in ventilator circuits. Cycling. The ideal ventilator. Ventilator terminology.

'All anaesthetists are bag-squeezers'
'All ventilators are bag-squeezers'
'Therefore all anaesthetists are ventilators.'

When an intubated patient is ventilated by hand with an Ambu-bag there are two main variables in the pattern of ventilation: (1) the rate at which the bag is squeezed and (2) the depth to which it is squeezed, corresponding to the respiratory rate and the tidal volume. It is also possible to produce a fast or a slow inspiration by rapid or slow compression of the bag, so the inspiratory flow rate may be considered to be a third but somewhat minor variable. Expiration, however, is a passive phase in virtually all methods of artificial ventilation, depending only on the elastic recoil of the patient's lungs.

REQUIREMENTS OF VENTILATION

Ventilator Requirements

Ventilators require some source of power, which may be either gas pressure or an electric motor. The gas used may either be compressed air, in which case this is used only to power the ventilator and plays no part in ventilating the patient's aveoli, or oxygen in various concentrations at either high or low pressure. Some ventilators (e.g. the Bird, Oxylog) effectively interrupt the high-pressure oxygen pipeline supply at intervals, thereby inflating the lungs. Low-pressure gas from an anaesthetic machine may be used continuously to fill a reservoir bellows which intermittently empties into an inflation bellows, thereby ventilating the patient as, for example, in the Manley ventilator.

Power for Cycling

There are four essential phases of ventilation: inspiration; inspiration to expiration cycling; expiration; and expiration to inspiration cycling. Each ventilator requires a method of cycling from one phase to the other. This is usually achieved by electromechanical means.

Patient Requirements

Whatever the method of ventilation used, the patient's requirements are simply those of fresh-gas flow—it is only while gas is flowing that the alveoli are expanded and gas is exchanged.

The commonest form of artificial ventilation uses the principle of intermittent positive pressure—that is to say, fresh gas is driven into the lungs under positive pressure, and leaves the lungs passively as a result of the elastic recoil. During normal breathing, inspiration is produced by creating negative intrathoracic pressure due to expansion of the rib cage, which is the opposite of the positive pressure produced during artificial ventilation. This may have serious effects on the cardiovascular system, because the negative pressure created in normal breathing helps to draw blood back into the chest, increasing the venous return and therefore the cardiac output. Intermittent positive pressure, on the other hand, produces the opposite effect and therefore often causes a small but significant fall in cardiac output.

VENTILATOR TYPES

As inspiration is the fundamental phase of any ventilator, it is possible to divide the different types of ventilators into two main groups, depending on how they produce inspiration.

Pressure Generators (East-Radcliffe, Manley)

These rely on compression of a bellows or bag of gas by a weight, usually resting on a hinged bracket above the bag (Fig. 22.1). When the weight is allowed to drop freely the bellows are compressed, the rate of compression depending on the resistance to inflation produced by the patient. As this resistance rises, the weight applied to the bellows must be increased to maintain the same inflation rate, and therefore this type of ventilator is suitable only for patients with relatively normal lungs. Those with stiff lungs (low compliance), or high airways resistance are

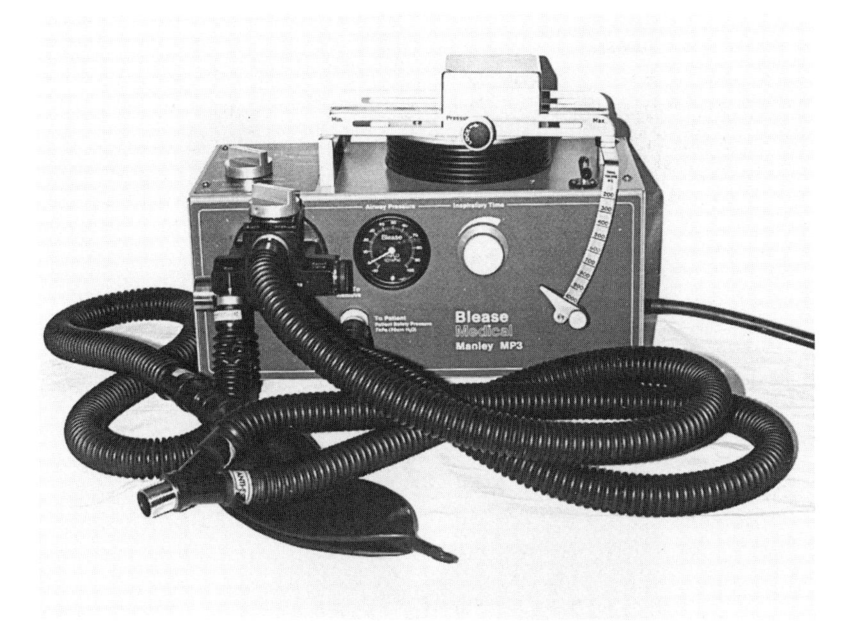

Fig. 22.1 Manley MP3 ventilator

usually unsuitable for a pressure generator, because if the resistance offered to ventilation is too high the bellows will hardly be compressed at all and the tidal volume will be inadequate.

Flow Generators

Many different ventilators can be included in this group, but they possess the same fundamental property, i.e. they are powerful enough to overcome lungs with low compliance or high airways resistance so that gas flow into such patients is maintained constant due to the reserves of power available in the ventilators. Flow generators may be subdivided into two main types.

1. *Those using high gas pressure.* This can be applied either directly or indirectly to the airway.

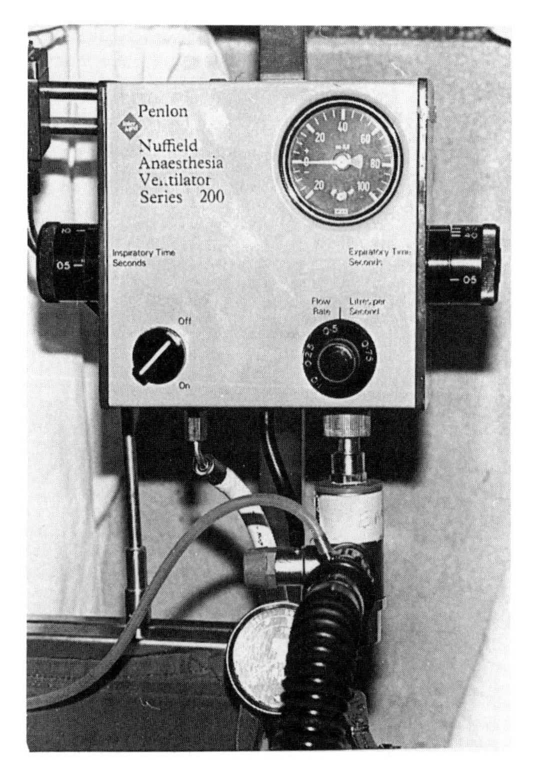

Fig. 22.2 Nuffield 200 ventilator

a. Direct application means that the high pressure gas is actually the fresh gas passing into the lungs, the flow being intermittently interrupted (e.g. Bird, Harlow, Oxylog ventilators).

b. Indirect use of high pressure gas as a driving force. In this case the high pressure gas is used to compress a bellows, which contains the fresh gas. The power of the driving gas, which could be compressed air, is such that the ventilator behaves as a flow generator. In the Penlon Nuffield 200 ventilator (Fig. 22.2), the high pressure driving gas is cycled via a fluid logic switching system and the ventilator is connected to the expiratory limb of a coaxial circuit, e.g. Bain or Lack (Chapter 9). Fresh gas enters the inspiratory limb of the circuit as normal and therefore the gas driving the ventilator never actually reaches the patient, provided the fresh gas flow is adequate.

In the case of the Servo 900 (Fig. 22.3), the ventilator functions at a gas pressure of 414 kpa (60 p.s.i.). The compressed gas expels fresh gas from a bellows, the power of the gas pressure being more than sufficient to overcome any airway resistance.

2. *Those using a powerful motor* to produce constant gas flow. In this situation the ventilator is equipped with a sufficiently powerful motor to produce a constant gas flow irrespective of the resistance offered by the lungs (e.g. Cape and Engström ventilators).

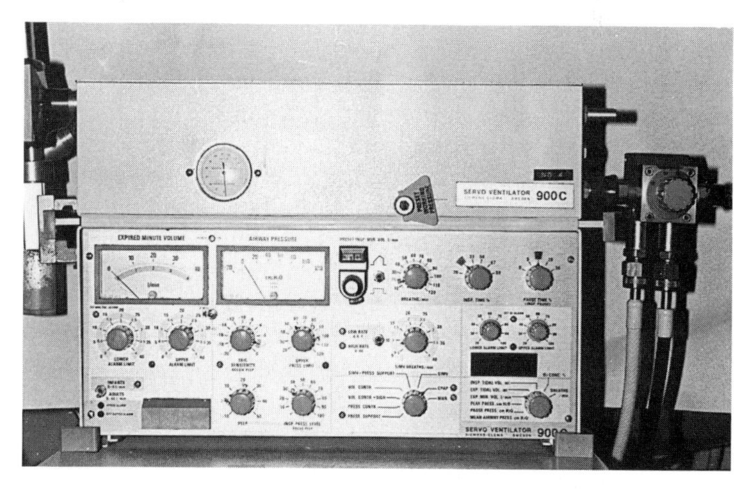

Fig. 22.3 Servo 900C ventilator

GAS FLOW DURING INSPIRATION

In summary, we can subdivide gas flow during inspiration into two types depending upon the ventilator used.

Pressure Generator

Here the flow into the lungs depends upon the compliance of the lung and the airways resistance. As the resistance to inflation produced by these rises, gas flow falls if constant pressure is applied. This type of ventilator is perfectly satisfactory for general use and is inadequate when the maximum possible generated pressure is not able to overcome the resistance offered by the lung.

Flow Generator

Here the flow into the lungs is maintained constant, the inflation pressure produced by the ventilator being more than adequate to overcome any resistance offered by the lung.

Gas flow into the lungs occurs while there is a pressure difference between the airway and the thoracic cavity which equals oesophageal pressure. The variations occurring in gas flow into the lungs in various conditions and types of ventilator are illustrated in Figure 22.4. This confirms that when using a pressure generator, in a patient with low lung compliance, as the ventilator pressure rises rapidly and quickly equals the resistance of the lung, gas flow ceases when the inspiratory phase continues for a fixed length of time. This does not occur with a flow generator. In the case of high airways resistance, gas flow into the lungs is continuously impeded, preventing the intrapulmonary pressure rising to equal the ventilator pressure before the inspiratory phase has finished. In this case therefore the tidal volume falls, although less so for the flow than for the pressure generators.

INSPIRATORY TIME

A short inspiratory time leads to increased physiological dead space. This occurs because the length of inspiration controls the

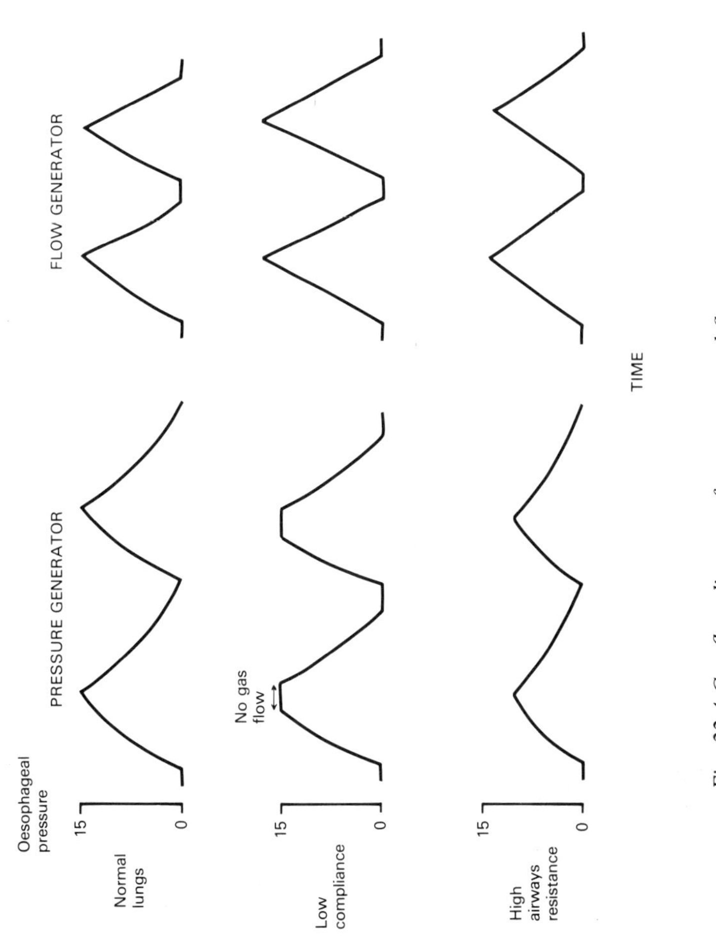

Fig. 22.4 Gas flow diagrams for pressure and flow generators

degree of gas exchange and mixing which occurs in the alveoli. If inadequate time is allowed for this to occur a number of alveoli will not take part in gas exchange and therefore remain as dead space. This is known as physiological dead space in contrast to the anatomical dead space of the conducting airways, which does not vary with ventilation. A long inspiratory time, however, does not improve gas distribution and merely allows the intrathoracic pressure to be elevated for an excessive time, resulting in further impairment of venous return and reduction in cardiac output.

EFFECT OF LEAKS OR OBSTRUCTION IN VENTILATOR CIRCUITS

Pressure Generator

Obstruction
Bellows cease to move as pressure is inadequate.

Leak
Bellows empty quickly and patient is not inflated. Ventilator sounds different.

Flow Generator

Obstruction
Pressure gauge shows increase in airway pressure, tidal volume falls. Pressure 'blow-off' if obstruction is complete.

Leak
No change in ventilator operation, but gauge pressure and tidal volume fall.

CYCLING

Cycling is the term given to the mechanism built into the ventilator which allows the inspiratory phase to change to the expiratory phase and back to inspiration, and may be subdivided into several types depending on the mechanism used.

Time-cycling

This is the commonest method used and essentially means that the change from inspiration to expiration, or the reverse, is produced by a timing mechanism that is not influenced by changes in the patient's lungs. The commonest form of time-cycling is an electromechanical method which occurs, for example, in the Cape, the Engström and the East-Radcliffe ventilators. It works in similar fashion to the time clock in a central heating system with a revolving disc driven by an electric motor which trips a switch to initiate and terminate both inspiration and expiration. A complete revolution of this disc represents one complete respiratory cycle.

Some ventilators also use time-cycling, operated electrically by a solenoid switch (e.g. the Barnet ventilator). This mechanism is far less common.

Pressure-cycling

This method is used both in the Harlow and Bird ventilators, i.e. those ventilators which allow inflation of the patient by intermittent interruption of a high-pressure gas source. In pressure-cycling, inspiration continues until the pressure in the lungs—which rises as more air enters them—reaches a predetermined value at which the ventilator cycles to expiration. When the pressure falls to zero again the ventilator cycles back to a further inspiratory phase.

Volume-cycling

Although some ventilators may appear to deliver a predetermined volume (e.g. the Cape) this in fact is time-cycled in the sense that the ventilator is so powerful that whatever tidal volume is set it will be delivered within a predetermined time. True volume-cycling means that the ventilator will not cycle until the preset tidal volume has been delivered, even if this takes many seconds in cases of high airways resistance. Volume-cycling is therefore relatively uncommon and unsatisfactory.

Flow-cycling

Some ventilators (e.g. the Bennett) are flow-cycled, meaning that they will cycle when no flow exists, either at the end of inspiration or at the end of expiration. Although this method is used on relatively few ventilators at present, it is still very satisfactory in some situations, particularly since no flow in the chest is of no benefit to the patient and merely dams back venous return.

Patient-cycling (Triggering)

Here the ventilator will cycle to the inspiratory phase when the patient generates a negative pressure by voluntary inspiration. When a predetermined pressure has been reached the ventilator will augment the patient's inspiratory effort and inflate him; hence this is a variable control which may be used to encourage patients to wean from a ventilator or when they hypoventilate to any extent. The Bird ventilator is one which includes a patient-triggering system and is often used by physiotherapists to encourage patients to breathe deeply.

THE IDEAL VENTILATOR

It is apparent therefore that the ideal ventilator for normal lungs in most conditions can be described simply as a 'bag-squeezer'. Such ventilators are cheap and easy to operate but are often unsuitable for ventilating patients with lung disease. Such patients with stiff lungs (low compliance) or high airways resistance require a ventilator with adequate reserves of power. This is usually one in which the tidal volume is preset and one which is able to produce a constant gas flow to deliver whatever tidal volume is set within a fixed inspiratory time.

VENTILATOR TERMINOLOGY

Inspiration/Expiration Ratio

On many ventilators this is a preset value, usually of 1:2, so that inspiration is half as long as expiration. This is satisfactory for most patients, although in some with obstructive airways disease expiration may need to be prolonged to allow adequate emptying of the lungs between breaths. In children, and especially neonates, this ratio usually approaches 1:1, but the cardiovascular consequences of this must not be forgotten.

Intermittent Mandatory Ventilation (IMV)

This technique is becoming popular in weaning patients from ventilators. Essentially it means that the patient receives a number of predetermined breaths per minute, usually about six, in between which they are able to breathe for themselves. The patients usually settle down to a rhythm, e.g. two of their own breaths to one ventilator breath and so on. The interval between mandatory breaths may be steadily increased allowing the patient to take over more of the respiratory function for himself. In synchronised IMV (SIMV) the ventilator constantly adjusts its ventilation rate to synchronise with the patient's own respiration.

Minute Mandatory Ventilation (MMV)

In contrast to IMV, this technique depends on the fact that the patient is required to breathe a predetermined volume of gas per minute. If he does this without help from a ventilator, no ventilation occurs. If, however, he is unable to exchange the amount of gas required, the ventilator will supplement his breathing with four to six large breaths a minute to make up the difference in the overall gas exchange.

Positive End-expiratory Pressure (PEEP)

PEEP maintains a continuously raised intrathoracic pressure during the expiratory pause, usually in the region of 5–10 cm water. Normal expiration occurs, brought about by the elastic recoil of the lungs, but instead of the intrathoracic pressure falling to zero it is maintained slightly above this level. This is intended to keep the alveoli expanded and filled with the gas mixture, which is oxygen-enriched. PEEP therefore increases gas transfer across the alveoli and consequently arterial blood oxygenation. It may also be used to prevent fluid leak across the alveolar capillary membrane which occurs in pulmonary oedema. Nevertheless, the haemodynamic effects of PEEP must not be forgotten, because continually raised intrathoracic pressure prevents venous return and may therefore reduce cardiac output.

Minute-volume Divider

This term is used to describe ventilators which operate off the low-pressure gas source from the anaesthetic machine (e.g. Manley). The minute-volume of gases entering the ventilator is preset on the rotameters of the anaesthetic machine. Having adjusted the tidal volume on the ventilator and predetermined the minute-volume, the number of breaths per minute is automatically determined by dividing the minute-volume by the tidal volume. Thus the ventilator acts as a minute-volume divider.

Servo Ventilator

A servo (self-adjusting) system (e.g. Siemens–Elema 900C) is one in which, in the case of a ventilator, an abnormally small breath is compensated for automatically by a corresponding increase in the volume of the next breath. The servo ventilator contains a system for measuring both inspiratory and expiratory gas flow and therefore volume. Predetermined minute- and tidal-volume settings on the machine are continuously monitored automatically. If the expired volume is inadequate the ventilator automatically compensates for this by temporarily increasing the tidal volume, so that the overall preset minute volume is achieved.

Continuous Positive Airway Pressure (CPAP) and Pressure Assist Modes

Although CPAP is available on most intensive care ventilators, e.g. Servo 900 series, its use is only applicable to spontaneous ventilation in an intubated patient. In the expiratory phase, CPAP produces a similar effect to PEEP, but the presence of a constantly elevated airway pressure during inspiration provides a small amount of assistance to supplement the patient's own inspiratory effort.

This is in contrast to the pressure assist mode where the patient's own inspiratory effort is supplemented by a preset inspiratory assistance from the ventilator. Unlike patient triggering, however, the tidal volume is determined by the magnitude of the patient's effort rather than by a predetermined ventilator setting.

23 Monitoring during Anaesthesia

Measurement of cardiac rate and rhythm. Measurement of blood pressure. Measurement of central venous pressure. Measurement of expired gas flow. Measurement of temperature. Measurement of cardiac output. Measurement of oxygen (oximetry). Measurement of carbon dioxide (capnography). Ventilator alarms.

Although it is essential for the anaesthetist to remain in close contact with the patient during induction, maintenance and recovery from anaesthesia, more complex anaesthetic techniques and the relative increase in the number of very ill patients being anaesthetised both require more complex monitoring equipment. If the anaesthetist can remain in physical contact with the patient throughout the anaesthetic, a good assessment is continually available of pulse, blood pressure, peripheral perfusion and general adequacy of anaesthesia. In many cases, however, due to the type of surgery being performed this contact is only partial and additional equipment is necessary.

MEASUREMENT OF CARDIAC RATE AND RHYTHM

ECG monitoring has been discussed in detail in Chapter 19, but it is also important to include this under the general heading of monitoring equipment. The ECG reflects changes in the electrical activity of the heart as impulses are transmitted through the excitable cardiac muscle, which then contracts. Although in routine 12-lead ECG recording different positions of the electrodes allow diagnosis of changing electrical activity in various parts of the heart, ECG monitoring during anaesthesia uses one chest lead (commonly CM5, chest, manubrium, V5) which gives a satisfactory display of all aspects of the cardiac cycle. In this lead three electrodes are used, the right arm (red) over the manubrium sternum, the right leg (yellow) over the left shoulder and the left arm (black) in the 5th intercostal space in the midclavicular line, the setting on the ECG machine being turned to lead 1. It is also possible to obtain a reasonable ECG by laying the patient on an electrode mat.

It is important to emphasise that ECG recording merely reflects electrical activity, and gives no indication of peripheral blood flow. ECG machines are usually coupled to a ratemeter giving an indication of the pulse rate.

Pulse rate is also frequently measured using a pulse meter, an instrument which depends on a light-sensitive photo-electric cell. The sensing device clips either on to the fingertip or earlobe, both of which normally have a good blood supply. This device contains a small light beam which shines through the fingertip or earlobe, changes in light intensity being sensed by the photo-electric cell. As blood flows into the fingertip, the light intensity will be reduced in a pulsatile manner. This change in intensity can then be assessed simply in terms of heart rate or can be displayed on an oscilloscope as a waveform reflecting blood flow. Measurement of peripheral flow, however, is severely reduced in vasoconstriction and this method is reliable only when blood pressure and flow are reasonably normal.

MEASUREMENT OF BLOOD PRESSURE

Accurate blood pressure measurement is an essential part of anaesthetic monitoring. Although palpation of the radial pulse gives an indication of satisfactory blood pressure, it is not possible to measure changes. Systemic blood pressure measurement involves either indirect intermittent recording or direct continuous measurement using an intra-arterial cannula.

Indirect Arterial Monitoring

The cuff method of measuring arterial blood pressure has been adapted in several forms for use during anaesthesia, particularly when access to the brachial pulse is impossible. In its simplest form, a single blood pressure cuff and stethoscope taped over the brachial artery allow auscultation of the Korotkov sounds corresponding to systolic and diastolic blood pressure in the conventional way. It is also possible to obtain an estimation of systolic blood pressure by using a pulse meter on the fingertip and a single cuff, systolic pressure being indicated when the pulse meter output ceases after inflation of the cuff, or reappears on deflating the cuff.

Indirect monitoring using the cuff principle has been adapted in two separate ways for anaesthetic use.

Oscillotonometer

This device (Figs. 23.1 and 23.2) consists of two inflatable cuffs enclosed in a single outer cuff which is placed around the upper arm. The upper of the two cuffs, or occluding cuff, corresponds to a normal blood pressure cuff, and the lower one, which is narrower than the upper, is the sensing cuff corresponding to a palpating finger or stethoscope. The instrument is first zeroed using knob 'A' and then, with valves 'B' and 'C' both closed, the cuffs are inflated to above the systolic pressure with lever 'D' in the closed position. Valve 'B' is then released slightly and lever 'D' is moved to the open position. This allows air to leak from the occluding cuff while the sensing cuff is maintained at the original pressure. When systolic blood pressure is reached blood will flow under the occluding cuff and produce pulsations in the sensing cuff which are transmitted to the needle on the dial. At this point level 'D' is returned to the closed position, equilibrating the pressure throughout the whole system and measuring the systolic blood pressure. This is the pressure achieved when the needle begins to flick. Movement of lever 'D' back into the open position allows further air to leak out of the occluding cuff and the needle oscillations gradually lessen and finally disappear. Release of lever 'D' then measures the diastolic blood pressure. This method is widely used and although somewhat inaccurate at the extremes of blood pressure is reliable at systolic blood pressures of about 60–160 mmHg.

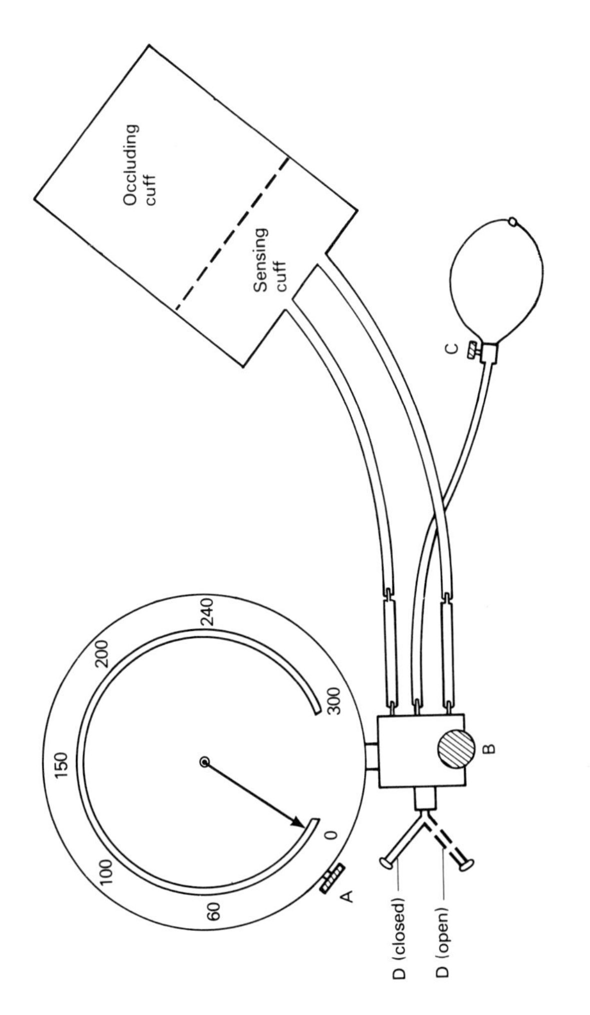

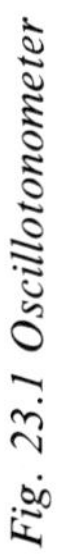
Fig. 23.1 Oscillotonometer

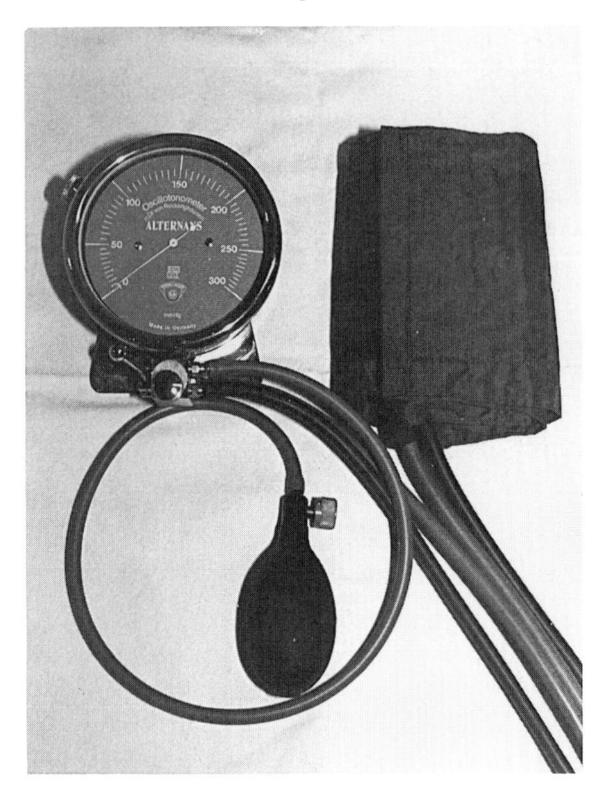

Fig. 23.2 von Recklinghausen's oscillotonometer

Other indirect cuff methods
Most other methods are semi-automatic or automatic adaptations of the oscillotonometer involving different methods of recording arterial pulsation from the sensing cuff. The Arteriosonde uses a small transducer (see below) instead of a sensing cuff which has to be placed over the brachial artery, while the Dinamap (Fig. 23.3) uses a sensing cuff whose changing pressure is then transmitted via a transducer. All these methods have similar limitations to the oscillotonometer.

Direct Intravascular Pressure Monitoring

Intravascular pressure, whether venous, systemic arterial or pulmonary, can be measured with the same system provided that

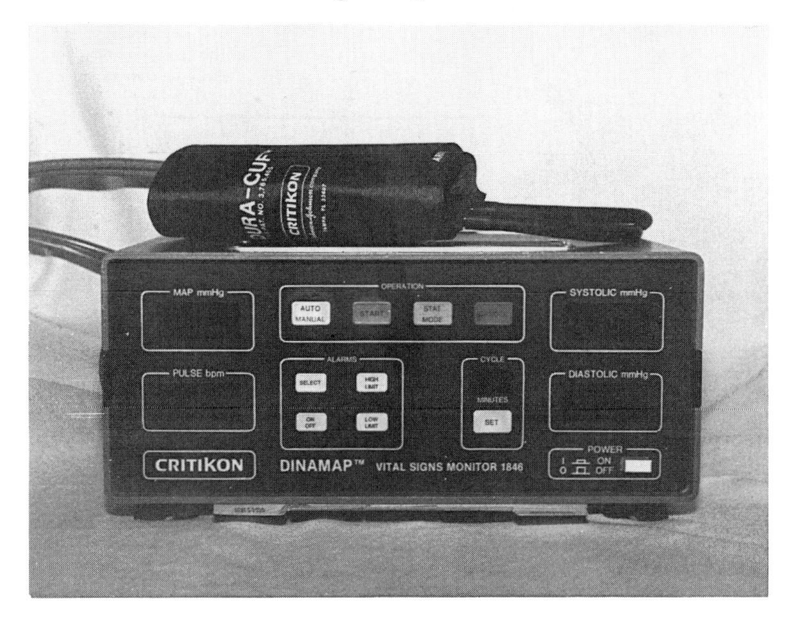

Fig. 23.3 Dinamap automatic blood pressure monitor

the instruments used are adjusted to respond to a suitable pressure range. Arterial pressure monitoring involves placing a cannula in a suitable artery, usually radial or brachial, and the transmission of the arterial pulse via a length of non-distensible manometer tubing to a method of pressure display. In its simplest form the pressure line may be connected to a pressure gauge or mercury manometer, provided that there is an air gap in the tube between the saline and the mercury. Although simple this method is not suitable for demonstrating pulsatile arterial flow, but merely gives a damped recording, providing an accurate measurement of mean arterial blood pressure.

Connecting the pressure tubing to a transducer and then to an oscilloscope will provide dynamic measurement of blood pressure. A transducer is simply a device that changes energy from one form into another, in this case, changing pulsatile movement of a column of fluid into electrical energy (Fig. 23.4).

Changes of pressure within the column of fluid cause movement of the diaphragm in the transducer and set up an electrical current which can then be transmitted and displayed on the oscilloscope. Inevitably, arterial blood pressure monitoring is

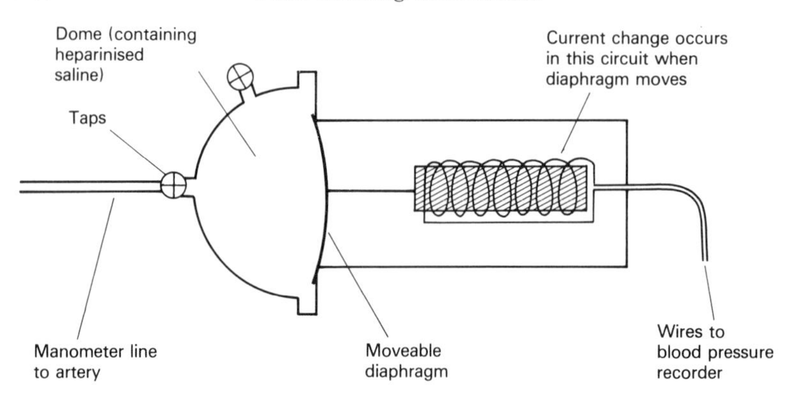

Fig. 23.4 Transducer

more accurate, particularly at the extremes of blood pressure, than any indirect form. Provided that the technique is used only when indicated, and arterial lines are only left in place for as long as they are needed and then removed, the morbidity is extremely low. Dangers, however, result from prolonged arterial cannulation, particularly in patients with peripheral vasoconstriction and also the inadvertent intra-arterial injection of certain drugs, particularly thiopentone.

MEASUREMENT OF CENTRAL VENOUS PRESSURE

The techniques of central venous cannulation have already been discussed in Chapter 20. As in direct arterial monitoring, central venous pressure can be displayed on a transducer and oscilloscope. However, the relatively lower pressures found in the venous system also permit the use of a fluid column to show venous pressure. Provided that the central venous cannula is in the chest (preferably in the right atrium), by connecting it to a column of fluid and zeroing the column at the level of the heart, the height of the fluid above zero will equal the pressure in the right atrium. Again, this method cannot respond to beat-by-beat change in pressure but gives an accurate measurement of mean central venous pressure. Balloon catheters (Swan-Ganz) are sometimes floated into the right atrium and then to the right ventricle and pulmonary artery to give a measurement of pulmonary artery blood pressure. As this is higher than central venous pressure it is necessary to use a transducer and oscilloscope to display the pressure, usually in the region of 25 mmHg systolic.

MEASUREMENT OF EXPIRED GAS FLOW

The Wright respirometer (Fig. 23.5) is commonly attached to a ventilator to provide a measurement of expired gas volume and therefore the adequacy of ventilation. This mechanical device measures gas volume as it passes over vanes within the respirometer, which rotate in the gas stream at a rate proportional to flow. It is inaccurate at low and high flows, though up-to-date versions are considerably better. The respirometer should not be left in circuit the whole time as continuous rotation of the vanes by humidified air causes them to stick and become inaccurate. An electronic version of Wright's respirometer is now available.

MEASUREMENT OF TEMPERATURE

Temperature monitoring is becoming increasingly useful, particularly during prolonged anaesthesia. Different temperature-

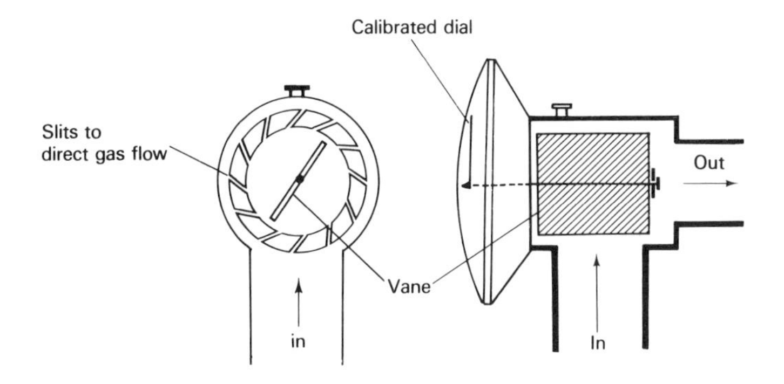

Fig. 23.5 Wright respirometer

sensing devices are available for use in various sites such as the skin, oesophagus, rectum and eardrum. They are all either thermistors or thermocouples, producing changes in electrical activity in response to temperature variation. The temperature can then be displayed on a gauge or by digital readout. It is useful to measure simultaneously both central temperature (usually either rectal or oesophageal) and skin temperature. Skin temperature reflects peripheral perfusion and the difference between central and peripheral temperatures indicates the degree of vasoconstriction or vasodilation, which may be important in assessing the adequacy of fluid replacement and metabolic state of the patient.

MEASUREMENT OF CARDIAC OUTPUT

Although cardiac output measurement is not used routinely except during cardiopulmonary bypass, its use in severely ill patients is increasing. Measurement involves the injection of a known quantity of either green dye or ice-cold saline into the right atrium and measuring either the dilution of the dye or the change in temperature of the blood in response to the cold saline injection after passing through the heart. The cardiac output is obtained by measuring the degree of dilution of the dye and then calculating the volume of blood into which a fixed quantity of dye must have diffused to obtain this dilution. Similar calculations apply to the use of ice-cold saline, the temperature change being sensed by a thermistor at the tip of a specially adapted Swan-Ganz catheter and the result passed to a dedicated cardiac output computer.

MEASUREMENT OF OXYGEN (OXIMETRY)

Within the Anaesthetic Circuit

Several devices are available for measuring the oxygen percentage in a gas mixture within the anaesthetic circuit. Those

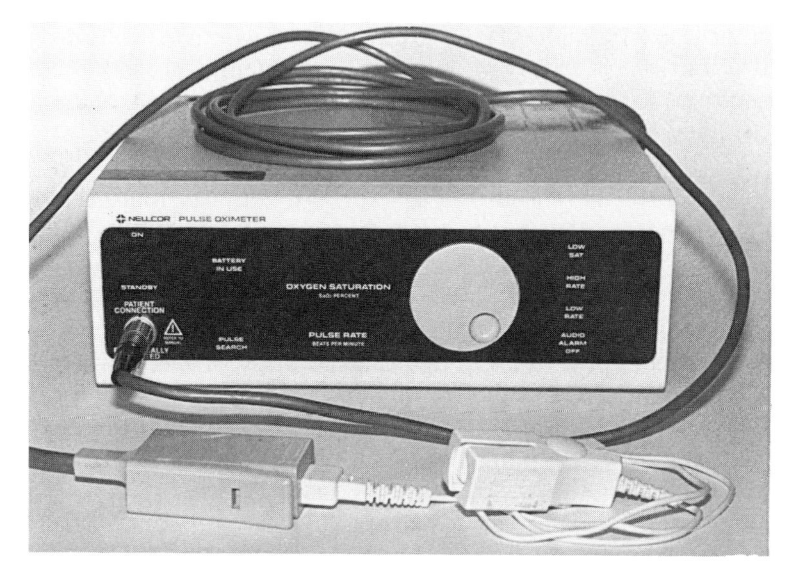

Fig. 23.6 Nellcor pulse oximeter

in clinical use utilise a fuel cell the electrical output of which is dependent upon the concentration of oxygen to which it is exposed. They also contain high and low alarms to increase their usefulness and are frequently now incorporated into standard anaesthetic machines. *They do however only measure the oxygen within the circuit and not within the patient.*

Within Blood

Although blood gas measurement is the definitive method by which oxygen concentration is estimated, it is invasive and only provides intermittent results (Chapter 2). Indwelling arterial oxygen electrodes are being developed to provide continuous estimation, but are not yet routinely available. Continuous non-invasive measurement of oxygen saturation, using devices such as the Nellcor pulse oximeter (Fig. 23.6) are becoming increasingly employed. Unlike the fuel cell within the anaesthetic circuit, the measurement made is of the *patient's* oxygenation. The method used is an adaptation of the finger plethysmograph trace, which depends upon shining a light through the finger and detecting the change in transmitted light related to the density of pulsatile arterial blood. They are accurate down to saturations of 70% but since they can make measurements on very small quantities of blood, should not be relied upon as an index of adequacy of blood flow.

MEASUREMENT OF CARBON DIOXIDE (CAPNOGRAPHY)

Measurement of the percentage concentration of carbon dioxide in expired air at the end of normal expiration is equivalent to the alveolar and therefore arterial CO_2 concentration. End-tidal CO_2 analysers depend upon the absorption of infra-red light by carbon dioxide, the higher the absorption, the less light is transmitted. They provide accurate, non-invasive, breath-by-breath measurement and as such monitor the adequacy of ventilation. *They do not measure oxygenation at the same time.*

VENTILATOR ALARMS

Ventilator alarms have now become routinely incorporated into most ventilator circuits on anaesthetic machines, if not into the

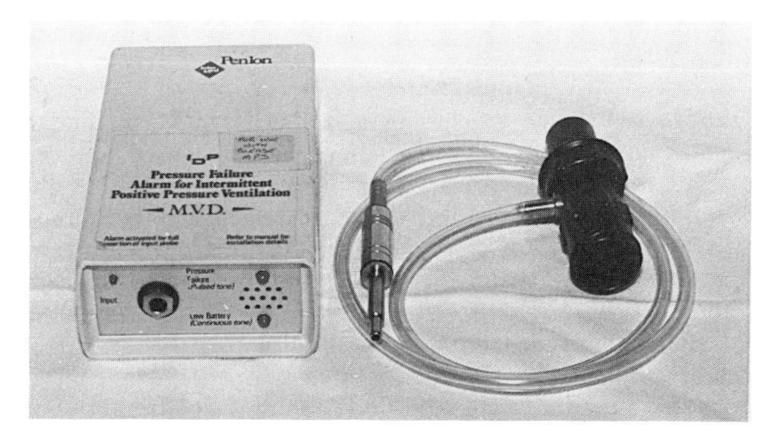

Fig. 23.7 Penlon IDP ventilator alarm

ventilators themselves (e.g. Servo 900, Chapter 22). Those used in theatre such as the Penlon IDP Alarm (Fig. 23.7) are pressure sensitive and contain both high (60 cm water) and low (12 cm water) settings. There is also a time delay in the region of 12 seconds built in to allow for the use of very slow respiratory rates. They are usually activated simply by being plugged in and can be tested by pressurising the anaesthetic circuit.

24 Complications of Anaesthesia: The Recovery Room

Respiratory system. Cardiovascular system. Awareness. Peripheral nerve injuries. Ophthalmic complications. Skin complications. Hypothermia. Hypersensitivity to anaesthetic drugs. Recovery from anaesthesia.

The possible complications of anaesthesia are legion, varying from minor and commonplace to serious and bizarre. The possible causes fall into various groups—e.g. anaesthetic equipment like laryngoscopes, endotracheal tubes, cannulae and needles inevitably produce a variety of complications. Another group is associated with the use of various anaesthetic agents, e.g. muscle relaxants. Some complications are more closely associated with the surgery than with the anaesthesia, although it is not unusual for the anaesthesia to be blamed: this group includes postoperative respiratory complications and venous thrombotic and embolic phenomena. Lastly, a group of complications—important because most of them are avoidable—arise simply because the patient is rendered unconscious. This is because anaesthesia causes the patient to lose various protective reflexes and it behoves the anaesthetist to look after these functions for him. These protective reflexes are found in various systems, e.g. the respiratory system, the eyes and the peripheral nervous system. From the extensive choice, this chapter selects some of the commoner and some of the more avoidable complications and sequelae.

RESPIRATORY SYSTEM

Obstruction

This is probably the commonest respiratory complication and may occur at any level of the respiratory tract and for many different reasons.

With the mouth closed, breathing occurs through the nose. If for some reason the nasal airway is obstructed breathing can occur only if the lips are separated. Thus there tends to be some degree of respiratory obstruction unless an oropharyngeal airway is used. It should be noted that in edentulous people the unsupported lips are much more mobile and the upper lip can be pulled right over the external nares when attempts are made to improve the airway by pulling the jaw forward. As the lips are also together, breathing is then completely obstructed.

Obstruction at pharyngeal level is most commonly due to the tongue falling back against the posterior wall of the pharynx. This occurs because the tongue is largely composed of muscle fibres, some of which arise from the mandible. The latter falls backwards as the unconscious patient relaxes, and the tongue goes with it. Extension of the head (and with it the mandible) frequently restores the airway, but there are times when this can be done only by pressing the thumbs or fingers directly behind the angle of the mandible and lifting it forwards.

Obstruction from the level of the larynx downwards is usually due to complications associated with endotracheal tubes, laryngeal or bronchospasm or to soiling of the respiratory tract with blood, vomit or secretions. Endotracheal tubes may be kinked or compressed at any level, including the nose and naso-pharynx. Occlusion of the distal end of the tube may occur if the bevel is pressed against the tracheal wall or if an overinflated cuff herniates over the end of the tube. Various problems associated with the faulty manufacture of endotracheal tubes and their cuffs have been reported in the past, but happily these are much less common with modern manufacturing standards.

Laryngeal spasm and bronchospasm may be precipitated by many factors, and are much more common in patients with irritable respiratory tract (e.g. heavy smokers, bronchitics and asthmatics). Common stimuli include the sudden inspiration of too high a concentration of almost any volatile anaesthetic, or reflex spasm occurring in response to a surgical stimulus at too light a plane of anaesthesia. The spasm usually resolves when the stimulus is removed. In recalcitrant cases laryngeal spasm (which is impossible, of course, if an endotracheal tube is in situ) will respond to a muscle relaxant because the laryngeal muscles responsible for this spasm are striated muscle. Bronchospasm may be slower to subside and may require bronchodilators.

Pre-existing Respiratory Disease and Anaesthesia

Pre-existing respiratory disease causes concern less often under general anaesthesia than might be expected. While laryngeal spasm or bronchospasm may be worrying, few intubated patients have much trouble during anaesthesia. This is not surprising because the ultimate treatment for respiratory failure nowadays is endotracheal intubation and ventilation.

The dangerous time for a patient with respiratory disease is in the postoperative period. The pain of the surgical incision, especially if it is an upper abdominal one, tends to make breathing shallow and coughing inefficient. Sputum retention tends to occur and atelectasis follows as the air is absorbed from the lung distal to the blocked bronchi. In the earlier days of anaesthesia these problems were accentuated by the prolonged drowsiness which followed deep levels of anaesthesia. With modern anaesthetic techniques these complications must be regarded as associated with the surgery rather than with the anaesthetic.

Hypoxia

Varying degrees of hypoxia may occur in association with many complications of anaesthesia. Even in normal circumstances, however, there is a tendency for hypoxia to occur during anaesthesia, and this may continue into the postoperative period. Most severe after abdominal operations, it nevertheless occurs to some extent after quite simple procedures and is believed to be caused by underventilation of the dependent parts of the lung.

A much shorter period of hypoxia occurs after any nitrous

oxide-based anaesthetic and is called 'diffusion hypoxia'. After the nitrous oxide has been turned off, large quantities of it leave the body through the alveoli. This nitrous oxide prevents the inspired oxygen in the air reaching the alveoli in its usually proportions and hypoxia ensues. This probably lasts less than ten minutes and is of no great significance in a healthy patient, but may add to the problems of the ill or debilitated patient who should always be given added oxygen during this period.

CARDIOVASCULAR SYSTEM

The commonest cardiovascular complications of anaesthesia are dysrhythmias and hypotension. A great variety of abnormal rhythms can occur under anaesthesia and some of these are described in more detail in Chapter 15. Not all dysrhythmias are serious, and the anaesthetist's main concern is whether they are or are likely to become life-endangering. Hypotension is never far away under general anaesthesia, as most anaesthetic agents tend to produce some degree of depression of the heart and peripheral vasomotor tone either directly or by their depressant action on the brain. With a fit patient under light anaesthesia, compensation is usually complete with a normal blood pressure. However, at deeper levels of anaesthesia or in older or debilitated patients some degree of fall in blood pressure is common.

Predisposing Factors

Various factors make dysrhythmias or hypertension more likely to occur under anaesthesia. These factors summate, and as some of them are avoidable it is important that by careful choice and execution of anaesthetic technique the anaesthetist reduces to a minimum the likelihood of these complications.

Pre-existing cardiovascular disease
The patient with cardiovascular disease is susceptible to complications during anaesthesia. The disease may be discovered at the pre-operative visit, but this is not always so. It is wise in this

context to regard no elderly patient as having a completely healthy cardiovascular system.

Anaesthetic agents
Some volatile anaesthetic agents, especially halothane, trichloroethylene and cyclopropane, have the propensity for producing dysrhythmias, some of them potentially serious. Halothane and enflurane are particularly likely to produce hypotension.

Increased catecholamine levels
Serious ventricular dysrhythmias are likely to occur in the presence of high circulating levels of catecholamines. These catecholamines, of which adrenaline is the most likely to produce dysrhythmias, may be exogenous (i.e. injected) or endogenous (i.e. produced within the body).

Hypoxia and hypercarbia
Both these factors tend to increase the incidence of dysrhythmias. They are usually due to faults in anaesthetic technique.

Direct or reflex stimulation
Direct stimulation of the heart at cardiac surgery or during operations nearby may produce abnormalities of cardiac rhythm. More commonly, dysrhythmias occur reflexly in response to stimulation of other areas of the body (e.g. the pharynx, the larynx, intra-abdominal mesenteries or traction on the extra-ocular eye muscles).

An example of several of these factors summating might be the administration of an adrenaline-containing solution to a patient spontaneously breathing a high concentration of halothane. (This technique is nearly always associated with some degree of hypercarbia.) The exogenously administered adrenaline, the halothane and the hypercarbia would combine to produce ideal conditions for generating serious ventricular dysrhythmia.

Air Embolism

Air may occasionally gain entry to the arterial side of the cardiovascular system at open-heart surgery. More frequently it enters the venous side, the commonest situation being when a vein is opened in an area where the venous pressure is low. This most commonly occurs at neurosurgical operations or other operations on the head and neck when the operation site is above the level of the heart. It can occur at other times, e.g. accidentally, at intravenous infusion. The air passes to the right ventricle where it is churned into froth. If of sufficient degree this may obstruct the pulmonary circulation. The air may also pass through the lungs or patent intracardiac defects and cause embolisation of the coronary or cerebral circulations.

Deep Vein Thrombosis and Pulmonary Embolism

Pulmonary emboli arise as fragments of thrombus occurring usually in the veins of the legs or pelvis. Neither usually occurs during the anaesthetic, but 3–14 days afterwards. Hence these complications are the province of the whole surgical team rather than the anaesthetist. Although the exact 'trigger' to the formation of venous thrombi is unknown, some of the factors associated with a high incidence are known and a certain amount of prophylaxis is possible. The incidence is highest in the middle-aged and elderly, with prolonged bed rest, after major and prolonged surgery especially of the lower abdomen, pelvis and hip-joint, and in patients with known coronary artery disease. In patients at risk it may be possible to improve venous return by raising the foot of the operating table or bed postoperatively, and pressure on the calves may be prevented by raising them off the surface of the operating table by sponge rubber supports under the heels. Venous pooling may be prevented by elastic stockings.

More active prevention includes subcutaneous heparin 5000 units 8-hourly for about five days starting two hours preoperatively, or 500 ml intravenous dextran-70 daily until the patient is mobile.

Although complications associated with anaesthesia may occur in many of the systems of the body, the ones discussed below belong to the group arising due to the loss of the patient's protective reflexes under anaesthesia.

AWARENESS

The effectiveness of the neuromuscular blocking agents has led to a new problem of general anaesthesia, unknown in the old 'single-agent anaesthesia' days: the problem of 'awareness' under anaesthesia. A patient under muscle relaxant anaesthesia may, if the anaesthesia is too light, be returning to consciousness but, on account of his paralysed muscles, be unable to communicate with the anaesthetist. The sense of hearing is usually the last to go on induction of anaesthesia and the first to return as anaesthesia lightens. Many of the reported cases of awareness are of conversations heard during the anaesthetic. Although pain is seldom complained of (probably a tribute to the efficacy of nitrous oxide as an analgesic) these incidents can be distressing to the patient and every anaesthetist must do his utmost to avoid them. It is now known that if only nitrous oxide and oxygen are used to maintain anaesthesia, even heavy premedication does not eliminate the possibility of awareness and, except in the case of very ill patients, an intravenous or inhalational adjuvant should be added to the anaesthetic. Even then, awareness is possible, especially with intravenous adjuvants—which are usually given as periodic increments rather than as a continuous infusion, so it is still possible for anaesthesia to become dangerously light as the time for the next increment approaches.

PERIPHERAL NERVE INJURIES

Injuries to peripheral nerves may arise as a result of compression against bony points or by tourniquets, from stretching of nerve trunks or plexuses in abnormal positions, by injection of irritant solutions (e.g. thiopentone) around nerves, or due to hypotension causing ischaemia. Examples of nerves susceptible to pressure injuries include the radial nerve as it winds around the shaft of the humerus, the ulnar nerve as it runs behind the medial epicondyle of the humerus, and the lateral popliteal nerve as it runs across the neck of the fibula. Traction injury probably occurs most commonly to the brachial plexus. The nerve most likely to be damaged by thiopentone injection is the median nerve in the antecubital fossa.

OPHTHALMIC COMPLICATIONS

The part of the eye most commonly damaged under anaesthesia is the cornea, which may ulcerate if it dries out as a result of the eye staying open during the anaesthetic, or it may become abraded by irritant vapours or antiseptic solutions. Central retinal artery thrombosis is a rare complication of anaesthesia and probably occurs only where there is hypotension in a patient already suffering from vascular disease.

Postoperative pain around the supra-orbital nerve has been reported and is probably due to prolonged pressure by a catheter mount over this nerve.

SKIN COMPLICATIONS

Ulceration of the skin over bony prominences (typically the sacrum) is always a danger in old or debilitated patients. This is more a problem of intensive care units, but is worth bearing in mind in such patients in the operating theatre, especially if surgery is prolonged.

HYPOTHERMIA

Significant falls of body temperature under anaesthesia are most likely to occur at the extremes of age, being particularly important in the neonate. The rate of fall of temperature is related to the temperature of the operating theatre. In normal adult patients heat loss is unlikely to be serious provided that the theatre temperature is kept above 21°C. Other causes of pronounced heat loss are the administration of large volumes of refrigerated fluids, especially blood, and irrigation of hollow viscera by fluids at below body temperature, e.g. the bladder during transurethral prostatectomy.

Postoperatively hypothermia may cause shivering with a distinct increase of metabolic rate and therefore of oxygen requirement. The patient feels uncomfortable and vasoconstricts.

The shivering commonly occurring after halothane anaesthesia does not seem to be associated with significant falls of temperature and is part of a generalised muscular spasticity. The masseteric spasm—frequently part of this syndrome—may be so fierce that if an oral airway is in place at this time the incisor teeth may be loosened.

HYPERSENSITIVITY TO ANAESTHETIC DRUGS

This became increasingly important with the extensive use of the intravenous induction agent Althesin, which has since been withdrawn. It was a relatively frequent problem (1 in 400 administrations), particularly when the drug was given repeatedly over a short space of time. All drugs given intravenously have the potential to cause adverse reactions either non-specifically, related to the pH of the drug, preservatives or histamine release, or specifically as part of an immune-mediated response. The intravenous route bypasses all the normal protective mechanisms of the body such as skin, mucous membranes, gut, etc., making the occurrence of severe reactions relatively common and unpredictable.

Of the intravenous induction agents currently available, neither etomidate, propofol (Diprivan) nor ketamine have been specifically associated with hypersensitivity reactions. The incidence of reactions to thiopentone is approximately 1 in 20 000 and to methohexitone 1 in 7000, although when these do occur, they are often severe, associated with bronchospasm and cardiovascular collapse. Neuromuscular blocking drugs such as d-tubocurarine, alcuronium and atracurium are frequently associated with non-specific histamine release, producing flushing, tachycardia, hypotension and sometimes bronchospasm.

The initial treatment of hypersensitivity reactions should include intravenous fluids to correct the relative hypovolaemia and intravenous antihistamines, e.g. chlorpheniramine (Piriton), and subcutaneous adrenaline to antagonise the effects of excessive histamine release and anaphylactic shock.

RECOVERY FROM ANAESTHESIA

The Recovery Room

The period of recovery from anaesthesia is undoubtedly one of the most dangerous times during a surgical patient's stay in hospital. Many factors contribute to this danger. The patient has to regain his protective reflexes, especially those protecting his respiratory tract. As anaesthesia lightens vomiting is likely and, with regurgitation an ever-present danger, it is a wise rule to turn all patients onto their sides as they recover from anaesthesia, or before extubation if an endotracheal tube has been used. Only rarely does the surgery make this impossible, e.g. when traction has been set up by means of a Steinmann pin through the tibia. Other adverse factors include possible hypoxia or hypercarbia as the patient tends to breath-hold in light planes of anaesthesia, or breathe inadequately as spontaneous respiration returns after muscle-relaxant anaesthesia. Extubation and pharyngeal suction may provoke serious dysrhythmias, especially if any of the above factors are present. Cardiac arrest may occur, but surrounded by trained medical and nursing staff and with resuscitation equipment to hand, there is a good chance of success if resuscitative measures are instituted promptly.

Until recently the standard of patient care after leaving the operating theatre fell dramatically. The patient was often transported semi-conscious and with inadequate nursing supervision straight back to the ward. There was an appreciable incidence of morbidity and even mortality on the journey from operating theatre to ward, and even care of the recovering patient in the ward was sometimes inadequate. Some sort of recovery room is included in all new theatre suite design, and many old theatre suites have been modified to include them. These units aim at providing an area where the patient may recover consciousness under the supervision of trained nurses with all the necessary resuscitation equipment and with the anaesthetist nearby. The pulse rate, blood pressure, respiration and temperature should be measured and charted and the recovery room personnel should also be expert at supervising other postoperative aspects of surgery, e.g. managing continuous bladder irrigation after prostatectomy.

While all recovery rooms should keep patients until they have regained their protective reflexes and achieved cardiovascular stability, whether the patient stays longer depends on the size and staffing of the recovery room. Most recovery rooms look after patients for only an hour or two at the most, but there is no doubt that longer-stay recovery wards have their advantages. One of these is safe and efficient postoperative pain relief by nerve-blocking techniques. The argument that recovery areas deprive nurses of experience of postoperative patient care is no longer acceptable; student nurses can be rotated through recovery wards where in a short time they will gain much better experience than they would obtain in months in a general surgical ward. The widespread introduction of recovery rooms in recent years has undoubtedly done much to increase safety for surgical patients.

25 Cardiac Arrest

Establishing the airway. External cardiac massage. Drug therapy. Defibrillation. Drug treatment of asystole. 'Crash box' contents. Defibrillators. Resuscitation of newborn.

Although cardiac arrest teams are routine in most hospitals, few doctors or nurses are regularly concerned with emergency resuscitation. It is vital, therefore, that the basic cardiac arrest procedure be uncomplicated, easily understood and memorised. Complicated drug regimens are sometimes necessary to achieve adequate resuscitation, but the fundamental procedures are more basic and may be divided into the A-B-C-D principle: A—Airway; B—Breathing; C—Cardiac massage; and D—Drug therapy.

ESTABLISHING THE AIRWAY

Cardiopulmonary resuscitation is doomed to failure in the face of inadequate oxygenation; and in many cases, maintaining a clear and adequate airway to allow oxygenation is all that the patient requires. Anaesthetists are often called to a cardiac arrest when the patient is simply suffering from respiratory obstruction, which inevitably leads to hypoxia and cardiac dysrhythmias. Forcibly lifting the jaw forwards will pull the tongue away from the posterior pharyngeal wall, since the tongue is attached to the inside of the mandible. This is best achieved by placing one's fingers behind the angle of the jaw just below the lobe of the ear and pushing strongly anteriorly. In response to this, many patients take a large breath and spontaneous ventilation begins. It may be necessary to use an oropharyngeal airway (size 3 for men and 2 for women) to maintain the position of the tongue. If the airway is filled with vomit or regurgitated fluid from the stomach it is important to suck this out as soon as possible. Small suction catheters, however, are not designed to remove solid matter and, if no Yankauer sucker is available, manual removal of obstructing material may be life-saving. Oxygen should be given to the patient as soon as possible through a face mask if he is breathing spontaneously, and with an Ambu-bag and mask if respiration has ceased. In most cases the resistance of the Ambu-bag and valve is too great to allow the patient to breathe spontaneously through this system for any length of time. Remember to ensure that the neck of the Ambu-bag (colour-coded blue) is connected to the inlet of the Ambu-valve (also colour-coded blue). Since the Ambu-bag is self-inflating, it is also important not to allow excess oxygen to flow into the bag causing the inflating valve to jam; an oxygen flow rate of 5 litres/min is usually adequate. It is also vital to check that the oxygen tubing connected to the Ambu-bag is the same oxygen tubing that is connected to the flowmeter on the wall!

If the patient is not breathing spontaneously and is unable to maintain his own airway endotracheal intubation is best carried out as soon as possible but the patient must be oxygenated first. Inflation of the lungs with oxygen should be accompanied by visible lung movement if this procedure is being adequately performed.

EXTERNAL CARDIAC MASSAGE

This procedure aims to compress the heart between the sternum and rib cage anteriorly and the vertebrae posteriorly and is successful only if adequate depression of the sternum is achieved. It is important not to attempt cardiac massage on a soft springy bed, but most modern hospital beds have a foam mattress resting on a firm surface. Unless one has immensely strong arms external cardiac massage is easiest and most efficient when kneeling at the same level as the patient's body, which enables one to keep the elbows straight and one hand over the other. Compression is carried out at the junction of the middle and lower thirds of the sternum at a rate of between 60 and 80 beats/min. Pressure too far down on the sternum may force the xiphisternum into the liver. It is important that a regular and synchronous rhythm of cardiac massage and ventilation is carried out. Once this has been achieved and a pulse is palpable, other procedures may be undertaken, but unless cardiopulmonary resuscitation is continued all other efforts are in vain. This may seem obvious but is all too often forgotten in the heat of the moment.

DRUG THERAPY

As soon as possible after the initial resuscitation it is important to diagnose the cardiac rhythm with an ECG and to set up a satisfactory intravenous infusion. Initial drug therapy should consist of 100 ml 8·4% sodium bicarbonate (i.e. 100 mmol) to correct the initial metabolic acidosis which invariably occurs. After this, intravenous infusion should be changed to 5% dextrose. The cardiac rhythm will commonly be found to be one of two types, asystole or ventricular fibrillation, and it is in those patients with ventricular fibrillation that the higher success rate of cardiac resuscitation occurs. In view of this, many people advocate emergency defibrillation before diagnosing the rhythm, because a fibrillating heart is easier to defibrillate immediately and one in asystole does not suffer from inadvertent defibrillation. Many qualified nurses on coronary care units are therefore trained to defibrillate as soon as circulatory arrest has been established.

DEFIBRILLATION

Initially the defibrillator is set to 100 joules for external electrode defibrillation and the paddles placed across the chest as far apart as possible. It is vital to ensure that there is no continuity of electrode jelly between the paddles as this may short-circuit the electric current. It is also essential that no member of the resuscitation team be in electrical contact with the patient. If a shock of this magnitude fails to defibrillate the patient, increasing current may be passed in increments of 50 joules. (It is also important to ensure that the rubber protecting caps usually placed over the paddles are removed before use!) Defibrillation often successfully restores normal cardiac rhythm and no further drugs are required.

DRUG TREATMENT OF ASYSTOLE

In asystole it is important to excite a flaccid heart—as opposed to calming an excited one, as is the case with ventricular fibrillation. This is achieved with intravenous adrenaline (1 ml 1:1000) and calcium chloride (10 ml 10%) and in most cases this will restore some sort of cardiac rhythm. However, it may well be ventricular fibrillation, in which case defibrillation is indicated. Further increments of adrenaline and calcium may be given but are seldom successful. Occasionally the rhythm which returns may be one of the sinus brachycardia, in which case atropine must be given to block the vagus nerve. In this event a full vagal blocking dose of atropine is about 2 mg. Occasionally ventricular tachycardia or numerous ventricular extrasystoles occur, necessitating the use of intravenous lignocaine (50–100 mg) to suppress the ectopic foci. The only other drug usually contained in crash boxes is isoprenaline, which is used only as an infusion to maintain heart rate and blood pressure, both as a result of β-adrenergic stimulation (Chapter 14). Although other drugs are sometimes used at cardiac arrests, those mentioned remain the backbone of this procedure; 100 ml 8·4% sodium bicarbonate is usually given at the start of resuscitation and again for every 10 minute duration of cardiac arrest to correct the metabolic acidosis. An acidotic heart is difficult to defibrillate.

'CRASH BOX' CONTENTS

Although these boxes often contain every conceivable resuscitative tool, they easily become unnecessarily complicated. In general, the following should be considered the essential contents:

Suction catheters and Yankauer sucker heads.
Oropharyngeal airways sizes 2 and 3.
Endotracheal tubes sizes 7 to 10 and connections. Smaller sizes should be available on wards with a paediatric responsibility.
An endotracheal tube introducer.
Ambu-bag, inflating valve and face masks sizes 3, 4 and 5.
Two working laryngoscopes.
Intravenous drip set and cannulae (it is unnecessarily muddling to have a wide range of these).
Intravenous fluids (8·4% or 4·2%) sodium bicarbonate and 5% dextrose.
Intravenous drugs (adrenaline, calcium chloride, atropine, lignocaine and isoprenaline). These drugs are now frequently available in the form of the IMS preloaded system (Fig. 25.1).

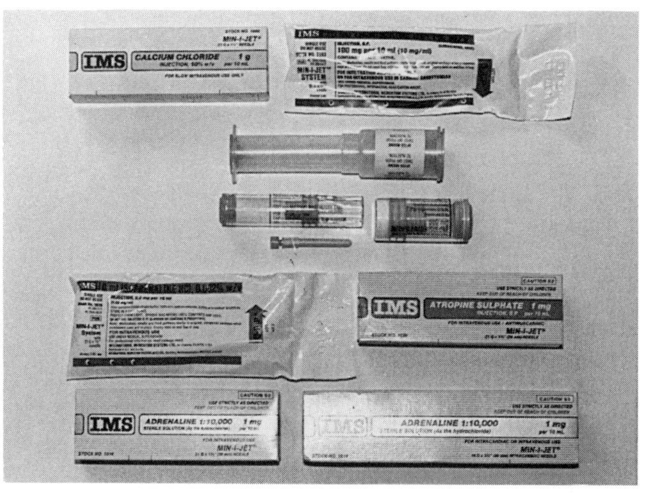

Fig. 25.1 IMS emergency drug system

This saves considerable time in the drawing up of drugs and eliminates many potential sources of error in the emergency situation.

Tape and bandage for fixing tubes and cannulae.

Many crash boxes contain far more equipment than this, but in practice most of it is unnecessary and prevents the resuscitator from rapidly finding the few essential items. The boxes should be checked each time they are used and also at weekly intervals to ensure that items such as laryngoscopes are in full working order.

DEFIBRILLATORS

These are commonly of the direct current (DC) type and are designed to pass an electric current across the heart in the form of a shock to alter the cardiac rhythm. This is commonly used to convert ventricular fibrillation back into sinus rhythm, but synchronised DC shock is also used to convert patients in atrial flutter or fibrillation back into atrial sinus rhythm. Most DC

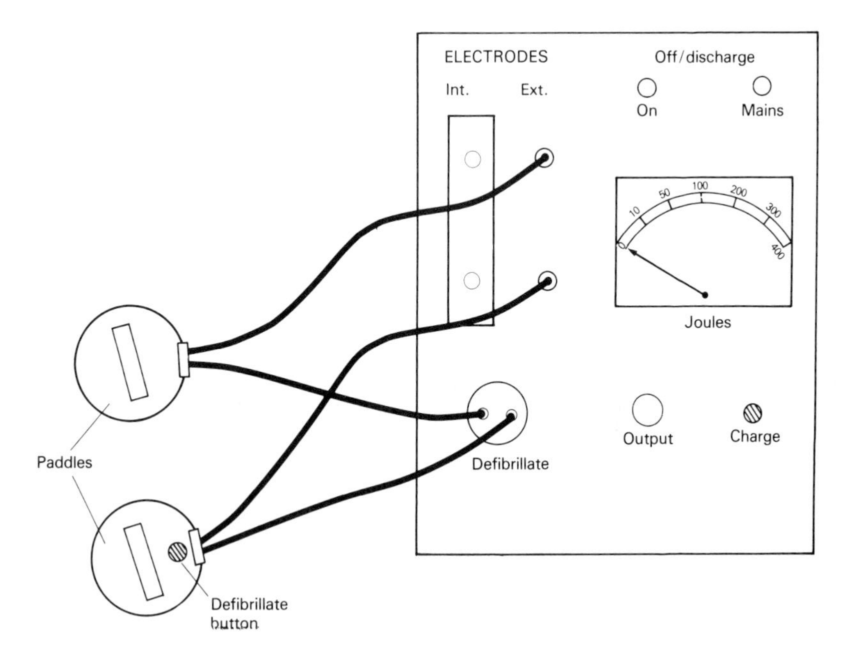

Fig. 25.2 Defibrillator

defibrillators may be used with either internal or external electrodes although, apart from patients undergoing open heart surgery, DC defibrillation is almost invariably carried out by the external route. Figure 25.2 illustrates a typical front panel from a DC defibrillator indicating the switch which allows the use of either internal or external electrodes. Other switches control on–off, charge, magnitude of charge (which is shown on the dial, measured in joules), and discharge. This last control is used to discharge the unit when it has been charged unnecessarily, or for test purposes. The usual charge employed for external defibrillation is between 100 and 400 joules while for internal defibrillation this ranges from 15 to 100 joules. Figures 25.3 and 25.4 show an older and more modern type of defibrillator, both working on the same principle described above. The newer models are more compact and easily portable.

RESUSCITATION OF NEWBORN

Although this is a specialist technique, it is important to understand the principles of resuscitation of the newborn for use

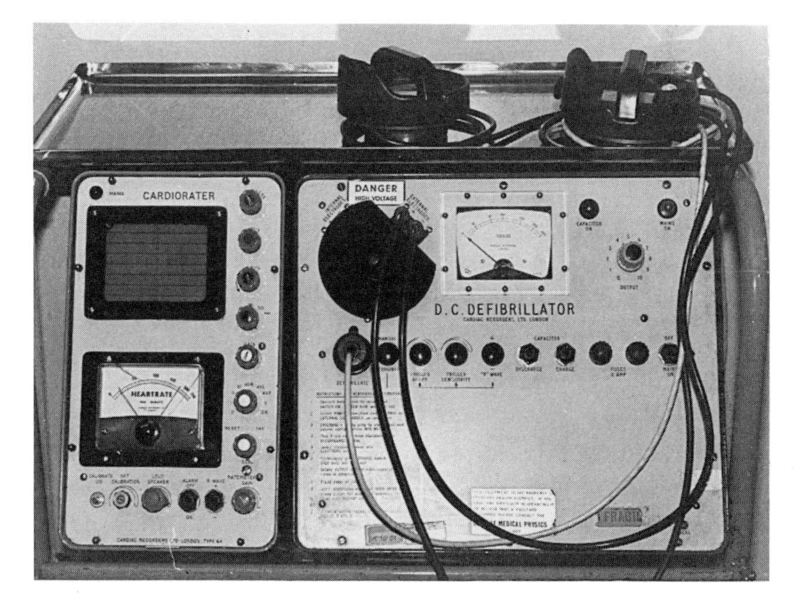

Fig. 25.3 Cardiac Recorders DC defibrillator (trolley mounted)

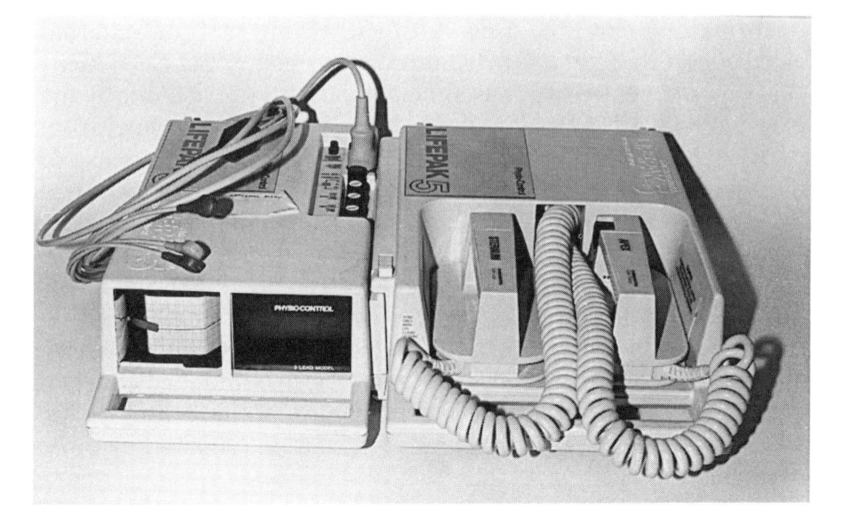

Fig. 25.4 Lifepak portable ECG/defibrillator with battery pack

in situations associated with anaesthesia in the obstetric unit. In normal circumstances the fetus is born cyanosed and begins to breathe rhythmically on birth. The fetal circulation can withstand a short period of hypoxia provided that the circulation to the brain remains adequate. Neonatal resuscitation involves: (1) clearing the upper airway, (2) administering small amounts of oxygen to reverse hypoxia, and (3) maintaining an adequate circulation.

In normal circumstances all that is usually required is nasopharyngeal and oropharyngeal suction with a sterile suction catheter and sputum trap to clear the upper airway and allow respiration to be established in the normal way. Excessive oral suction, however, may produce laryngospasm and cyanosis. If the newborn infant is drowsy or flaccid as a result of prolonged hypoxia or drug therapy, further measures may be necessary. Provided that respiration is established suction and minimal oxygen therapy will usually restore the situation, but where this is insufficient orotracheal intubation may be necessary. This procedure often stimulates the infant to breathe spontaneously, although gentle positive pressure ventilation for several minutes may help recovery and in particular allow an adequate pulse rate to be maintained (bradycardia being the most sensitive sign of neonatal hypoxia). The usual orotracheal tube used is about 2·5 or 3 mm internal diameter and often has a shoulder separating the tracheal from the pharyngeal part of the tube (Warne neonatal tube).

If there is any doubt about the adequacy of the circulation, external cardiac massage with one or two fingers only, placed over the sternum, should be instituted until a pulse is palpable. Again, this often returns within a few seconds of adequate resuscitation. If drug-induced respiratory depression is suspected, an opiate antagonist may be used. Neonatal naloxone has now superseded both levallorphan and nalorphine for this purpose and often has remarkable results in a depressed infant. Hypoglycaemia and acidosis, together with hypothermia, may all cause residual depression and flaccidity and prolonged neonatal resuscitation must take account of all these possibilities by the administration of glucose, bicarbonate, and by keeping the infant warm on a special resuscitation table.

26 Emergency Anaesthesia

Vomiting and regurgitation. Fluid and electrolyte depletion. Local analgesia. Anaesthesia after major trauma. Pre-operative procedures. Shock lung.

The term 'emergency' implies an urgency which prevents the full and careful preparation of the patient that would be possible and desirable before an elective procedure. Few surgical emergencies are so dire that a full history and physical examination are not possible. The degree to which laboratory and radiological investigations are considered essential in the individual case will depend on many factors, including regional, national and economic factors. Few anaesthetists in the UK would anaesthetise an elderly, bronchitic patient with several days' history of intestinal obstruction without full biochemical and haematological information and a chest x-ray examination, but the same anaesthetist might have to proceed without the advantage of any of these investigations if presented with a similar patient in the Himalayan foothills or the African bush. On the other hand, to request extensive investigations on every fit young patient who has suffered an uncomplicated limb fracture would waste time and money. Each anaesthetist and each surgical team will know the environment in which they work and should strive for as good pre-operative assessment as circumstances allow.

There are other circumstances, usually associated with uncontrollable bleeding, where there may just be time to obtain laboratory information but full resuscitation of the patient is impossible before operation has to be carried out to save his life. Rapid transfusion of blood (which may have to be un-crossmatched Group O Rh-negative) and other fluids may effect temporary improvement in the patient's condition, but this usually worsens again as increased blood pressure produces further bleeding. Examples of such cases are bleeding from a duodenal ulcer or a badly ruptured ectopic pregnancy.

VOMITING AND REGURGITATION

Probably the most important factor common to all emergency procedures is the possibility that the stomach will contain undigested food or fluid material which may be vomited or regurgitated into the pharynx, whence it may find its way into the lungs.

The gastric contents are usually derived from one of two sources: undigested food and alimentary canal secretions.

Undigested Food

Any patient being presented for anaesthesia may have undigested food in his stomach. Before elective procedures all food and fluid are withheld for a long enough time for the stomach to have emptied. This period is usually taken as about four hours for liquids and six hours for solid food. In emergency anaesthesia there are two reasons why the stomach may not have emptied. Firstly, the surgical treatment may be considered to be of such urgency that it is not possible to wait for several hours, and secondly (and probably more importantly), in most emergencies gastric digestion is greatly slowed or may even cease. Where the patient has had an accident, it is wise to calculate from the time the patient last ate until the time of the accident rather than from the last meal until the induction of anaesthesia.

Less obvious trauma than broken bones, e.g. the psychological stress of being admitted unexpectedly to hospital, may delay gastric emptying in many patients; only in the least urgent of emergency procedures is it reasonable to regard the stomach as being empty.

Alimentary Canal Secretions

Variable amounts of liquid gastric contents are common when there is stasis in the alimentary tract, whether in the stomach itself or further down the intestine. In these circumstances, the presence of fluid in the stomach is inherent in the condition, and the situation will not improve (and indeed will probably become worse) by delaying.

Differences between Vomiting and Regurgitation

Vomiting is an active process involving contraction not only of the smooth muscle of the upper alimentary canal but also of the striated muscle of the diaphragm and abdominal muscles. It occurs only in light planes of anaesthesia which are usually seen only at induction of and emergence from anaesthesia. It cannot occur when a patient has been effectively paralysed by a neuromuscular blocking agent and cannot occur under deep anaesthesia.

Regurgitation, on the other hand, is a passive process and simply implies the flowing of fluids under the influence of gravity. It is more likely to occur under deep anaesthesia or in patients who have been paralysed, because some striated muscle from the diaphragm forms loops around the angle between the stomach and the oesophagus, which probably help to support the smooth muscle of the gastro-oesophageal (cardiac) sphincter. Normally the tone in the cardiac sphincter is high enough to prevent the passage of gastric contents into the oesophagus, but certain factors (e.g. hiatus hernia, pregnancy or the presence of an oesophageal or gastric tube) make the sphincter less competent. Other factors may raise the intragastric pressure to a height at which it overcomes even a competent sphincter. Such conditions include intestinal obstruction, the gravid uterus near term, the fasciculation of the abdominal muscles caused by suxamethonium, or by items of anaesthetic equipment, or even the patient's arms left resting on the epigastrium at induction of anaesthesia.

Prevention

Nasogastric and orogastric tubes
Where the gastric contents are thought to be liquid (as in most cases of intestinal stasis) a small tube (size 12 or 14 French gauge) passed into the stomach will serve to aspirate the gastric contents. The additional benefit of passing a wider-bore tube when the gastric contents are expected to be solid or semi-solid is debatable, because the eyelets of even the largest tubes are easily blocked by particulate matter.

The disadvantages of these tubes are that they cannot be guaranteed to empty the stomach and, by their presence, tend to make the cardiac sphincter less competent. Opinion is divided but, having emptied the stomach, most anaesthetists would remove the tube before inducing anaesthesia.

General Anaesthesia

The patient's airway is only safe under general anaesthesia when a cuffed endotracheal tube is in place. The danger period is between induction of anaesthesia and inflation of the cuff on the tube. With modern anaesthetic techniques it is usually possible to reduce this period to a few seconds, and various methods of inducing anaesthesia (given below) have been devised to reduce the danger to a minimum.

Induction of anaesthesia supine with a head-up tilt
The theory behind this technique is that if the patient is in a steep enough head-up position the hydrostatic pressure in the stomach will not be great enough to force gastric contents up as high as the pharynx. Unfortunately, to achieve sufficient height of the pharynx over the stomach a head-up tilt of about 45° is necessary; hence the anaesthetist has to stand on a stool to intubate the patient. At the same time, the head-up posture may dangerously accentuate the hypotensive effects of the agent used for inducing anaesthesia. Lastly, if gastric contents should enter the pharynx in this position it is difficult to prevent their entry into the larynx. Because of these disadvantages this technique has largely gone out of favour.

Head-down tilt in the lateral position
The rationale behind using this position is that, although regurgitation is more likely, it is hoped that the gastric contents will run out of the nose and corner of the mouth instead of into the larynx. With practice, intubation in the left lateral position is remarkably easy with the tongue falling away from the laryngoscope, but in a patient who is difficult to intubate the manoeuvre may be more difficult in this position than in the more familiar supine position.

Supine horizontal position
This position has only become acceptable since the introduction of Sellick's manoeuvre or cricoid pressure. This involves pressure on the cricoid cartilage as the patient is going to sleep. This squeezes the lower end of the pharynx against the sixth cervical vertebra thus preventing the regurgitation of fluids into the pharynx. In addition to performing the cricoid pressure with the forefinger and thumb of the right hand, it is important to place the left hand behind the patient's neck and lift forwards. If this is not done, the pressure of the right hand may undo the flexion of the cervical spine on the thoracic spine which is the best position for laryngoscopy and intubation. The pressure is maintained until the endotracheal tube is passed and its cuff inflated. It is important to mark the cricoid cartilage with a pen as it is not always easy to find, especially in women—where the cartilage is smaller. The reason for using the cricoid cartilage is that it is the only complete ring of cartilage in the respiratory tract so that its firm posterior part is more effective at occluding the pharynx. While effective at preventing regurgitation, it is said that if active vomiting occurs while cricoid pressure is being applied the pressure should be released or oesophageal rupture may occur. Faced with the choice between the 'devil' of oesophageal rupture or the 'deep blue sea' of inhalation of gastric contents, most anaesthetists would probably opt for the deep blue sea, but there is no doubt that a few would prefer to join the devil!

Cricoid pressure is also a useful adjunct to induction of anaesthesia in either of the other two postures described above.

Induction of anaesthesia
Before inducing anaesthesia, secure access to a vein is essential. A winged needle is just about acceptable, but if an intravenous infusion via a cannula is not already running when the patient

arrives in the anaesthetic room it is probably wise to set one up.

The anaesthetic equipment must be (as always) carefully checked and must include two laryngoscopes. Particular attention must be paid to the adequacy of the suction apparatus and to checking the ease with which the trolley or table can be placed in the head-down position.

It is wise to pre-oxygenate the patient for at least three minutes. This increases the amount of oxygen in the lung alveoli so that the continuing circulation of blood through the pulmonary capillaries will continue to pick up oxygen and maintain arterial PO_2 while the patient is apnoeic. Active inflation of the lungs by squeezing the reservoir bag—the practice at elective procedures—is dangerous for two reasons. Firstly, inadvertent inflation of the stomach will increase the likelihood of regurgitation and, secondly, it simply increases the period at risk between induction of anaesthesia and inflation of the endotracheal tube cuff.

Most anaesthetists would probably induce anaesthesia with an intravenous induction agent scaled down to allow for the patient's debility, and intubate with the help of suxamethonium. Thiopentone is the induction agent with which most anaesthetists have the greatest familarity. Carefully used, it is safe, but it should be remembered that it has a depressant effect on the myocardium. Other intravenous agents may be used and a few anaesthetists would use an induction with cyclopropane in oxygen provided that they were familiar with the technique and happy with the antistatic precautions, cyclopropane being readily detonable.

Maintenance of anaesthesia

Maintenance of anaesthesia for abdominal emergencies is usually by controlled respiration with a muscle relaxant, using nitrous oxide and oxygen with a small amount of inhalational or parenteral adjuvant. The muscle relaxant may be additional small increments of suxamethonium or the same drug used as an infusion. However, as the total amount of suxamethonium used increases, the neuromuscular block it produces tends to develop the characteristics of a 'dual block' (Chapter 12). If this happens the patient may not breathe adequately at the end of the operation.

Most anaesthetists would probably use a non-depolarising relaxant, but there also, especially in abdominal emergencies, breathing may not be adequate at the end of the operation due to apparent incomplete reversal of the relaxant by adequate doses of neostigmine.

With the widespread introduction of intensive therapy units, the discussion as to the possible causes of inadequate breathing at the end of operation has now become somewhat academic. It is now realised that instead of watching the still-intubated patient anxiously to decide whether his breathing is adequate, it is much safer to leave him intubated and ventilated for a few hours during which time the problem almost invariably resolves spontaneously.

Spontaneous respiration anaesthesia is satisfactory for most peripheral operations (e.g. orthopaedic procedures) but as the patient can be kept more lightly anaesthetised with muscle-relaxant anaesthesia, it is increasingly common to paralyse patients undergoing emergency procedures even when not strictly necessary to provide good surgical operating conditions. It is safer for the patient (and more comforting for the anaesthetist) to be in full control of his protective reflexes before returning to what may be indifferent recovery facilities, especially at night.

Emergence from anaesthesia

The likelihood of vomiting is greatest, and the risk of regurgitation has not entirely passed, as the patient is recovering consciousness. The patient should be turned on his side breathing oxygen and the mouth and pharynx carefully sucked out. The endotracheal tube should be left in place with the cuff inflated until the patient shows signs of coughing on the tube. Extubation should be carried out with reasonably firm pressure on the reservoir bag which helps both to inflate atelectatic alveoli and to blow out any liquid which may have collected in the larynx above the endotracheal tube cuff, where it is beyond the reach of the pharyngeal sucker.

FLUID AND ELECTROLYTE DEPLETION

Many patients presenting for emergency anaesthesia are suffering from some sort of fluid and electrolyte depletion. The nature and severity of the fluid loss will depend on the cause and its duration. The fluid required may, for example, be blood in cases of haemorrhage, blood and plasma after burns and scalds, plasma in peritonitis, and various electrolyte-containing fluids with different levels of intestinal obstruction. A careful history and clinical examination of the patient will give a good idea of what is required and this is confirmed by haematological and biochemical investigation. At least partial restoration of the patient's fluid and electrolyte balance adds greatly to the safety of the whole procedure, but as mentioned earlier, resuscitation in cases of severe bleeding may be only partially successful.

LOCAL ANALGESIA

It may seem tempting to pass an endotracheal tube after topical analgesia of the upper respiratory tract so that the cuff of the tube can be inflated before general anaesthesia is induced. However, there are disadvantages with this technique. In the first place, it is less pleasant and more exhausting for the patient. Secondly, and more important, the method is not as safe as it might appear. If the patient should vomit or regurgitate after the larynx has been anaesthetised, but before the endotracheal tube has been passed, he may have great difficulty in coughing effectively enough to prevent aspiration of the vomitus into his lungs. This risk is especially great in the frail and elderly.

Another approach to the problem of emergency anaesthesia is to perform the operation under local analgesia, thus eliminating the dangers of vomiting and regurgitation. For peripheral operations these techniques have much to recommend them. The fact that they are not used routinely for these procedures in the UK is probably a reflection of the fact that the usually high standard of general anaesthesia has led most patients to expect (and most anaesthetists to provide) general anaesthesia for most operations. There are signs, however, that there is an increasing use of regional techniques for emergency operations on the limbs. This may be associated with higher standards of training of anaesthetists, the description of new regional techniques and the introduction of more reliable and longer-acting local analgesic drugs, e.g. lignocaine and, more recently, bupivacaine.

The usefulness of the more central regional techniques, i.e. spinal and epidural analgesia for emergency surgery, is more debatable. They may be more reliable than multiple peripheral blocks, e.g. combined sciatic and femoral blocks for leg operations, but any central block providing analgesia above the level of the knee, i.e. the third lumbar segment, leads to some degree of sympathetic blockade. The higher the block the more vasodilation is produced and the less able is the body to compensate for any reduction in circulating blood volume from whatever cause.

It is now accepted that with even uncomplicated fractures of long bones of the legs there is the loss of some 500–1000 ml of blood into the surrounding tissues. Unless great care is taken to replace this fluid the induction of spinal or epidural analgesia to quite modest levels may be accompanied by hypotension.

Providing spinal or epidural analgesia for abdominal surgery is more hazardous and may be difficult to make effective. The implications of this sort of analgesia for abdominal surgery are discussed in Chapter 33. It will be remembered that if abdominal viscera are not distended or their mesenteries pulled upon they can normally be cut, ligated or burnt without pain. Unfortunately, this is not true for inflamed or near-gangrenous bowel, the handling of which can cause great distress. The afferent impulses are carried not only in the sympathetic nerves (which can be blocked by analgesia extending up to the 5th thoracic segment) but also in the branches of the vagus nerves, which run no part of their course with the spinal cord and are therefore unaffected by these forms of analgesia. Bilateral vagal block requires either a coeliac plexus block or the infiltration of local anaesthetic round the vagal trunks as they lie on the oeosophagus in the highest part of the abdomen. This area is inaccessible through most surgical incisions.

As always, the anaesthetist is safest using the techniques with which he is most familiar, and it is safer for his patient if he uses a well-tried technique in an emergency rather than experimenting with some unfamiliar method.

ANAESTHESIA AFTER MAJOR TRAUMA

Anaesthetics after major trauma are now given more and more often, particularly as a result of car and motor-cycle accidents.

Although many of the injuries may look extensive it is important to resist the temptation to take the patient to theatre before adequate diagnosis has been made and resuscitative treatment carried out. Several important procedures which are an extension of first aid must be carried out before the patient is in a fit state to be anaesthetised: (1) oxygenation and intubation, (2) restoration of circulating blood volume, (3) assessment of level of consciousness, (4) analgesia, and (5) correction and avoidance of hypothermia.

Oxygenation and Intubation

With the exception of patients with severe chest trauma, endotracheal intubation following extensive injuries is confined to those patients who are unable to protect their own airway, usually as a result of unconsciousness or severe faciomaxillary damage. A patient who actively resists all efforts to intubate him does not require intubation. Nevertheless, following major trauma all patients should be given supplementary oxygen whether or not they appear to need it and whether or not they are prepared to tolerate it, because the dangers of cerebral, hepatic and renal hypoxia in this condition are appreciable.

Restoration of Circulating Blood Volume

It is important to avoid hypovolaemic shock (where there is evidence of severe blood loss) by the early administration of intravenous fluids and plasma expanders. These should be replaced as soon as possible with whole blood, since although the plasma expanders such as dextran or Haemaccel will maintain blood pressure, they do not carry oxygen, and filling the circulation with them may prevent subsequent blood transfusion without causing fluid overload.

Assessment of Level of Consciousness

As soon as the patient is in a fit state to be questioned it is important to obtain any relevant medical history of illness or drug treatment. It is also important to know whether the patient has received anaesthesia uneventfully in the past, and whether he suffers from any drug or other sensitivity. If this is impossible for any reason, the patient's belongings should be checked to see if they carry a medical warning card—for example to indicate diabetes mellitus or steroid therapy.

Analgesia

Following major trauma, patients may suffer extreme pain and unless they are completely unconscious it is unreasonable to withhold all forms of analgesia. Intravenous opiates provide the most satisfactory and efficient form of analgesia, but their use is contraindicated in patients with head injuries or respiratory difficulty. Entonox has been used with some success in such cases, but most neurosurgeons prefer codeine phosphate for analgesia in patients with head injury to avoid the masking of neurological signs.

Correction and Avoidance of Hypothermia

After a major accident many patients will have been exposed on the roadside for some time and hypothermia complicates resuscitation and makes estimation of circulating blood volume difficult.

Successful immediate resuscitation of patients suffering from major trauma must be followed by a detailed assessment of their injuries. It is vital that this is done in a logical sequence as follows.

1. *Head injury*
Examination for skull fractures must be accompanied by assessment of the level of consciousness, of pupil size and reactivity and other evidence of raised intracranial pressure due to bleeding.

2. *Facial injuries*
These are often extensive and may well prevent normal laryngoscopy and intubation. It is important to avoid displacing facial fractures, which is easily done during emergency intubation.

3. *Cervical spine injuries*
If there is any suspicion of spinal fractures it is vital that no movement occurs in this region, because transection of the cord may result in quadriplegia. Immobilisation of the cervical spine under local anaesthetic with traction may be necessary if other injuries permit.

4. *Chest injuries*
Injuries to the chest include injuries to the trachea and bronchi as a result of tear or rupture of the air passages, tears of the major thoracic vessels or heart, and injuries to the chest wall and lung. Blood in the tracheobronchial tree usually indicates direct lung trauma. Chest injuries range from isolated rib fractures—which may involve underlying lung contusion or pneumothorax—to flail chest injuries resulting from individual ribs fractured in two places. Stove-in chest is often complicated by ruptured viscera, haemopneumothorax and damage to intrathoracic structures. After immediate resuscitation it is important to establish the severity of such injuries by x-ray examination and possibly angiography.

5. *Abdominal and pelvic injuries*
These again are usually a combination of fractures, commonly of the pelvis, together with ruptured or contused viscera, particularly the liver, the spleen and the small bowel. Acute gastric dilation may occur after a severe accident and may produce abdominal swelling suggesting severe haemorrhage. Vigorous transfusion without adequate diagnostic procedures may result in pulmonary oedema even in fit young people.

6. *Peripheral fractures*
It is important to assess each fracture for potential blood loss and temporary immobilisation of them may be adequate until after the treatment of more severe injuries. Major fractures are associated with a surprisingly large concealed blood loss—e.g. femur 2–3 units, pelvis 3–4 units, tibia and fibula 1–2 units.

Subsequent treatment of patients suffering severe trauma is based on the maxim of getting everything into perspective. For example, a ruptured spleen is more important than a fractured ankle despite the fact that the peripheral fracture may be obvious while the intra-abdominal injury may be concealed. A detailed examination of the patient together with a chest x-ray, an abdominal and pelvic x-ray and any other relevant x-ray examinations—e.g. skull and spine—should be done immediately, possibly with a four quadrant abdominal tap to exclude intra-abdominal bleeding. Detailed x-ray examination of peripheral fractures may be carried out at a later date.

The initial problem is to *correct the potentially fatal conditions.*

PRE-OPERATIVE PROCEDURES

Whenever possible it is essential for the patient to be visited pre-operatively by the anaesthetist, not only to assess the degree of injuries and therefore the special measures which may be necessary during the operation but more especially to allay the inevitable anxiety. Many patients will be in severe pain and may also be confused or semi-conscious. Premedication with analgesia has usually already been given if the patient has been treated in the casualty department, but the possibility of the patient having a full stomach may necessitate the administration of pre-operative antacids. Intravenous atropine is usually given in the anaesthetic room. Further details of emergency anaesthesia have already been discussed on pp. 270–277.

Once the patient is asleep and the injuries can be examined more closely, it is important to plan the surgical treatment according to what the patient can withstand at that time and to anticipate prolonged postoperative ventilation by carrying out tracheostomy at the time of operation. Major trauma cases benefit enormously from postoperative care in an intensive-care unit where their fluid balance, blood replacement and other requirements can be closely monitored. Many will require a period of postoperative ventilation and also the attention of many different specialists such as neurosurgeons, orthopaedic surgeons, anaesthetists and general surgeons. An intensive care unit is the best place to coordinate this treatment.

SHOCK LUNG

After major trauma, and many other conditions, impaired gas exchange in the lung may arise insidiously. This is usually manifested by a decrease in arterial oxygenation without, in the initial stages, a rise in carbon dioxide concentration. This is because the essential lesion in shock lung is a diffusion defect which affects oxygen transfer to a greater extent than carbon dioxide, the more readily diffusible of the two gases. Shock lung may be caused by numerous injuries and insults, particularly haemorrhagic hypotension, direct lung and chest wall trauma, aspiration of gastric contents and fluid overload. There are also many other causes not associated with major trauma, but the essential pathology is similar in all cases.

The lesion in shock lung includes damage to the alveolar capillary endothelium resulting from micro-emboli, platelet aggregates, bacterial toxins and chemical mediators, such as serotonin, bradykinin and 5-hydroxytryptamine (5HT). This damage produces an alveolar capillary leak which, in turn, increases the pulmonary extravascular water. A picture develops of a decrease in functional residual capacity (FRC) and a decrease in compliance (the lungs becoming stiff and more difficult to inflate). The end-result of this process is a diffusion defect which is more marked for oxygen than carbon dioxide, resulting in inadequate oxygenation of the blood as it passes through the lungs.

Clinical Course

The clinical course of shock lung may be divided into four discrete phases.

Phase 1: Fluid leaking extravascularly
Although this produces mild hypoxia, compensated for by hyperventilation and an increase in the work of breathing, there is little change seen on the chest x-ray and many patients are not diagnosed at this stage.

Phase 2: More fluid leak
At this stage alveoli begin to collapse, hypoxia becomes more severe and there is a decrease in surfactant (the agent produced in the lung to maintain alveolar surface tension). Restlessness and oliguria may occur and the chest x-ray shows pulmonary oedema, pleural effusions and lung collapse.

Phase 3: Unconsciousness
At this stage patients become unconscious and symptoms are severe, although the full extent of the condition is often not realised until this stage.

Phase 4: Death
Increased carbon dioxide concentration and acidosis, together with severe hypoxia, lead to a bradycardia and then renal and hepatic failure with death resulting from hypoxia.

Treatment

The pathology of shock lung would appear to be relatively clearly defined. The treatment depends on a high index of suspicion together with early diagnosis and may be divided into three sections.

1. Treatment of the cause
This includes microfiltration of blood and blood products, rapid treatment of any haemorrhage and the avoidance of overtransfusion.

2. Block of the mediators of capillary damage
High dose steroids (30 mg/kg prednisolone) have been advocated in this condition although their efficacy, except when given immediately after the insult, is still in doubt.

3. Reversal of the pathology
This includes symptomatic treatment ranging from artificial ventilation together with positive end-expiratory pressure, sedation and paralysis, to cardiac support with digitalis and diuretics, and finally to general circulatory support. The avoidance of hypoxia must be accompanied by avoidance of hyperoxia since exces-

sively high inspired oxygen concentrations may also cause lung damage.

Although the morbidity in shock lung is high, early diagnosis and treatment may produce a survival rate of up to 50%, which is all the more important because many patients suffering major trauma are teenagers or young adults.

27 Principles of Intensive Care

Concepts of intensive care. Monitoring techniques. Equipment. Medical and nursing complement. Daily intensive care. Sedation in intensive care. Problems in intensive care.

Most hospitals in the UK, with any responsibility for acute medical care, now contain an intensive-care unit, although many such units are conversions of existing wards rather than purpose-built. These hospitals usually also contain a coronary-care unit, which may be either part of the intensive-care complex or separate. Although a mixture of coronary care and intensive care within the same unit is far from ideal, this may have advantages from the nursing, and particularly the teaching and training, point of view.

Intensive care itself is mainly concerned with acute respiratory, cardiac and metabolic treatment, and the commonest types of case admitted to a general hospital intensive-care unit are as follows.

1. *General medical cases:*
   (a) overdoses
   (b) renal failure
   (c) neurological
   (d) respiratory failure.

2. *Major trauma.*

3. *General surgical cases* (usually postoperative care):
   (a) vascular

(b) massive haemorrhage
(c) coagulation problems
(d) airway problems
(e) endocrine
(f) nutritional.

Other cases which may require intensive care depending on specialist surgery are: (a) cardiothoracic, (b) neurosurgical and (c) renal dialysis.

CONCEPTS OF INTENSIVE CARE

Seriously ill patients require intensive medical care, intensive nursing care and the use of specialist equipment both for monitoring and treatment. It is far more logical and economical to concentrate these facilities in one unit to which the patient is brought, rather than to nurse such patients in general medical and surgical wards, necessitating reduplication of manpower and equipment. Much of the success in intensive-care units is attributable to the accurate and scrupulous care of the patients made possible by a high nurse to patient ratio, in contrast to the routine care available in the general wards. At the same time it is important for the clinician running an intensive-care unit to realise that it is impossible to be an expert in all aspects of intensive care. He must act both as decision maker and coordinator, able to bring together skills necessary to treat a particular case.

MONITORING TECHNIQUES

By concentrating all seriously ill patients in a single unit, more extensive monitoring of the patient is possible, both from the point of view of the skills of the staff and the time available. In general, all patients are monitored regularly and frequently in terms of blood pressure, ECG, temperature, pulse rate and central venous pressure. It is essential that adequate and accurate records are kept, minute by minute if necessary, of the patient's condition, particularly in relation to when drugs are given, to assess the effects of both the drug and the dose on the patient concerned; this can be achieved only with adequate medical and nursing care. In addition, detailed intensive-care charts allow accurate estimation of fluid input and output which is often critical in seriously ill patients and in whom there is no room for inaccuracies or missing data—which inevitably occur on general wards. More extensive monitoring of the patients depends on the particular condition being treated, but may include monitoring of direct arterial blood pressure, pulmonary artery pressure, left atrial pressure and intracranial pressure. In addition, other advanced techniques such as electro-encephalography may be necessary and available.

Although the patients may be heavily sedated or apparently unconscious, it is important to remember that as they recover they require a great deal of encouragement and even orientation, many of them having been admitted to the unit as an emergency and waking up totally unaware of their surroundings. The importance of 'tender loving care' cannot be overemphasised in this often horrific situation and indeed the patients' relatives may be subjected to far more stress and strain than the patients themselves, who may be largely unaware of what is going on or how seriously ill they are. It is necessary for the relatives to speak as frequently as they wish with members of both the medical and nursing staff. They should be kept fully informed of all events, and be free to come and go as often as they wish, provided that they do not interfere with intensive therapy.

EQUIPMENT

The ideal number of beds for a general hospital intensive-care unit is probably 1% of the total hospital bed complement, although this may need to be increased when specialist units are being considered. It is impossible to estimate the cost of intensive care but it is about ten times the cost of a normal hospital bed per day. The equipment that is available in intensive-care units is both specialised and variable. The enormous expense of individual items of equipment is one of the basic reasons for concentrating intensive-care equipment on one site and bringing the patient to it, where both doctors and nurses have been specially trained in using the equipment. Although the ECG is usually displayed at the bedside of each individual patient, remote display is often useful, particularly in coronary care where it is distressing for patients to be 'observed' continually by the bedside. The unit should contain its own defibrillator together with other essential pieces of equipment such as ventilators, drip counters and oxygen analysers. The use of special intensive-care beds often allows both x-ray examination and weighing of the patient in bed, which may be a considerable advantage. Each bed station should have its own supply of piped oxygen, compressed air, nitrous oxide and suction, together with adequate electrical outlets. Most purpose-built intensive-care units also contain their own facilities for blood gas and electrolyte determinations together with haemoglobin and other essential investigations. This is important as these factors may need to be measured at frequent intervals during the day, making transport to routine laboratories impracticable.

MEDICAL AND NURSING COMPLEMENT

An intensive-care unit ideally requires one nurse continually assigned to each patient, together with one nurse per shift to carry out administrative and other duties, and any unit which possesses such a complement during the day and is reduced to ordinary ward staffing at night cannot be called an intensive-care unit, as this requires 24-hour patient care. A resident junior doctor, usually an anaesthetist or a physician, together with regular ward rounds and consultations with more senior members of the medical staff, are both essential to the intensive medical care necessary to improve the condition of patients and to enable the unit to run smoothly.

DAILY INTENSIVE CARE

This combination of general and specialised nursing care ranges from washing and turning the patient, to ventilator care, haemodialysis, etc. This daily nursing care must be accompanied and augmented by daily medical care, which consists of examination and investigation of the patient. It is important to do more than merely view that patient and his charts from the end of the bed, as investigations can only supplement clinical medical knowledge. The patients should be examined by the resident doctor as often as necessary, depending on their condition, and further specialist attention sought if needed. Detailed attention should be paid to both fluid and electrolyte balance, which are accurately charted on the input and output charts. Routine investigations include chest x-ray, ECG, haemoglobin, full blood count, urea and electrolytes, blood gases and specific bacteriology. Other investigations, depending on the patients concerned, might include blood sugar, liver function tests, clotting factors, plasma cortisol, which may be done at intervals during the week rather than every day. Although patients in intensive care are looked after continuously and become familiar to the doctors and nurses, it must not be forgotton that unless the patients' condition improves and they progress daily, they are not getting better.

SEDATION IN INTENSIVE CARE

Intravenous sedative techniques are widely used in intensive care both in ventilated patients and those breathing spontaneously. It is important to assess the relative needs for sedation and analgesia, since opiate infusions may be required in addition to pure sedation. Benzodiazepines, particularly midazolam and diazepam, are frequently used to provide continuous sedation, but unlike the short-acting intravenous induction agents, their action may be considerably prolonged following cessation of infusion. They provide good cardiovascular stability and anxiolysis and in addition are potent amnesics, which may be of considerable advantage in the intensive-care situation.

Neuromuscular blockade may also be required in the restless head-injured or multiple trauma patient, but should only be given together with adequate sedation and analgesia. In patients with severe respiratory problems, in whom oxygen transfer is critically impaired, heavy sedation and neuromuscular blockade may be required to reduce oxygen consumption to a minimum.

PROBLEMS IN INTENSIVE CARE

Most problems occurring in intensive care, apart from the initial pathology, concern three main systems—cardiovascular, respiratory and renal. Neurological and alimentary problems may also occur but are less common. Cardiovascular problems may involve hypotension together with reduced cardiac output and may require supportive drug therapy and other measures to improve the peripheral circulation. Respiratory problems are largely concerned with respiratory failure and may lead to a decision to employ artificial ventilation or other forms of respiratory supplementation. These are often avoided by vigorous and regular physiotherapy, which is another benefit available in intensive care. Renal problems may necessitate fluid restriction, peritoneal or even haemodialysis, and siting an intensive care unit near the renal unit is logical.

Alimentary problems are mainly concerned with malabsorption resulting from nasogastric feeding and other nutritional problems which may require temporary parenteral feeding. Many of the neurological problems which occur, such as confusion, are often minimised by adequate communication with the patient in ways other than verbally. Nevertheless, many patients become very agitated by their lack of ability to communicate with those looking after them. Specific neurological lesions due to pressure on nerves, or corneal abrasions are not uncommon but are usually avoidable.

The coexistence of other diseases and previous drug treatment complicating the patient's condition must not be forgotten. These are often not available when the patient is initially admitted and it is important to consult relatives or the patient's own general practitioner as soon as possible to ascertain any potentially complicating additional pathology.

Other problems that occur in intensive care include those of coagulation, particularly in relation to disseminated intravascular coagulation following massive haemorrhage, shock lung or fat embolism (Chapter 26). Many patients in intensive care receive long-term intravenous therapy necessitating the use of central venous catheters, which are best maintained in a sterile condition in intensive care (Chapter 44). Some patients may require tracheostomy if prolonged ventilation is contemplated, and although the enthusiasm for this fluctuates between hospitals and countries, it is still a widely used technique.

Finally, it should not be forgotten that patients who are admitted to intensive care as a result of trauma and who are apparently untreatable may still become potential organ donors, an important factor when one considers the benefits of transplantation to the remainder of the population.

28 Anaesthesia for Ear, Nose and Throat Surgery

Surgical access. Other general principles. Individual operations.

The particular problem of operations on the nose and throat is that these operations take place on the upper respiratory tract. The anaesthetist must give the surgeon the best possible access, yet at the same time protect the lungs from soiling by blood and debris arising from the operation.

SURGICAL ACCESS

There are several techniques by which the anaesthetist can provide the surgeon with good access to the operation site.

Endotracheal Intubation

Where possible, a cuffed oral tube is used, but at times a nasal tube may be indicated. In addition to the cuff a throat pack helps to protect the upper larynx from blood and secretions.

Local Analgesia

This was formerly very popular in nose and throat surgery, many operations (e.g. tonsillectomy, nasal polypectomy, Caldwell–Luc operations and even laryngectomy) being possible under regional techniques. Most modern surgeons regard most of these operations as requiring considerable heroism on the part of the patient if carried out in this way, and now request general anaesthesia. However, the upper respiratory tract is highly vascular, and to reduce bleeding it is quite common to inject vascoconstrictor solutions, or to apply topical vascoconstrictor agents, e.g. liquid cocaine 5–10% or cocaine paste BPC 25%.

Some operations, especially on the larynx, may be carried out under general anaesthesia with, in addition, the topical spraying of a local analgesic solution on the operation site. The larynx is extremely sensitive, and this technique allows the use of lighter general anaesthesia.

Insufflation Anaesthesia

This involves blowing a gaseous anaesthetic mixture into the patient's upper respiratory tract. The patient breathes spontaneously, and dilutes the mixture with an amount of air depending on his tidal and minute volumes and the volume of anaesthetic mixture being provided. This was a popular method for administering nitrous oxide, oxygen and ether for tonsillectomy, the mixture usually being given via a side-tube on the Boyle-Davis gag.

A more modern version of this technique is sometimes used for laryngeal microsurgery by administering the anaesthetic through a small tube, e.g. a 12 or 14 FG suction catheter passed through the vocal cords so that the tip lies somewhere between the larynx and carina. With modern emphasis on atmospheric pollution by anaesthetic gases, this technique verges on the unacceptable.

Deep Anaesthesia

Another way to leave the operating field clear for the surgeon is to induce anaesthesia and deepen it to a plane depending on the operation to be carried out. The face mask is then removed and the surgeon performs his task as anaesthesia is lightening. Used in conjunction with topical analgesia of the larynx and trachea this gives the surgeon several minutes of excellent conditions to perform, for instance, a laryngoscopy. Used without the local analgesia this technique was also favoured when guillotine tonsillectomy was in fashion.

Injectors

The injector system described in Chapter 35 on p. 348 may be modified for use at laryngoscopy.

OTHER GENERAL PRINCIPLES

Premedication for nose and throat operations should be appropriate to the patient's needs. It is probably wise to err on the side of conservatism so that the patient more rapidly regains the ability to protect his own respiratory tract from soiling by blood or debris.

It is sometimes said that topical analgesia should not be applied to the larynx during ENT anaesthesia in case the patient inhales material from the pharynx at the end of the operation. Even so, it is obviously impossible to adhere strictly to this rule because anaesthesia in some cases depends to a greater or lesser degree on topical analgesia. Fortunately, once they have recovered from the general anaesthesia most patients seem to have a protective cough reflex arising from areas lower in the respiratory tract than those reached by the topical analgesia. For example, after thorough application of topical analgesia for bronchoscopy, the problem when the patient is wakening is to stop rather than start him coughing. On the other hand, there seems no point in routinely spraying the larynx with local analgesic solution for every nose and throat operation (e.g. for tonsillectomy) as satisfactory anaesthesia does not depend on it.

Patients who have undergone endotracheal anaesthesia should have regained their protective reflexes before extubation and it is important after throat and nose operations that all patients should recover in the lateral or semi-prone position.

Many ENT operations are performed with reduced theatre lighting, the patient's face usually being partly or completely hidden by surgical drapes. This makes careful observation of the patient's colour and vital signs more difficult than in many other anaesthetics and the anaesthetist must be particularly vigilant. Monitoring (Chapter 23) should be as comprehensive as possible, and at least for major cases, oximetry and capnography are desirable.

Induction and maintenance of anaesthesia should be smooth and rapid, straining and hypercarbia being prevented. The head and neck is a very vascular region, and any engorgement produced by coughing or a rise in PCO_2 may take many minutes to subside, with a prolonged deterioration of operating conditions. A wide choice of spontaneous or controlled respiration techniques is satisfactory for most ENT surgery but the surgeon may request hypotensive anaesthesia for some middle-ear or laryngeal operations.

INDIVIDUAL OPERATIONS

Tonsillectomy and Adenoidectomy

The (at times) near-barbaric guillotine tonsillectomy performed on the unsuspecting and often unpremedicated child has to most anaesthetists' relief largely given way to dissection tonsillectomy. For this the patient should come to the anaesthetic room adequately premedicated and anaesthesia be induced by the intravenous (or less commonly, the inhalational) route. Suxamethonium is usually used to introduce an orotracheal tube in younger children and a nasotracheal tube in older children and adults. A nasotracheal tube is contraindicated if adenoids are to be curetted. Maintenance is commonly with nitrous oxide, oxygen and halothane with spontaneous respiration, but other agents and controlled respiration are also satisfactory.

When diethyl ether was the common inhalational agent, an insufflation technique using a side-tube on the Boyle-Davis gag or a hollow hook in the corner of the mouth was most popular. If halothane—a much more powerful and insidious agent than ether—is used in this way, so great is the contamination of the air round the patient's face that some surgeons are scarcely fit to drive their cars after a morning of such cases!

Local analgesia is now seldom used for adult tonsillectomy. After the patient had sucked a local anaesthetic lozenge further topical analgesia of the oropharynx and tonsillar region was carried out with a 5% cocaine spray. Local analgesic solution was then injected into the posterior and anterior pillars of the tonsil with a special, curved 'tonsil' needle and, finally, injection lateral to the tonsil made with a straight needle. It could be a most satisfactory technique—but required the fortuitous meeting of the right patient, the right anaesthetist and the right surgeon.

Bleeding tonsil

Even after the careful technique of dissection tonsillectomy, a small proportion of the patients bleed a few hours after the operation. These patients (usually, but not invariably, small children) present one of the most frightening emergencies to face the anaesthetist and must be approached with the utmost care.

The child has usually lost a significant proportion of his blood volume, and much of this may be present in the stomach. An intravenous drip must always be set up, blood crossmatched and, if necessary, a blood transfusion started pre-operatively. Anaesthesia should be induced on the operating table with the child carefully held on his left side and the table about 15° head-down. An inhalational induction with nitrous oxide, oxygen and halothane is probably safest and usually very easy, the weak, often heavily sedated and exhausted child making little protest. Efficient pharyngeal suction must be instantly available. If vomiting or regurgitation occur, the face mask is removed, suction carried out and anaesthesia allowed to lighten until the episode has passed. Orotracheal intubation is carried out under the nitrous oxide, oxygen and halothane when anaesthesia is deep enough.

Some anaesthetists prefer a more typical 'crash induction' with thiopentone and suxamethonium after pre-oxygenation. The problem with this technique is that when the mouth is open the anaesthetist is often met with a confusing 'curtain' of blood and mucus and anxious moments may pass before he can see to pass the endotracheal tube.

Nasal Operations

The most common operations confined to the nose are the removal of nasal polyps and submucuous resection of the nasal septum (SMR). These operations are now usually carried out under general anaesthesia using an endotracheal tube and pharyngeal pack. In addition, it is usual to improve surgical access and reduce bleeding by the topical application of cocaine spray 5% or cocaine paste 25%—always taking care to stay within the safe dose of that drug.

Both these operations can be performed under local analgesia alone and various techniques have been described for applying liquid cocaine 5% to the points of entry of the nerves supplying the nasal cavity. For submucuous resection, whether under general or local analgesia, it is usual to inject a small amount of local analgesic with vasocontrictor deep to the mucous membrane of the septum to aid the dissection and reduce bleeding.

Operations on the Paranasal Sinuses

The same general anaesthetic technique as employed for nasal operations is used. The commonest sinus operation is the Caldwell–Luc operation on the maxillary antrum. For this operation, besides the general anaesthetic, cocaine spray or paste is applied to the nose as for nasal operations, as a drainage hole (antrostomy) is made between the sinus and nasal cavity. In addition, vasoconstrictor solution is injected into the gum over the canine fossa, this being the site of the surgical incision.

Even these quite extensive operations can be carried out under local analgesia. The nasal cavity is prepared as already described and, in addition, nerve blocks of various branches of the trigeminal nerve supplying the paranasal sinuses are required. Few modern surgeons, and even fewer patients, would contemplate these operations under local analgesia with the high standards of general anaesthesia now available.

Ear Operations

Many of these operations are now carried out with an operating microscope. The surgeon requires a quiet, uncongested operating field. A smooth, spontaneous respiration anaesthetic with the patient a few degrees head-up will often provide these conditions, but it is probably more reliable to avoid hypercarbia by controlled respiration.

Sometimes the surgeon may require hypotensive anaesthesia. Again a variety of techniques can provide this, but it must be remembered that a hypotensive patient in the reduced lighting conditions and under concealing drapes requires meticulous anaesthetic monitoring.

Microsurgery of the Larynx

Two of the techniques used for this surgery—insufflation anaesthesia through a small tube such as a suction catheter, or intermittent inflation using the Venturi principle—have already been mentioned. A third method involves the use of a special type of cuffed endotracheal tube, e.g. a Pollard tube. This tube, which is of latex with a reinforcing nylon spiral, is 10 mm wide in its proximal part. The distal part which passes through the vocal cords has a narrower diameter, giving the surgeon better access to the larynx and vocal cords. The cuff prevents blood and tissue entering the trachea from the operation site.

Lasers are now sometimes used to diathermy nodules on the vocal cords. If the beam comes in contact with the endotracheal tube it will cause it to ignite, and to prevent this eventuality it is necessary to wrap the tube in aluminium foil.

Tracheostomy

Tracheostomy (Chapter 35) may be an urgent life-saving procedure, or it may be done as a more elective operation to ensure long-term ventilation. In cases of dire emergency the surgeon may carry out the operation with no anaesthesia, but in less urgent cases local analgesia is satisfactory.

If upper respiratory obstruction is not too severe, the operation is more comfortably carried out under general anaesthesia. It is usually claimed that an inhalational induction and intubation is the safest, but if the lungs can be inflated after thiopentone induction by squeezing the reservoir bag it is safe to administer suxamethonium. A variety of sizes of endotracheal tubes with introducers should be available as the larynx may be narrowed or distorted.

Laryngectomy

The anaesthetic management of these cases depends on whether the patient has already had a tracheostomy performed. If so, the anaesthetist must replace the silver tube with a cuffed tracheostomy tube and then administer the anaesthetic by that means.

If the patient has not already had a tracheostomy, endotracheal anaesthesia is induced in the same way as described in the previous section. A problem may arise when the larynx is divided from the trachea and the anaesthetic system has to be transferred from the endotracheal tube to the newly inserted cuffed tracheostomy tube at the permanent tracheostomy site. It is vital that choice of sterile tracheostomy tubes and catheter mounts for connection to the anaesthetic machine be available and tested before the incision is made in the larynx. If the patient is breathing spontaneously, and if the trachea has been sprayed with local analgesic at induction, the transfer is usually straightforward. However, if IPPR is used, there may be some anxious moments when the endotracheal tube is partially withrawn from the larynx until the surgeon succeeds in replacing it with the cuffed tracheostomy tube.

It should also be borne in mind that the blood loss at these operations may be quite heavy, especially if there are lymph glands to be dissected out. Some of the patients may be very frail and careful monitoring is essential.

29 Anaesthesia for Eye Surgery

Intra-ocular pressure. Oculo-cardiac reflex. Other special features. Local analgesia. General anaesthesia. Common operations.

Although the most localised of all branches of surgery, there are nevertheless certain special features of anaesthesia for eye surgery that merit special consideration.

INTRA-OCULAR PRESSURE

The sclera and cornea together form the globe of the eye (Fig. 29.1), the contents of which are referred to as being 'intra-ocular'. The intra-ocular space is divided unequally into a smaller anterior part containing aqueous humour and a larger vitreous body containing vitreous humour. There is a constant production and removal of aqueous humour and in the important disease glaucoma, where the drainage of aqueous humour is obstructed, there is a pathological rise in intra-ocular pressure.

Factors Raising Intra-ocular Pressure

Two drugs whose mydriatic (pupil-dilating) action causes obstruction to free drainage of aqueous humour from the angle of

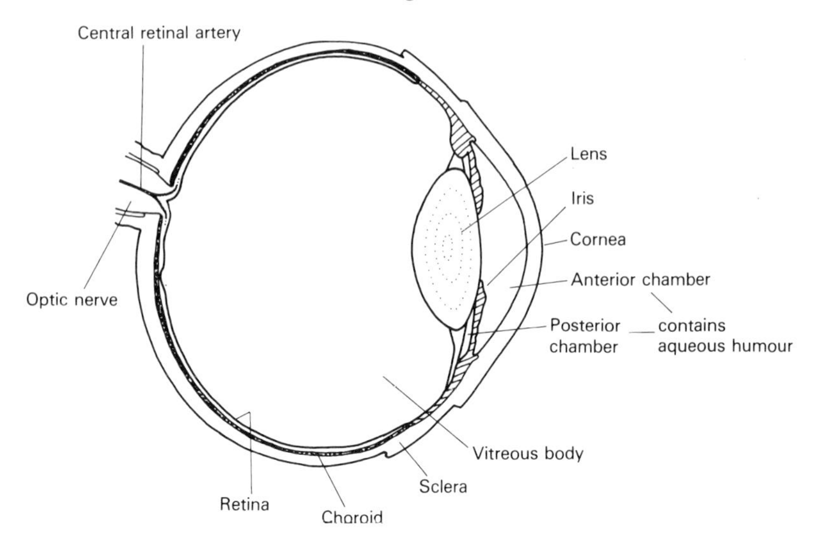

Fig. 29.1 The eye

the anterior chamber, thereby increasing intra-ocular pressure, are atropine and cocaine. These agents should therefore not be applied locally to the eye in glaucoma. Parenterally administered atropine is not considered to cause a significant increase in intra-ocular pressure.

The other anaesthetic agent in common use which causes a rise in intra-ocular pressure is suxamethonium. The rise is pressure in this case is caused by the extra-ocular muscles of the orbit squeezing the globe during their suxamethonium-induced fasciculation.

Other anaesthetic factors increasing intra-ocular pressure are venous engorgement due to coughing, vomiting, straining or a head-down tilt, hypoxia and hypercarbia. Extra-ocular causes are a peri-orbital haematoma produced when performing a retro-ocular block, and the pressure on the eye produced by the orbicularis oculi muscle when the patients screws up his eye—as might happen on wakening from an anaesthetic.

Factors Decreasing Intra-ocular Pressure

Falls in intra-ocular pressure tend to be less dramatic and are caused by most narcotic analgesics and general anesthetic agents.

Hypotension, hypocarbia and a head-up tilt are other factors decreasing the intra-ocular tension.

OCULO-CARDIAC REFLEX

Traction on the extra-ocular eye muscles (as inevitably occurs in squint operations) may cause cardiac dysrhythmias, bradycardia or even cardiac asystole. These reflex effects may be abolished by administering intravenous atropine in a dose of about 1 mg for an adult with a proportionately smaller dose for children. Subcutaneous or intramuscular atropine given as premedication does not reach a high enough blood level to give protection against these adverse effects.

OTHER SPECIAL FEATURES

Eye surgery, like ear, nose and throat surgery, is performed exclusively on the head and neck. Although the anaesthetist is not vying with the surgeon for the same area, the airway is somewhat inaccessible and the head and neck largely obscured. Particular vigilance is therefore required in monitoring the patient. Another feature of eye anaesthesia is that on no other operating list is the anaesthetist so likely to meet the extremes of age in one session. It is not unusual on one list to have patients ranging from small babies to the frail and elderly, the latter usually having cataract operations.

Ecothiopate Iodide

These are eye drops sometimes used in glaucoma and have a powerful anticholinesterase activity. A prolonged response to suxamethonium has been described after its use in patients using ecothiopate eye drops.

LOCAL ANALGESIA

Surface analgesia of the eye for operations on the conjunctiva and cornea is easily produced by local analgesic eye drops. Probably the most popular of these are the rather short-acting proxymetacaine (Ophthaine) 0·5%, amethocaine 0·5%, and lignocaine 4%, none of which dilate the pupil. Cocaine 2%, although it causes transient cloudiness of the cornea and dilation of the pupil, is still used at times because its powerful vascocontrictor action is useful for reducing oozing during operations on hyperaemic eyes.

Local infiltration with 0·5% lignocaine in 1:200 000 adrenaline gives excellent analgesia for operations on the eyelids. For intraocular operations good analgesia is readily obtained by topical analgesia of the conjunctival sac associated with a retro-ocular block using 2 ml local analgesic solution injected behind the eyeball.

If possible patients for eye surgery under local analgesia should be well sedated. Nevertheless, it must be remembered that many of these patients are frail and elderly and great care must be taken when prescribing drugs that may depress the cardiovascular or respiratory systems. It may be best to give a relatively modest premedication in the ward (e.g. small dose of pethidine and phenothiazine, or diazepam) and add tiny increments of further sedation intravenously in the anaesthetic room or operating theatre if required.

GENERAL ANAESTHESIA

As one of the most important factors in general anaesthesia for eye surgery is the avoidance of postoperative nausea and vomiting, many anaesthetists routinely include an anti-emetic in the premedication.

Provided that the considerations mentioned are taken into account various spontaneous and controlled ventilation anaesthetic techniques give excellent operating conditions for eye surgery. It is good practice to spray the vocal cords with topical local analgesic to minimise coughing at extubation or the possibility of straining on the endotracheal tube if anaesthesia is too light. With spontaneous respiration techniques the depth of anaesthesia must be sufficient for the eye to remain stationary.

COMMON OPERATIONS

Squint

These operations are nearly always carried out on small children, who should be well premedicated. Most anaesthetists would intubate after a thiopentone and suxamethonium induction, and maintain anaesthesia with nitrous oxide, oxygen and halothane. There are no other special features about these cases apart from taking precautions to suppress the oculo-cardiac reflex, as already discussed (p. 303).

Cataract Extraction and Lens Implant

The procedure of cataract extraction is now frequently accompanied by the implantation of a plastic replacement lens at the same operation. These patients are invariably elderly and surgery can be safely carried out under local analgesia. In addition to the technique described above, it is a wise routine to block the terminal branches of the facial nerve to the orbicularis oculi muscle. This avoids the possibility of the dangerous rise in intra-ocular pressure caused by the patient screwing up his eyes during or after the operation.

General anaesthesia must be carefully and gently given, taking into account the patient's age and any intercurrent disease. Intubation may be carried out with suxamethonium as the rise in intra-ocular pressure, which it causes, passes off in a few minutes. It should not be used again during the course of the anaesthetic. Maintenance of anaesthesia may be with spontaneous respiration or with a non-depolarising muscle relaxant. Alternatively, intubation and maintenance of anaesthesia may be carried out under a non-depolarising relaxant. Apart from spraying the larynx with local analgesic solution at intubation to prevent coughing when the endotracheal tube is removed at the end of the operation, it is also wise to keep anaesthesia deep enough at the end of the operation for extubation to be performed without inducing coughing. This is easier where a spontaneous respiration technique has been used.

While good anaesthetic technique and the use of anti-emetics postoperatively should minimise the extent of coughing, nausea and vomiting, fortunately, with modern improvements in surgical instruments and especially in suture materials, the danger of extrusion of intra-ocular contents has been much reduced.

Perforating Eye Injuries

These cases combine the danger of extrusion of the intra-ocular contents, should intra-ocular pressure rise, with the risks of vomiting and regurgitation inherent in any emergency anaesthetic. Probably most anaesthetists would feel that the safest compromise would be to intubate with suxamethonium and cricoid pressure but to give a small dose of a non-depolarising muscle relaxant first to reduce the rise in intra-ocular pressure caused by suxamethonium.

30 Dental Anaesthesia

Anaesthesia for out-patient dentistry. Chair anaesthetic techniques. Anaesthesia for in-patient dentistry.

ANAESTHESIA FOR OUT-PATIENT DENTISTRY

Many thousands of general anaesthetics are given every year in dental surgeries, mainly for extractions although some dentists undertake extensive conservation work under general anaesthesia. Many of these anaesthetics are given by general practitioners or other part-time anaesthetists who are often highly skilled at dental anaesthesia. Quite correctly, however, they are reluctant to treat anyone except the completely fit, and for this reason a great many of the patients referred to hospital dental departments are those thought unsuitable for chair anaesthesia in the dental surgery.

Successful and safe dental anaesthesia depends on using essentially simple techniques. Nevertheless, both the pre-operative preparation of the patients and the equipment available are often relatively inadequate. The anaesthetist takes on trust the fact that the patients are starved, and occasionally children have been given food or fluid early that morning by well-meaning parents despite instructions to the contrary. Resuscitation equipment in dental surgeries is often inadequate or absent and when present is used so infrequently that many of the drugs are out of date, or items of equipment such as laryngoscope batteries do not function.

CHAIR ANAESTHETIC TECHNIQUES

Patients anaesthetised in the dental chair are now usually anaesthetised supine, although some anaesthetists and dentists still prefer the patients in the sitting position. This may predispose to a vasovagal attack under anaesthesia, the consequences of which may be serious, if not fatal, when an acute fall in blood pressure goes unrecognised; for this reason the supine position is becoming more popular. It is essential to ensure that the patient can open his mouth sufficiently and has an unobstructed airway. Dental abscess with swelling leading to inadequate mouth opening may prove an extremely difficult problem when the patients are anaesthetised and relatively relaxed. If induction of anaesthesia is achieved intravenously, methohexitone, etomidate or Diprivan are commonly used, because all these drugs wear off quickly enough to allow the patient to leave the surgery shortly afterwards. Many children receive a gaseous induction, often only with nitrous oxide and oxygen if the extractions planned are expected to take 2–3 minutes. For prolonged anaesthesia halothane or enflurane are used to supplement the anaesthetic technique. Maintenance of anaesthesia, in almost every case, is therefore accomplished with nitrous oxide/oxygen and halothane or enflurane when necessary. Nasotracheal or orotracheal intubation in out-patient dental practice is uncommon and patients requiring such manoeuvres should normally be admitted to hospital. The use of nasal anaesthetic masks leaving the mouth free for operation is usual and a pharyngeal pack of either gauze or absorbent sponge should be used to prevent inhalation of blood or tooth fragments. It is vital to ensure that the pack is removed at the end of the procedure before the patient wakes up.

Invariably, patients are allowed to recover lying in the dental chair and are then usually returned to a nearby waiting room. Recovery areas are a rare luxury in out-patient dental anaesthesia except in purpose-built surgeries. Although not ideal, the patients are often allowed home within a short time of the anaesthetic, and for this reason must be accompanied by a responsible adult and encouraged to rest at home. They should not be allowed to go on public transport, drive a car, or do anything which might be dangerous as a result of relatively impaired judgement.

Continuous Intravenous Anaesthesia

Some dentists employ either continuous or intermittent administration of methohexitone, diazepam, or in some cases Diprivan, for either anaesthesia or sedation during prolonged periods of conservative dental treatment. Although they are often very skilled in these procedures, fatalities have occurred, largely before it was accepted that two experienced people needed to be present, one to carry out the dental treatment and the other to administer the anaesthetic agents and look after the airway. If this technique is to continue it is vital that adequate medically qualified staff are present.

Relative Analgesia

Many dentists now employ relative analgesia for sedation during dental treatment, particularly in children. Entonox (50% nitrous oxide, 50% oxygen) is administered through a nasal mask providing sedation and analgesia for extractions and conservation work. This is often augmented by local anaesthetic techniques. The dentists take considerable trouble to train children to tolerate relative analgesia, emphasising that with this technique they will not go to sleep. If the child is then subjected to a general anaesthetic involving gas induction, which to them is identical with relative analgesia, the fact that this technique has then been used to put them to sleep may well make them intolerant of relative analgesia in future. For this reason, perhaps intravenous inductions should be used more commonly for children in the future.

ANAESTHESIA FOR IN-PATIENT DENTISTRY

As already indicated, in-patient dental treatment is often necessary in patients who are either unfit for chair anaesthesia or who require extensive treatment. The commonest cases are multiple extractions, dental clearances, surgical removal of particularly difficult teeth, e.g. wisdom teeth (8s), and apicectomies or conservative dental treatment. Extensive operations such as mandibular osteotomy are often performed in major dental units. Many of these cases require prolonged anaesthesia and nasotracheal intubation is commonly used. In a hospital the patients are pre-operatively prepared in the standard fashion and benefit from full premedication, their operative treatment usually being too major for them to be treated as day cases. It is important also to examine the patients pre-operatively to ensure an adequate degree of mouth opening.

Anaesthetic Technique

Most patients presenting for in-patient dental treatment are young or middle-aged adults and for this reason intravenous induction is usually employed. Thiopentone, methohexitone or Diprivan are usually followed by suxamethonium to facilitate nasotracheal intubation. This may often, however, be achieved in a spontaneously breathing patient by the blind nasal technique. Most anaesthetists prefer a plain uncuffed nasal tube for dental treatment, resorting to the cuff only when major oral work or maxillofacial work is required. A good pharyngeal pack is essential and the patients are then commonly allowed to breathe nitrous oxide/oxygen and halothane or enflurane spontaneously for the duration of the operation. Intravenous infusion is not usually employed except during extensive surgery, e.g. osteotomy, although an indwelling needle is essential. The use of hypotensive anaesthetic techniques and the precautions necessary when the jaws are wired together postoperatively, are discussed in Chapter 31.

Extubation is carried out with the patient lying on his side, the nasotracheal tube being withdrawn into the oropharynx to provide an adequate airway until the patient is fully recovered. Several problems may occur in the immediate postoperative period. Patients often feel nauseated and may vomit, so anti-emetics are widely used. After extractions (particularly of the molar teeth) which are often traumatic, soft tissue swelling and inability to open the mouth is common. This may be a particular problem in a patient who requires to be re-anaesthetised after extractions. Postoperative pain is often considerable and the patients require adequate analgesia. Some oral surgeons are now infiltrating the empty sockets with bupivacaine 0·75% to provide prolonged analgesia after surgical extraction, to good effect. It is also possible to dislocate the lower jaw during intubation or operative treatment and it is important to check that this has been reduced before the patient is allowed to recover from the anaesthetic.

In some centres, day-case oral surgery is becoming popular, particularly with the advent of short-acting drugs such as Diprivan, alfentanil and isoflurane. Although unpremedicated, full general anaesthesia with nasotracheal intubation and pharyngeal packing is necessary, together with full recovery facilities. The patient may require anything up to six hours to recover fully and even then facilities must exist for overnight admission if he or she is unfit to return home.

Several patients presenting for in-patient dental treatment do so because they suffer from medical conditions that make them unfit for out-patient dentistry. Dental clearance is common in patients with congenital or acquired heart disease before operative correction under cardiopulmonary bypass, and anaesthesia in these cases may require specialised techniques. Pre-oxygenation and very small doses of intravenous induction agents are essential if hypoxia and hypotension are to be prevented.

Mentally retarded or psychologically disturbed patients are often referred for in-patient hospital treatment and, apart from the problems in communicating with these patients and in getting them to accept dental anaesthesia, it is important to consider their mental condition and consequently the drug therapy that they may be receiving. Many may be epileptic, in which case methohexitone is contraindicated, or may be on several psychiatric drugs, for example tricyclic antidepressants or monoamine oxidase inhibitors, the latter being contraindicated in anaesthesia (Chapter 16). Children with Down's syndrome or other congenital abnormalities may also have heart disease and it is important to have adequate documentation of such patients before anaesthesia. Patients with other congenital conditions, such as blood coagulation defects and blood disorders such as sickle cell disease, also present for in-patient dental anaesthesia, and again adequate pre-operative screening is essential if disasters are to be avoided.

31 Anaesthesia for Plastic and Maxillo-facial Surgery

Plastic surgery. Microvascular surgery. Maxillo-facial surgery. Cranio-facial reconstruction.

PLASTIC SURGERY

Although general anaesthetic techniques for plastic surgery do not differ greatly from those commonly used, additional drugs and manoeuvres are often employed specifically to reduce blood loss. While plastic surgery on the limbs is often carried out under tourniquet, a small amount of bleeding in an operation on a highly vascular area (e.g. the face) can be extremely troublesome. Elective drug-induced hypotension during anaesthesia is discussed in Chapter 15, but certain additional techniques are often employed during plastic surgery. These are mainly designed to reduce the possibility of venous congestion in the operative site, and also to a certain extent to reduce systemic blood pressure. A smooth anaesthetic technique which avoids coughing, straining or other manoeuvres likely to raise venous pressure during induction is vital. Where possible the operative site is placed at a higher level than the heart, e.g. in facial surgery the patient is tilted foot-down. Carbon dioxide, being a potent vasodilator, must not be allowed to accumulate and for this reason the patients are often either ventilated or allowed to breathe spontaneously round a circle system containing soda-lime to absorb the carbon dioxide produced.

The drugs used are commonly those which produce a slow fall and rise in systemic blood pressure, since rapid alterations may well produce reactionary haemorrhage and bleeding under the skin flaps towards the end of the operation. The surgical technique may include local infiltration of solutions containing adrenaline to produce localised vasoconstriction and therefore reduction in bleeding, and it is important to monitor the patients for possible dysrhythmias which may result from inadvertent intravenous injection of adrenaline.

The techniques of intubation and pharyngeal packing for plastic surgery operations may require considerable skill, particularly in patients with facial deformities or those in whom misplacement of the larynx may make conventional direct laryngoscopy impossible. Blind nasal intubation is often carried out for such procedures and it is important to have an adequate range of endotracheal tubes, both nasal and oral, available. Intra-oral or intra-nasal haemorrhage will require control by oropharyngeal packs, which are inserted at induction and which must be checked for removal before the patient is extubated. These may either be of absorbent gauze or sponge and are used in conjunction with both cuffed and uncuffed nasal intubation.

The anaesthetic requirements of emergency maxillo-facial and other plastic surgical operations on the head and neck are similar. The importance of a smooth induction and maintenance of anaesthesia are rightly emphasised, but a stormy and partially obstructed recovery phase may be equally detrimental. A smooth and gradual return of blood pressure to normal levels helps to prevent reactionary haemorrhage, and a clear airway prevents respiratory obstruction, venous congestion and carbon dioxide retention.

MICROVASCULAR SURGERY

Recent advances in the use of operating microscopes and surgical techniques have led to many operations being performed in which free musculo-cutaneous flaps are grafted, together with anastomosis of their blood supply. Such operations, both elective and emergency, following trauma, are extremely time consuming, particularly if several microvascular anastomoses are being performed as in reconstructive surgery following traumatic digital amputation.

Anaesthesia for these cases requires special attention in two main areas. The prolonged use of certain anaesthetic drugs and gases may lead to tolerance or to toxic effects such as bone marrow defression from nitrous oxide or pulmonary atelectasis and collapse due to denitrogenation. Secondly, the physiological problems of fluid balance, temperature regulation, humidification, posture and pressure sores must be specifically treated since such operations may last in excess of 12–18 hours.

MAXILLO-FACIAL SURGERY

Although most maxillo-facial operations are carried out electively some time after acute trauma, it is important to ensure that the patient has an empty stomach, particularly where there is a possibility of them having swallowed blood or other foreign bodies. In many cases the operative technique involves wiring together the upper and lower jaws to stabilise fractures, and postoperative vomiting could be disastrous. For this reason, a pre-operative anti-emetic is frequently prescribed. Some anaesthetists also employ metoclopramide to help with gastric emptying immediately before anaesthesia. In patients whose postoperative airway maybe in doubt, elective intra-operative tracheostomy may well be considered, and in patients in whom severe facial swelling and oedema or other injuries may be involved (e.g. cervical fractures), pre-operative tracheostomy may be necessary. In such cases premedication is avoided to guard against the dangers of respiratory depression, but most other patients benefit from pre-operative sedation and drying of the mouth. Since some of these patients may require a hypotensive anaesthetic, premedication with atropine, which may cause tachycardia, is best avoided.

As in plastic surgery, it is vital to achieve a smooth induction and maintenance of anaesthesia, avoiding carbon dioxide retention and venous congestion. A longer-acting intravenous induction agent (e.g. thiopentone) is usually most satisfactory, although in patients whose airway is in doubt, and hence where a transient apnoea caused by thiopentone may be dangerous, gaseous induction of anaesthesia is usually safer. Muscle relaxation using suxamethonium before intubation is again used only when there is no doubt about the possibility of being able to ventilate the patient artificially with a mask and airway should intubation prove impossible.

As it is usually important that the patient be awake at the end of the operation immediately before extubation, particularly when the jaws have been wired together, most anaesthetists favour a relaxant and fentanyl technique using IPPV. This technique not only allows the patient to be awake in the immediate postoperative period, but also prevents excessive rises in CO_2 and reduce the possibility of venous congestion. The patient is placed on the table in the head-up position, which again helps to reduce venous pressure in the operative field. A streamlined cuffed nasal tube is usually used to intubate patients for maxillo-facial surgery, since this not only allows artificial ventilation, which is relatively difficult through an uncuffed nasal tube with the correspondingly large leak, but also seals the airway and, together with a good pharyngeal pack, prevents aspiration of blood and other debris.

Considerable blood loss may occur during maxillo-facial surgery, despite the use of hypotensive techniques in conjunction with a conventional and impeccable anaesthetic. It is important to set up a good intravenous infusion because the patient may need blood transfusion. Direct arterial blood pressure monitoring may be extremely useful in these operations, which are often prolonged and during which elective hypotension may be employed.

Postoperatively the patients should be looked after in a recovery room or intensive-care unit for several hours, as the not uncommon postanaesthetic complications of nausea and vomiting, restlessness and hypotension may all be much more difficult to deal with in a patient in whom the jaw has been wired together. It is important that the nurses be made aware of which wires link the upper and lower jaw and are supplied with a pair of wirecutters with which to separate the upper and lower jaws in an emergency.

CRANIO-FACIAL RECONSTRUCTION

Cranio-facial reconstruction for the treatment of severe anatomical abnormalities, usually congenital in origin, is now becoming a more widely used technique, although only in specialised centres. It combines all the problems of maxillo-facial surgery and neurosurgery, together with those related to prolonged anaesthesia for microvascular surgery. The patients are frequently children, often with other congenital abnormalities and cardiac defects and may be technically extremely difficult to anaesthetise and intubate. The surgical techniques involved are unique and the requirements of each operation related particularly to airway management must be discussed with the surgeon on an individual basis.

32 Anaesthesia for Patients with Renal and Hepatic Disease

Renal disease. Renal failure and renal transplantation. Hepatic and renal function related to anaesthesia. Patients with hepatic failure.

RENAL DISEASE

Routine urological surgery does not normally require specialist anaesthetic techniques, but many patients presenting for prostatectomy and other urological procedures are elderly and suffer from other diseases, particularly of the cardiovascular and respiratory systems. Careful pre-operative assessment is important to ensure their fitness for anaesthesia and particularly their ability to tolerate mildly hypotensive techniques which are commonly used for prostatic surgery. Lumbar extradural or spinal anaesthesia is often used to decrease intra-operative blood loss and hypotense the patient mildly. Patients with a history of cardiovascular or cerebrovascular disease are unsuitable for such procedures. Papillary carcinoma of the bladder is usually treated by repeat cystoscopy and cystodiathermy, and as these patients have a high incidence of repeat anaesthesia, the possibility of hepatotoxicity from multiple exposures to halothane must also be borne in mind.

Operations on the upper urinary tract and kidney involve

careful positioning of the patient in the lateral position, and breaking the table to permit maximum exposure of the loin. Other problems of urological anaesthesia relate to specific features of renal disease. These may be summarised as impaired or absent excretion of water, electrolytes, urea and many drugs. This may be accompanied by reduced production of erythropoietin, which controls the formation of red blood cells, and excess production of renin, which through the renin-angiotensin mechanism controls arterial blood pressure (Chapter 2). Excess renin production produces hypertension, renin release being stimulated by a fall in renal perfusion, the reflex being designed to maintain kidney blood flow. Abnormal renin production may occur as a result of renal artery stenosis.

RENAL FAILURE AND RENAL TRANSPLANTATION

Impaired or absent renal function produces not only disorders of fluid and electrolyte balance but also alteration in the levels of renally produced hormones. The patients are therefore anaemic, acidotic and often hypertensive and may present considerable problems during anaesthesia.

Pre-operative Considerations

The patients are often extremely nervous and used to hospitals because they have had many previous admissions. In addition, the excitement of a possible transplant after many years on dialysis leaves them far from calm.

Cardiovascular problems may include hypertension—often treated by β-blockade and α-methyldopa or ACE inhibitors, e.g. captopril (Chapter 14)—mild congestive cardiac failure and sometimes even pulmonary oedema. It is important to control potential cardiovascular problems by pre-operative dialysis to remove excessive fluid.

Metabolically, the problems of uraemia, acidosis and hyperkalaemia must be controlled pre-operatively by dialysis if anaesthesia is to be uneventful. As postoperative dialysis includes locally heparinising the patient, this is best avoided until the second or third postoperative day to prevent possible haemorrhage at the operative site resulting from systemic absorption of the heparin. Immediate pre-operative treatment is therefore essential. Increased calcium excretion and secondary hyperparathyroidism may also result from renal disease.

Routine drug therapy in patients with renal disease may include antihypertensives, diuretics and in some cases steroids, which must be maintained intra-operatively in the normal way (Chapter 16). The anaemia which results from renal disease is chronic, resulting from a decreased production of erythropoietin. These patients can compensate for their chronic anaemia in several ways, and the combination of anaemia and acidosis, in particular, maintains tissue oxygen delivery. For this reason, it is essential for patients to maintain their mild acidosis during operation, as correction to normal values will impair tissue oxygenation.

Pre-operative Information

Although many patients in renal failure will be starved and pre-operatively prepared in the usual way, certain information is important. Details of the time when the patients last ate or drank, the time of their last dialysis and their current drug therapy, are all essential. It is important also to have measurements of their current urea and electrolytes and haemoglobin after their last dialysis treatment, together with their age, post-dialysis weight and blood pressure. Many patients are often given a resonium enema pre-operatively to reduce their serum potassium concentration, as hyperkalaemia is probably the most serious intra-operative complication. If major surgery is planned, pre-operative crossmatching, usually involving red cells specially prepared for the patient, must be carried out well in advance and the site of the patient's arteriovenous dialysis fistula must be known so that blood flow through it can be protected.

Anaesthetic Technique

Oral premedication is usual in these patients, since intramuscular injections may produce haematomata following systemic absorption of the local heparinisation used during dialysis. Intra-operative steroid cover may also be necessary in certain cases. Intravenous induction is carried out using an intravenous infusion of normal saline placed under local anaesthetic in the back of the hand, saline being preferred to 5% dextrose. It is important to avoid using forearm or anticubital veins because these may be needed later for dialysis treatment. Pre-oxygenation is followed by a thiopentone, fentanyl, relaxant sequence, usually with atracurium. The introduction of this non-depolarising neuromuscular blocking drug, which is uniquely metabolised in plasma and the duration of action of which is therefore independent of renal function, has contributed considerably to the anaesthetic technique in these patients. Suxamethonium is usually avoided as it produces a rise in serum potassium following muscle fasciculation, although it may be specifically indicated in certain circumstances where the patient is inadequately prepared or starved.

IPPV maintaining the $P\text{CO}_2$ at the patient's normal level is used to avoid alterations in the chronic metabolic acidosis which facilitates oxygen delivery to the tissues.

Routinely, 66% nitrous oxide in oxygen is used, although some anaesthetists may supplement this with a small dose of halothane or isoflurane, and indeed may ventilate the patient with a volatile agent without using relaxants. Non-depolarising muscle relaxants tend to be partly metabolised in the liver and partly excreted unchanged in the kidneys; for this reason their action may be excessively prolonged in patients with renal failure. However, the patients are usually reasonably fit and require an adequate dose of relaxant to achieve muscle relaxation. It is important therefore to administer relaxants only at the beginning of the operation, since it is usually incremental administration during the procedure which results in inadequate reversal at the end unless atracurium is used. Central venous pressure monitoring may also be used, particularly in anephric patients, unable to excrete fluid load, because postoperative fluid balance may be critical for maintaining an adequate blood flow through the fistula.

The arteriovenous fistula is the patient's lifeline to dialysis: flow must therefore be maintained to avoid clotting. Avoiding hypotension due to hypovolaemia or cardiac depression is essential. Local techniques include wrapping the arm in warm gamgee or a stellate ganglion block to increase blood flow to the arm.

Intra-operative monitoring should include ECG—particularly to detect hyperkalaemia (peaked T waves)—and measurement of arterial blood pressure. This should always be by an indirect method as the use of arterial lines, particularly in the arm, may damage an artery potentially suitable for fistula formation.

HEPATIC AND RENAL FUNCTION RELATED TO ANAESTHESIA

Many drugs administered as part of routine anaesthesia undergo some metabolism in the liver before being extracted by the kidneys. The link between adequate hepatic and renal function is therefore important when considering the doses of drugs to be given and their normal duration of action. Non-depolarising muscle relaxants, in particular, demonstrate this balance between metabolism and excretion, and if one or other organ's function is impaired then the other will compensate. This means that additional hepatic metabolism will occur in renal failure and vice versa, although both processes may take considerably longer.

The liver is not only involved with metabolising drugs, but also in generating and maintaining adequate concentrations of plasma proteins, these having many functions including the binding of certain drugs (Chapter 3). The degree of protein binding influences the potency and duration of the action of various drugs, and inadequate hepatic function may produce hypoproteinaemia and thus impaired protein binding.

The liver also synthesises prothrombin, and hepatic failure may be complicated by disorders of coagulation.

Inadequate renal function inevitably produces problems of fluid and electrolyte excretion, as well as influencing the duration of action of various drugs that depend on renal excretion in the unchanged form. It is particularly important during anaesthesia to ensure that there is no renal failure as a result of hypovolaemia, as this may mimic renal failure in the patient with normal renal function.

PATIENTS WITH HEPATIC FAILURE

The importance of the liver in drug metabolism, plasma protein synthesis and blood coagulation has already been discussed. Nevertheless, as the liver is normally capable of regeneration and therefore ultimately of regaining normal function, it is essential that any anaesthetic technique should not produce more hepatic damage. Careful use of drugs, particularly induction agents, analgesics and muscle relaxants—all of which are metabolised to a greater or less degree in the liver—is essential. However, the most important factor is to maintain an adequate hepatic blood flow and therefore oxygen supply.

The liver receives two-thirds of its blood supply from the portal vein arising from the splanchnic circulation, and one-third from the normal arterial supply. Normal portal blood flow and oxygenation is therefore an important factor in avoiding further hepatic damage during operation. Catecholamine release, which is produced by several anaesthetic agents, will produce splanchnic vasoconstriction and a reduction in portal flow, whereas other agents which produce splanchnic vasodilation (e.g. halothane, enflurane and isoflurane), are more likely to maintain normal oxygenation of the liver. This is in strange contrast to the normally held view that halothane is toxic to the liver and emphasises that hepatotoxicity is an extremely rare phenomenon, and that in normal circumstances halothane is a good maintainer of hepatic blood flow.

Hepatic failure sometimes results in renal failure, thought to be caused by the need to excrete high levels of bilirubin. Hepatorenal failure may occur in jaundiced patients and for this reason diuretics, particularly mannitol, are often given together with a fluid load immediately pre-operatively to protect against the development of this syndrome.

33 Anaesthesia for Abdominal and Gynaecological Surgery

Anatomy. Techniques of anaesthesia. Postoperative nausea and vomiting. Gynaecological surgery.

A chapter devoted mainly to anaesthesia for abdominal surgery is justified because it embraces a high proportion of elective and emergency anaesthesia; some of the special features of emergency anaesthesia are discussed in Chapter 26. The triad of anaesthesia—narcosis, analgesia and muscular relaxation—is referred to in Chapter 1 and it is during anaesthesia for abdominal surgery that provision of good muscular relaxation is of paramount importance to aid surgical access. The methods of achieving this are described below.

ANATOMY

The skin and muscles of the abdominal wall are supplied mainly by the lower intercostal nerves. However, it is more important to have some knowledge of the segmental levels of the spinal cord which supply the various almost horizontal strips of skin, called 'dermatomes', at the various levels. Figure 33.1 shows that the skin in the region of the xyphisternum is supplied from the 6th

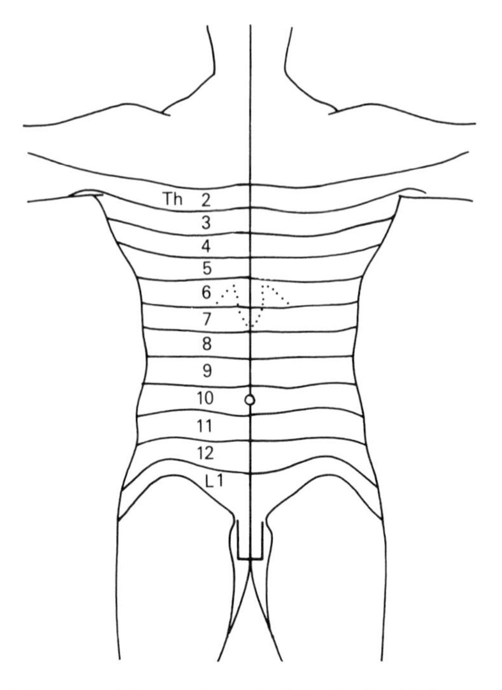

Fig. 33.1 Segmental innervation of abdominal wall dermatomes

thoracic segment, the umbilical level is innervated from T10 and it is not until the suprapubic region that the 1st lumbar segment is involved. The reasons for this perhaps surprising innervation of the anterior abdominal wall by thoracic nerves is that these intercostal nerves follow the ribs until the latter swing upwards in the form of their costal cartilages or, in the case of the lower ribs, end floating freely. The intercostal nerves continue forwards in the line of their earlier pathway in company with the posterior part of the ribs, and this leads them round onto the front of the abdomen where they supply almost horizontal dermatomes. The innervation of the abdominal wall by thoracic and the 1st lumbar segments of the spinal cord means that for any spinal or epidural block to be effective for surgery on the abdomen, some sympathetic nerve fibres must also be blocked with vasodilation and a tendency to hypotension.

The peritoneum is a serous membrane consisting of two layers resembling a deflated plastic bag. The anterior layer (the parietal peritoneum) lines the inner aspect of the anterior abdominal wall, while the posterior layer (the visceral peritoneum) closely invests the viscera which protrude into it from behind. If they protrude far enough into the peritoneum it meets again behind them to form a mesentery. The parietal and visceral layers of peritoneum are usually closely applied to each other, being separated only by a little serous fluid. The potential space between the two layers is readily converted into a real one by the entry of air at operation, or by the injection of carbon dioxide or other gas through a needle into the closed abdomen—as occurs during laparoscopy.

The parietal peritoneum is supplied by nerve fibres from the same segments that supply the overlying skin. Like the underlying viscera the visceral peritoneum is normally insensitive to cutting or burning, but the nerve endings in the viscera and mesenteries do register pain in response to inflammation and stretching.

Sensory Innervation of the Viscera

Sensory nerve fibres from the abdominal viscera are carried along two pathways—the sympathetic and the parasympathetic. The sensory nerves which run with the sympathetic nerves pass through the coeliac plexus and then in the greater, lesser and least splanchnic nerves to the sympathetic chain and thence to the spinal cord at the T5–12 segments (Figs 33.2 and 41.1).

The parasympathetic component travels in two parts—a larger vagal part carrying sensation from most of the abdominal viscera, including the alimentary canal down to the transverse colon and a smaller pelvic part carrying sensation from the rest of the bowel and the pelvic organs via the pelvic splanchnic nerves to the 2nd, 3rd and 4th sacral segments of the spinal cord. The vagal component (like the sympathetic) passes through the coeliac plexus, but then passes through the thoracic cavity and neck to the brain without ever joining the spinal cord. Thus, while spinal or epidural analgesia to the level of the 5th thoracic segment will produce complete block of the sympathetic component of intra-abdominal sensation, it has no effect on the vagal component, which can be blocked only by infiltration of local analgesic into the coeliac plexus, or into the vagal trunks higher in the abdomen or in the neck.

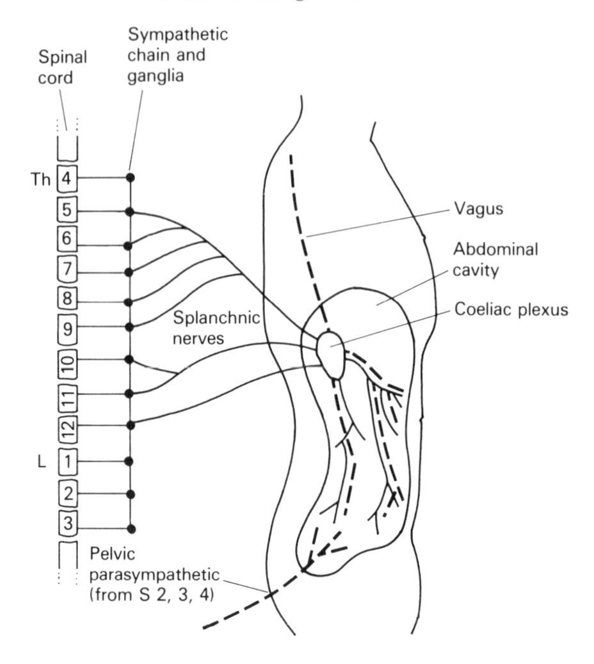

Fig. 33.2 Pathways of abdominal sensory nerves

In summary, the nature and distribution of sensory nerves within the abdominal cavity allows gentle handling, cutting and suturing of uninflamed viscera, provided that no tension is put on mesenteries, without either sympathetic or parasympathetic blockade. Rougher handling, or surgery on inflamed viscera, requires full blockade of both sympathetic and parasympathetic pathways.

TECHNIQUES OF ANAESTHESIA

Most abdominal surgery is made easier by (indeed, some operations are impossible without) good muscular relaxation. The only common exceptions are elective operations for inguinal or femoral hernia repairs. For these, the mild degree of relaxation associated with a spontaneous respiration anaesthetic using nitrous oxide, oxygen and about 1% halothane should be sufficient and is preferred by some anaesthetists.

Like all striated muscle that of the abdominal wall musculature tends to be in a state of less than full relaxation: this is called muscle tone. This tone in the muscles may be raised to much stronger levels of contraction in response to noxious stimuli sending large numbers of impulses up the sensory nerves to the spinal cord. There, the information is transmitted to the motor side of the spinal cord, whence impulses are carried down the motor nerves and across the neuromuscular junctions to the muscle fibres. This sensory-to-motor reflex arc has to be broken to produce muscular relaxation and this can be done on the sensory side, the motor side or both of them or, nowadays, most effectively at the neuromuscular junction. Some of the techniques of anaesthesia producing relaxation are discussed below.

Spontaneous Respiration Anaesthesia

Spontaneous respiration anaesthesia with single agents (e.g. chloroform, ether, or, more recently, cyclopropane) was the classical method of providing anaesthesia for abdominal surgery. Unfortunately, good muscular relaxation with these agents is produced only in the deepest planes of anaesthesia—indeed, only when the patient is near respiratory arrest. For prolonged upper abdominal surgery such as a gastrectomy, so great was the necessary 'soaking' with these powerful agents that the patients tended to be drowsy and sick for hours afterwards, with a high incidence of respiratory and venous embolic phenomena. As a result, and as anaesthetic techniques improved, this type of anaesthesia for abdominal surgery has largely disappeared from the medically advanced parts of the world. However, in less well-endowed areas, it may still be acceptable to use one of these agents (di-ethyl ether) because it is so safe. Even then, it may often be possible to administer it from an accurate and temperature-compensated vaporiser like the EMO (Chapter 10).

Muscle Relaxant Anaesthesia

Muscle relaxants transformed anaesthesia for abdominal surgery, great depths of anaesthesia no longer being necessary. Excellent operating conditions may be obtained with the lightest of general anaesthesia from which the patient quickly recovers. With the possible exception of herniorrhaphies, as mentioned above, it is customary to perform endotracheal intubation for most abdominal operations and this may be done with either suxamethonium or one of the non-depolarising relaxants. Relaxation is usually maintained by using one of the latter group. The question is, how light should the general anaesthesia be? If only nitrous oxide and oxygen are used for maintaining anaesthesia, the patient may be aware at some stage during the operation. There is no doubt, therefore, that the nitrous oxide should be supplemented with additional anaesthetic either as a trace of an inhalational agent, or a parenteral analgesic like fentanyl or pethidine. However, even with the anaesthesia deepened in this way some patients show varying degrees of pallor, sweating, or bradycardia which suggests that noxious stimuli are being produced by surgical manipulations, especially traction on mesenteries. How much harm this causes the patient is impossible to assess, but it is customary in these circumstances to give additional analgesia or atropine or both. Atropine abolishes the bradycardia by blocking the cardiac vagus and stops the sweating because the nerves to the sweat glands, although sympathetic, are cholinergic.

Regional Techniques

As methods of producing muscular relaxation for abdominal surgery, spinal and epidural analgesia have been much less used since the advent of muscle relaxants. Both techniques tend to produce relaxation by blocking the sensory side of the reflex arc. The local analgesic agents for producing spinal block are usually powerful enough to produce motor block, so that side of the reflex arc is also broken. The drugs used for epidural analgesia, on the other hand, do not usually produce such intense motor block so that more muscle tone may remain, especially in response to painful impulses being carried up the unblocked vagal pathways. This problem may be overcome if light general anesthesia is added to the regional blockade and excellent operating conditions may be provided in this way, especially for operations requiring muscle relaxation combined with some degree of hypotension, e.g. Wertheim's hysterectomy or abdominoperineal resection of the rectum.

Abdominal relaxation may also be achieved by more peripheral nerve blocks, e.g. multiple, bilateral intercostal blocks. This method needs supplementation with light general anaesthesia because neither the sympathetic nor parasympathetic (vagal) fibres are blocked by these injections.

POSTOPERATIVE NAUSEA AND VOMITING

Inclusion of this subject in this chapter does not imply that the problem is confined to abdominal surgery.

The aetiology of postoperative nausea and vomiting is complicated, with a great many contributing factors. These include the personality of the patient, his pre-operative state, the nature and extent of the operation, premedication, anaesthetic agents and postoperative drugs. Postoperative vomiting has by no means disappeared with modern anaesthetic techniques but the incidence, severity and duration have been reduced.

Prevention and Treatment

In patients known to have suffered from postoperative vomiting in the past, prevention starts with a carefully taken history of previous anaesthetics and, if possible, a perusal of the notes to try to identify some premedicant drug or anaesthetic agent which is associated with the problem. Avoiding this trigger may be all that is necessary, but if no definite cause can be found it may be wise to be sparing with pethidine or opiates in the premedication, or to give an anti-emetic with the premedication, during the operation or in the early postoperative period. It must be remembered that all anti-emetics tend to produce drowsiness and therefore will delay full recovery from the anaesthetic. They also tend to produce hypotension and may have other undesirable side effects (see below).

Treatment should never be started until it has been established that there is no surgical cause for the nausea or vomiting. Most anti-emetics in common use are phenothiazine derivatives and they are usually given by injection. Examples with adult dosage are perphenazine (Fentazin) 2·5–5·0 mg, metoclopramide (Maxolon, Primperan) 10 mg and prochlorperazine (Stemetil) 12·5 mg. At times all these drugs have been reported as causing untoward side-effects which are extrapyramidal in nature. These include oculogyric crises, in which the eyes roll upwards and only the whites are visible, trismus and spasm of the back muscles which may be severe enough to cause opisthotonus. The spasms may be severe enough to cause hypoxia and, with the trismus, are often mistaken for tetanus. Fortunately, if correctly diagnosed this condition is readily treated by injecting an anti-parkinsonian agent like benztropine (Cogentin) 1–2 mg intravenously. Anti-emetic drugs are considered individually in Chapter 13.

These reactions are commoner in teenagers and younger children, so it is wise to use anti-emetics sparingly in these age groups. Even in adults it is advisable to prescribe only two or three doses before reviewing the effect. If persistent nausea or vomiting continues another cause should be sought, and if none is found a change to a different anti-emetic made.

GYNAECOLOGICAL SURGERY

This consists essentially of lower abdominal and vaginal surgery. The anaesthetic techniques required for abdominal gynaecological surgery do not differ from those for other abdominal procedures. The possible exception is Wertheim's hysterectomy, where the haemorrhage associated with the extensive dissection of pelvic lymph glands may be reduced by a hypotensive technique. Of the various methods available the classical (and still possibly the best) method is a high spinal block with light general anaesthesia.

For vaginal surgery a wide choice of techniques using spontaneous or controlled ventilation are acceptable. Major vaginal operations, however (e.g. vaginal hysterectomy) may be haemorrhagic, especially in premenopausal patients, and the surgeon may request hypotensive anaesthesia.

Also included in the vaginal operations are the various operations associated with abortions, both spontaneous or therapeutic. In these cases it must be remembered that bleeding from the cavity of the uterus may occur for the same reasons as mentioned in Chapter 39 on obstetric anaesthesia, and that halothane in particular should be avoided.

One real gynaecological emergency is a ruptured ectopic pregnancy. The bleeding varies in extent, but at its most severe may be one of the most frightening emergencies with which an anaesthetist has to deal. Attempts must always be made to resuscitate the patient, but in the most severe cases proper restoration of the blood pressure cannot be achieved until laparotomy is performed and salpingectomy carried out on the side from which the bleeding is occurring.

Laparoscopy

Laparoscopy has been increasingly used in recent years in general surgery and gynaecology, both for diagnostic and therapeutic purposes. In gynaecology one of its diagnostic uses is in the differential diagnosis of an acute abdominal emergency thought to be an ectopic pregnancy, and its commonest use is for laparoscopic tubal sterilisation.

The basis of the technique is to introduce gas into the peritoneal cavity with a needle, so that the abdominal or pelvic viscera fall away from the anterior abdominal wall. The laparoscope can then be more safely passed and the abdominal contents visualised. Some of the complications, e.g. damage to a blood vessel by the needle, are directly related to the technique, but there are others which are related more to the anaesthetic.

The gas generally used is carbon dioxide, or less commonly nitrous oxide. The reason for choosing one of these gases is that they are highly diffusible and so are rapidly absorbed into the circulation and excreted by the lungs. Unfortunately, carbon dioxide in large quantities in the bloodstream can cause hypotension or cardiac arrhythmias, especially if halothane or enflurane are used. Nitrous oxide on the other hand, while safer when absorbed into the bloodstream, can at least theoretically support combustion and most surgeons are not happy to use it when employing diathermy within the peritoneal cavity.

In gynaecological laparoscopy, the patient is usually placed steeply head-down so that the pelvic contents may be seen more easily. Diaphragmatic descent, already hindered by the weight of the abdominal contents in this position, is made even more difficult by the intra-abdominal pressure exerted by the gas. For this reason, controlled ventilation is usual to maintain adequate ventilation and especially elimination of carbon dioxide. However, if high intrathoracic pressures have to be applied, a point may come where blood is dammed back from entering the chest and heart, so that cardiac output and blood pressure fall. This condition may be worsened by a vena-caval occlusion effect similar to that seen in obstetrics as the high intra-abdominal pressure compresses the inferior vena cava. It is therefore important that the anaesthetist monitors the patient's blood pressure, especially as abdominal distention becomes pronounced.

Postoperatively the patient's cardiovascular system must be monitored carefully for arrhythmias and for hypotension. She should probably be kept in the recovery room for at least half an hour after the release of the gas from the peritoneal cavity. By no means all the gas is released in this way, and blood gas measurements have shown that the $P\text{CO}_2$ sometimes does not reach its maximum level until 30 minutes after gas release.

A perhaps surprising postoperative symptom after laparoscopy is the occurrence of shoulder tip pain. This is believed to be caused either by gas under the diaphragm, or more likely by blood or other fluid running up to the lower surface of the diaphragm in the head-down position. Lower abdominal pain also occurs, especially after gynaecological procedures such as sterilisation, and probably results from Fallopian tubal spasm.

34 Anaesthesia for Vascular Surgery

General considerations. Pre-operative assessment. Preparation for anaesthesia. Extracranial vascular surgery. Vascular radiology.

GENERAL CONSIDERATIONS

In the past 30 years improvements in surgical techniques and equipment (especially suture materials), in methods of diagnosis (especially vascular radiology) and in anaesthesia have led to the steady expansion of vascular surgery as a surgical sub-speciality.

While a small proportion of treatable arterial disease is caused by congenital abnormalities or by syphilis (once an important cause of arterial disease) the major cause of occlusive vascular disease is now atherosclerosis. This generalised disease affects all the arteries in the body, including the coronary, cerebral and renal arteries. Vascular surgery has now progressed to the stage where even the arteries to the vital organs may be operated on, but even in peripheral vascular surgery (e.g. of the legs) it is important to remember that the widespread nature of the disease indicates that the blood supply to the vital organs is imperfect and that anaesthesia must be carefully planned and carried out to reduce complications.

Other serious conditions are often associated with atherosclerosis, the commonest being hypertension. Most drugs used for this purpose produce some degree of sympathetic blockade, leaving a vagal preponderance, so that many patients on anti-hypertensive therapy show some degree of bradycardia. These patients, like patients with sympathetic blockade produced by spinal and epidural analgesia, have difficulty compensating for factors that may produce hypotension, e.g. sudden blood loss or a head-up tilt. For this reason it was formerly thought that therapy should be stopped pre-operatively, but it is now believed that these risks are less than those of myocardial or cerebral damage during anaesthesia and surgery when anti-hypertensive drugs have been withdrawn.

The other serious disease most commonly associated with atherosclerosis is diabetes mellitus. It has been estimated that 20% of all patients with occlusive vascular disease of the legs suffer from this condition and in particular it affects young patients suffering from vascular disease.

Cigarette smoking is closely correlated with the incidence and severity of vascular disease. While patients coming for elective vascular surgery will have stopped or greatly reduced their consumption, some patients coming for emergency surgery may be heavy smokers.

It is common for surgeons to induce regional heparinisation in the vascular distribution of an artery being operated on to reduce the incidence of thrombosis during arterial clamping. This is achieved by using a dilute solution of heparin in saline, e.g. 5000 μg/500 ml, which does not usually produce complete systemic anticoagulation. If it does, however, the problems produced are more likely to be surgical than anaesthetic, although they would certainly deter the anaesthetist from using, for example, continuous epidural analgesia as a method of post-operative pain relief.

PRE-OPERATIVE ASSESSMENT

In some vascular surgical cases haste may be so imperative that thorough pre-operative assessment may have to be curtailed to save the patient's life. Given time, however, the generalised nature of the atherosclerosis necessitates thorough pre-operative evaluation. The history-taking, for instance, should inquire particularly about chest pain indicating angina or previous myocardial infarction, for the presence of intermittent claudication, for blackouts indicating severe cerebrovascular disease, for breathlessness due to cardiac or respiratory disease or ankle oedema, which may be due to right-sided cardiac failure. Most patients will be on some type of long-term medication, e.g. anti-hypertensive drugs, digoxin, anti-arrhythmics, diuretics, anticoagulants or insulin or oral hypoglycaemics. Use of these drugs over the operative period will have to be decided upon.

Laboratory investigations should include a full blood count, a full biochemical profile, including renal and liver function tests, 12-lead ECG, a chest x-ray examination and sometimes blood gas analysis or other long function tests.

PREPARATION FOR ANAESTHESIA

As already mentioned, most patients undergoing vascular surgery are suffering from generalised degenerative arterial disease. Younger, healthier patients may be suffering from acute hypovolaemia (as from a stab wound) or from the effects of multiple injuries (as after a road traffic accident). In addition, most vascular operations are lengthy and sudden rapid blood loss may occur. Consequently, for all major vascular surgery the following are required:

1. At least one large bore (14G or 12G) venous cannula. This venous line must also be provided with a blood microfilter, a warming coil and thermostatically controlled water bath and some means of speeding the blood transfusion.
2. A central venous pressure line.
3. An arterial pressure line.
4. An ECG.
5. A means of measuring core body temperature.
6. A thermostatically controlled water blanket for use during the operation.
7. A urinary bladder catheter.
8. A nasogastric tube, many of these patients suffering from some degree of postoperative ileus.

It is essential that at least the arterial pressure and the ECG are recorded continuously on an oscilloscope.

Ruptured Abdominal Aortic Aneurysm

The rupture of an abdominal aneurysm, whether into the peritoneal cavity, retroperitoneally or into the bowel is potentially lethal and carries a high mortality. Death occurs either from massive blood loss or from the associated hypotension which is poorly tolerated by patients with arteriosclerosis. These may be extreme surgical emergencies where resuscitation is not possible until the abdomen has been opened and the aorta clamped.

It has been suggested that the muscular fasciculations associated with suxamethonium may cause further bleeding from the aneurysm. These may be reduced or avoided by preliminary administration of a small dose of a non-depolarising relaxant or by intubation with one of this group of relaxants, e.g. pancuronium. Unfortunately the reduction in intra-abdominal pressure resulting from muscular relaxation can also cause renewed bleeding and in most cases it is wise to anaesthetise the patient on the operating table with the surgeon ready to start. These patients are all at risk from inhalation of gastric contents at induction of anaesthesia and 'intestinal obstruction-type' precautions should be taken before intubation. After careful pre-oxygenation this involves cricoid pressure, which may be difficult but not usually impossible to perform efficiently when intubation is being carried out under a non-depolarising relaxant.

Maintenance of anaesthesia is with nitrous oxide and oxygen and muscle relaxants, with narcotic adjuvants or possibly low concentrations of halothane if there is a tendency to hypertension. The patient's cardiovascular status is carefully monitored and blood or other intravenous fluids given as appropriate. Many anaesthetists favour the administration of substantial amounts of Hartmann's solution, as this often reduces the severity of 'de-clamping shock' which tends to occur on removal of the aortic clamp to restore the aortic flow in this or other operations on the abdominal aorta. Impaired coagulation may be seen due either to depletion of clotting factors caused by the massive blood transfusion, or occasionally due to disseminated intravascular coagulation.

These patients should almost always be electively ventilated for several hours postoperatively.

Dissecting Aneurysm of the Aorta

This is not a true aneurysm, but a break occurring in the intima that allows blood to escape from the lumen of the aorta and to track longitudinally between the layers of the aortic wall, sometimes for a considerable distance. If rupture occurs through the outer coats of the aorta the outcome is quickly fatal. If this does not occur various complications may result from occlusion of various branches of the aorta which may occur if the dissection spreads as far as their points of origin from the aorta. Thus, renal or spinal cord ischaemia may result from occlusion of the renal or lumbar arteries.

Treatment is usually conservative with attempts to relieve the severe pain associated with the condition and induced hypotension to try to contain the dissection. Thoracic epidural analgesia is one method of achieving both these aims. Surgery is sometimes performed to provide a re-entry ostium to relieve the pressure occluding the important renal or lumbar arteries. Dissection usually starts in the thoracic aorta, and to prevent the marked rise in blood pressure which occurs on clamping the aorta it is necessary to induce hypotension, e.g. with sodium nitroprusside.

Elective Aorto-Iliac Surgery

This is commonly for elective repair of an aortic aneurysm or for the relief of occlusive aorto-iliac disease, the latter usually by grafting or by endarterectomy. This is major surgery but there is less urgency and, as a result, more time for pre-operative investigation and preparation of the patient. In slowly progressive occlusive disease there is time for a collateral circulation to develop so that clamping and unclamping of the aorta tend to produce less dramatic fluctuations in blood pressure.

Femoro-Popliteal Surgery

Surgery on arteries distal to the inguinal ligament is still on relatively large-bore arteries in patients with generalised cardiovascular disease, but the problems of surgery itself are considerably less. Should haemorrhage occur it is more easily controlled than in the abdomen and clamping and de-clamping problems are minimal, not only because these arteries are smaller but because they have usually been occluded, or relatively occluded, for some time. The commonest operations are femoro-popliteal bypass using a strip of the patient's own long saphenous vein, or endarterectomy.

Peripheral Vascular Emergencies

These may be caused by trauma, embolism or sudden extension of a thrombus. Trauma usually occurs in younger patients who are basically fit, unless they are suffering from multiple injuries. In these cases anaesthesia has the usual potentially dangerous implications of any emergency anaesthesia, but otherwise is largely concerned with the appropriate correction of blood loss. Emboli usually arise either from a fibrillating atrium, from a mural thrombus associated with myocardial infarction, or less commonly as a detached vegetation from a heart valve in subacute bacterial endocarditis. In all these conditions the patient may be seriously ill from the underlying disease, but fortunately the operations can often be easily carried out under local infiltration analgesia. Rapid occlusion of an artery may also occur with thrombus formation, although this is not usually as dramatic as in the case of trauma or embolism.

Whatever the cause, the sudden nature of the arterial obstruction tends to produce vasospasm in the surrounding small vessels. This reduces the adequacy of any collateral circulation past the obstruction. Sympathetic nerve block (e.g. lumbar sympathetic chain block) may improve the peripheral circulation by relieving the spasm.

Microvascular Surgery

See p. 313.

EXTRACRANIAL VASCULAR SURGERY

This type of surgery is designed to restore the blood supply in the arteries carrying the oxygen supply to the brain. The commonest operations are bypass grafting or endarterectomy. As the arterial disease is generalised, clamping of the vessel to be operated on may result in acute cerebral ischaemia. For this reason, many surgeons insert a temporary arterial bypass from the common carotid artery proximally to the internal carotid beyond the occlusion. Many patients are treated hypertensives and, as a sudden rise in blood pressure may lead to cerebral haemorrhage and a fall in blood pressure to a reduction in cerebral blood flow, it is important during anaesthesia to maintain the blood pressure as near their treated level as possible.

Many of the requirements of neurosurgical anaesthesia (Chapter 37) apply also to anaesthesia for surgery on the arteries supplying the brain. For example, anything but very mild degrees of hypercarbia or hypocarbia should be avoided and only very low concentrations of halothane used, if at all.

On emergence from anaesthesia, about one-third of patients develop severe hypertension, with the threat of cerebral haemorrhage. An infusion of trimetaphan (Arfonad) or the slow injection of propranolol, sometimes with hydralazine have been suggested as a means of controlling blood pressure at this time.

VASCULAR RADIOLOGY

Most vascular radiological investigations can be carried out under local analgesia except in children and uncooperative adults. Injection of the radio-opaque dye is not exactly painful, but produces a somewhat unpleasant burning sensation which may cause the patient to move and spoil the quality of the films. For this reason, in less cooperative patients better results are likely to be obtained under general anaesthesia.

The investigation in this branch of radiology which is most commonly carried out under general anaesthesia, is translumbar aortography. For this the patient lies prone on the x-ray table and a long needle is inserted through the lumbar region into the aorta. Dye is then injected forcibly into the aorta and the table moves so that the x-ray camera can take sequential pictures of the dye as it passes down the lower limbs. Once again, anaesthesia is being carried out in patients with less than perfect cardiovascular systems—this time in the prone position. In this position, even with supports under the patient's hips and chests, carbon dioxide is likely to be retained if respiration is allowed to be spontaneous, and for this reason controlled ventilation is preferred.

35 Anaesthesia for Thoracic Surgery

Endobronchial and one-lung anaesthesia. Pneumonectomy or lobectomy. Bronchopleural fistula. Oesophagectomy. General anaesthesia for bronchoscopy. Local anaesthesia for bronchoscopy. Tracheostomy. Chest drains. Postoperative thoracic care.

The thorax contains both the lungs and pleura, the trachea and bronchi, the oesophagus, the heart and the great vessels. This chapter deals with anaesthesia for surgery of the lungs, trachea, bronchi and oesophagus, cardiac surgery being dealt with in Chapter 36.

The lungs are each surrounded by two layers of pleura—the parietal pleura attached to the chest wall, and the visceral pleura which invests the lung surface itself. The negative pressure existing within the pleural space is responsible for maintaining the lung in the expanded position, even in expiration. An increase in negative intrapleural pressure brought about by thoracic wall expansion during inspiration, together with the two layers of pleura remaining adherent due to surface tension, is responsible for lung expansion. If the pleural space is exposed to atmospheric pressure caused by air entering it from inside via the bronchi (broncho-pleural fistula) or externally due to chest wall injury, the resulting pneumothorax allows the lung to collapse. This collapse is further enhanced by the negative pressure created during inspiration, but can be prevented by positive pressure inspiration—in other words, artificial ventilation. IPPV is therefore an essential part of thoracic anaesthesia, maintaining the lungs in an expanded state during the operation with the chest open. This equal expansion of both lungs also prevents 'mediastinal flap', which results from uneven inflation of the lungs during normal breathing in the presence of a pneumothorax and may result in severely impaired venous return.

Thoracic anaesthesia in the presence of an open chest is comparatively straightforward provided that artificial ventilation is employed; an identical anaesthetic technique to that employed for abdominal laparotomy is perfectly suitable for thoracotomy provided that the surgeon is able to work with both of the patient's lungs expanded. Many of the complications of thoracic anaesthesia result from the need to collapse one of the lungs in order to provide surgical access for lung or oesophageal resection. Most anaesthetists therefore employ a nitrous oxide/oxygen, relaxant, analgesic anaesthetic technique, using IPPV. Although in the past a considerable amount of thoracic anaesthesia, particularly in patients with tuberculosis, was carried out under local or regional anaesthesia, this has now been largely superseded by general anaesthetic techniques.

ENDOBRONCHIAL AND ONE-LUNG ANAESTHESIA

If the surgeon is happy to operate on a moving lung, thoracic anaesthesia is possible with an endotracheal tube, but many surgeons prefer to operate on a still lung or to be able to retract the lung away from the operative field in, for example, oesophagectomy. Selective intubation of either the right or left main bronchus (Fig. 35.1) allows independent ventilation of either right or left lung while the other lung is allowed to collapse.

Double-lumen endobronchial tubes are now widely used for this purpose and consist of two separate tubes lying side by side, either in the anterior–posterior or lateral plane, one of which is long, cuffed and designed to fit in either the right or left main bronchus while the other terminates in the trachea (Fig. 35.2). Such tubes allow independent ventilation of either the right or left lung and for this reason it is usual to use a left-sided tube where possible, thereby avoiding placing a bronchial cuff in the

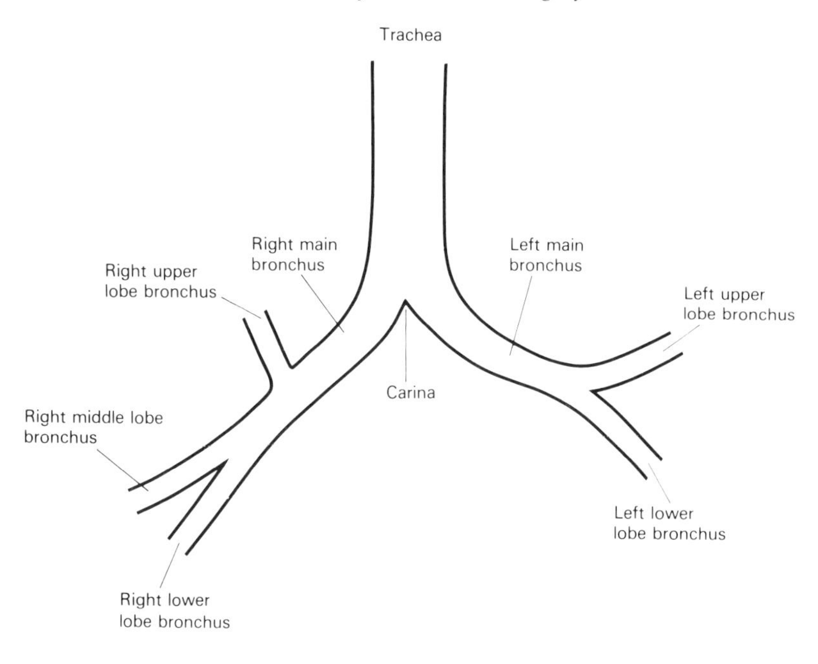

Fig. 35.1 The bronchial tree

upper part of the right main bronchus and possibly occluding the right upper lobe bronchus. Occasionally the right upper lobe bronchus arises from the trachea rather than the right main bronchus and in both these situations right upper lobe collapse may occur, although an abnormal right upper lobe bronchus should have been detected by bronchoscopy before intubation. In addition to allowing independent ventilation of right and left lung, endobronchial anaesthesia also isolates an infected lung from its 'clean' partner. In cases of chronic lung infection—such as bronchiectasis or bronchopleural fistula with an empyema —inadvertent spillage of pus from the bad to the good lung may result in severe postoperative complications. Before the advent of double-lumen tubes, a bronchus blocker was often inserted under direct vision through a bronchoscope into the main bronchus of the infected lung, thereby preventing spillage and allowing the good lung to be intubated with an endobronchial tube.

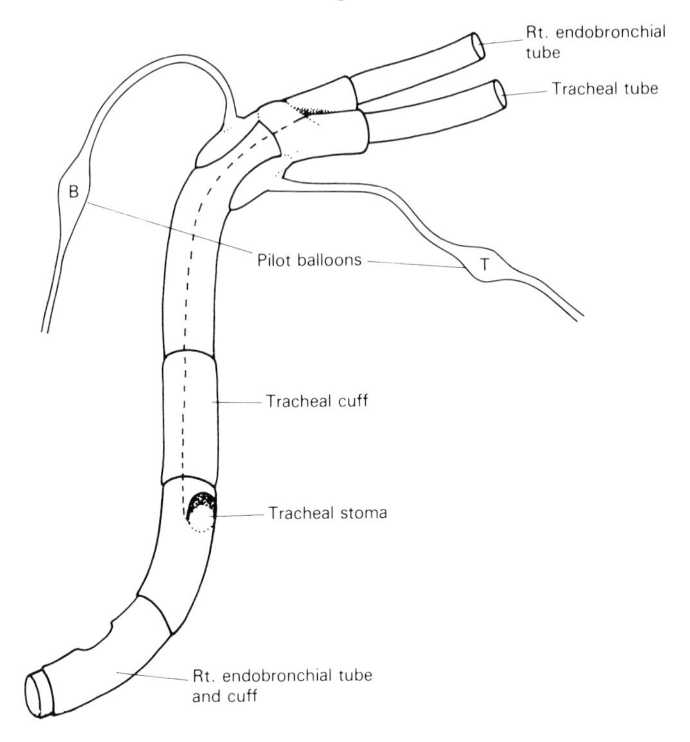

Fig. 35.2 Robertshaw endobronchial tube

PNEUMONECTOMY OR LOBECTOMY

Resection of all or part of one lung is usually performed for either neoplastic disease or bronchiectasis, a chronic inflammatory condition of the lung which usually affects the bases and produces severe destruction of lung tissue. Many of the patients presenting for lung resection are severely incapacitated and breathless but nevertheless tolerate operations reasonably well. By the nature of the disease they are often heavy smokers and may already have a limited exercise tolerance. Diagnosis has usually been made by pre-operative bronchoscopy but, if there is any doubt, anaesthetic induction should allow for a further bronchoscopy before intubation. An intravenous infusion is set up under local anaesthesia, the patient is pre-oxygenated for a full five minutes and anaesthesia is then induced with intravenous analgesia, thiopentone and a muscle relaxant, either suxamethonium, later to be followed by pancuronium, or pancuronium in the first instance. A range of endobronchial tubes should always be available, a large and medium Robertshaw for a man and a medium and small Robertshaw for a woman. Some anaesthetists prefer the Carlens or White tubes as an alternative and other varieties are available. The position of the tube is checked by first inflating the endobronchial cuff until there is no leak back past it when positive pressure is applied solely down that half of the double-lumen tube. Auscultation then confirms that only that lung is being inflated (with special attention to the right upper lobe with right-sided tubes) and lastly the tracheal cuff is inflated and ventilation of the other lung confirmed. The correct functioning of the tube should be re-checked when the patient has been positioned on the operating table. This check should be repeated when the patient has been positioned in the full lateral position for the operation, because the tube may slip during turning.

Anaesthesia may then proceed in the usual way until the chest is opened and it is necessary to collapse the upper lung. It is important to realise at this point that in normal circumstances while blood flow occurs predominantly to the dependent part of the lung, gas flows to the top of the lung, and if the upper lung is collapsed an imbalance will develop between gas and blood supply to the dependent lung. This is known as a ventilation/perfusion imbalance and may result in relative hypoxia. It is therefore essential to increase the inspired oxygen concentration during one-lung anaesthesia, and this may be achieved either by using 50 % oxygen in nitrous oxide together with supplementary analgesia, or 100 % oxygen and a volatile agent, e.g. halothane. The former technique has the advantage that the patient wakes easily at the end of operation and is able to sit up and breathe deeply in the early postoperative period.

One-lung anaesthesia should not be undertaken if, when the lung is collapsed, the patient is unable to maintain adequate oxygenation even with supplementary oxygen during anaesthesia, as he will never be able to lead a normal life when breathing air. Other indices of inadequate oxygenation during one-lung anaesthesia are a rising pulse rate or blood pressure occurring soon after the lung has been collapsed. In any of these

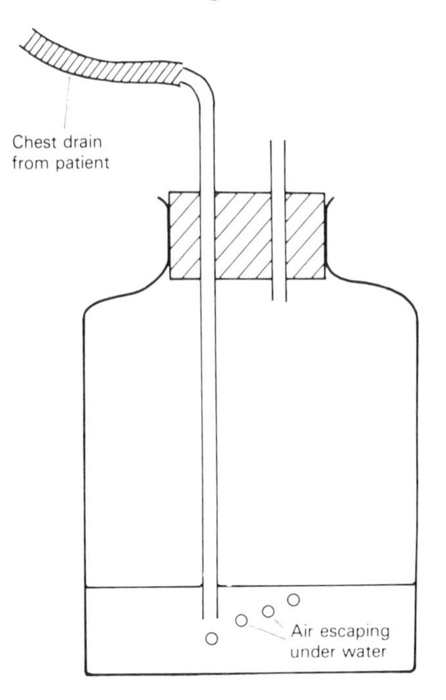

Fig. 35.3 Underwater seal bottle

events the anaesthetist and surgeon should consult before proceeding with the operation.

If the lung has not been totally resected, it is important at the end of the operation to ensure its complete re-expansion, which requires considerable pressure on the reservoir bag of the anaesthetic circuit. The thoracic cavity must be drained after all operations to avoid accumulation of either air or blood which may impede lung expansion. Air is drained through an apical thoracic drain and blood through a basal one, both linked to underwater seal bottles (Fig. 35.3).

These allow air and blood to leave the chest but prevent air being sucked into the chest during the negative inspiratory phase. When satisfactory lung expansion has been achieved and the chest wall is closed, muscle relaxation is reversed and the patient sat upright in bed and given supplementary oxygen. An early postoperative chest x-ray is essential to ensure adequate expansion of the remaining lung and also the correct placement of chest drains. During transfer of the patient, if the drains are raised from the floor their tubing should be clamped to prevent the water being siphoned back into the chest.

Postoperative analgesia is often a problem after thoracotomy, and intercostal blocks at the time of operation may considerably help to relieve pain. Systemic analgesics are often relatively ineffective and the recent introduction of epidural anaesthesia, particularly using morphine or other opiates, may be a considerable advantage.

BRONCHOPLEURAL FISTULA

A fistula between the lung and the pleural cavity allows free flow of air in and out of the pleural space. Provided that a valvular system does not exist the affected lung will collapse and external chest drainage will only permit re-expansion so long as the chest drain remains in position. If the pleural contents, usually fluid, become infected and form an empyema, surgical treatment is usually indicated: however, a normal induction and endobronchial intubation would result in severe complications. In the presence of a bronchopleural fistula IPPV results in increased intrapleural pressure and therefore the creation of a tension pneumothorax; for this reason patients with bronchopleural fistulae must be allowed to breathe spontaneously until endobronchial intubation has been accomplished. In addition, if infection is present either as an empyema or as chronic bronchiectasis, before induction the patient should be positioned so that spill of the infected material into the opposite lung does not occur. Induction of anaesthesia should ensure that the patient does not stop breathing, and for this reason an inhalational induction in the sitting position is usually thought to be ideal. Once intubation of the opposite lung has been achieved a normal one-lung thoracic anaesthetic technique may be used and pus from the offending lung can be aspirated up the opposite endobronchial tube lumen.

OESOPHAGECTOMY

In oesophagectomy endobronchial and one-lung anaesthesia are employed simply to facilitate operative dissection and anastomosis of the oesophagus in the chest. For the lower third of the oesophagus a left thoracotomy is usual, though for higher lesions a right-sided approach is more convenient. In either situation the overlying lung is usually collapsed during the operative procedure, although as lung resection is not involved, straightforward re-expansion of the lung without subsequent problems is generally achieved. Postoperative pain seems to be greater than sometimes occurs with pneumonectomy, and considerable care is necessary to avoid postoperative chest infections.

GENERAL ANAESTHESIA FOR BRONCHOSCOPY

Bronchoscopy is used either for diagnostic or therapeutic purposes, and with the advent of the fibre-optic bronchoscope many procedures do not now require full general anaesthesia. Rigid bronchoscopy, however, is still carried out in many centres, particularly before thoracic work, as it is often easier directly to visualise and biopsy tumours with this technique. The anaesthetic requirements are that the patient should be relatively lightly anaesthetised, oxygenated and able to wake quickly postoperatively, to maintain his own airway and to cough up any blood and other secretions which have accumulated during the procedure. An indwelling needle is essential and pre-oxygenation is followed by an incremental thiopentone/suxamethonium technique supplemented by artificial ventilation with a Venturi system using oxygen attached to a side limb of the bronchoscope. High-pressure Entonox is sometimes used in place of oxygen to provide a greater depth of anaesthesia and possibly reduce the risk of awareness during this procedure. It is important to ensure adequate oxygenation at all times as many patients have considerable cardiovascular or other problems exacerbated by the hypoxia which may result from a severe coughing spasm.

High-frequency oscillation and high-frequency jet ventilation are two newer ventilatory techniques which are particularly suitable for use during rigid bronchoscopy. They rely upon very rapid small volume oscillations of gas flow in and out of the lungs with minimal changes in airway pressure. As such, they provide adequate alveolar ventilation, arterial oxygenation and carbon dioxide extraction without significant lung movement, making them ideally suited to this procedure. They have also been used in patients with bronchopleural fistulae and severely reduced pulmonary compliance, such as shock lung and pulmonary contusion to prevent the development of high airway pressures. They are not widely available at present and are still considerably more expensive than conventional ventilators.

Fibre-optic bronchoscopy seldom requires general anaesthesia, although if required a thiopentone/nitrous oxide/oxygen and halothane technique using a small endotracheal tube—which allows the fibre-optic instrument to be passed alongside—is usually found to be sufficient.

LOCAL ANAESTHESIA FOR BRONCHOSCOPY

This is a relatively unpleasant procedure, but some patients are suitable only for a local anaesthetic technique for bronchoscopy. In this event premedication is often used and the patient's mouth and pharynx are then anaesthetised by encouraging them to suck an amethocaine lozenge. The overall amount of local anaesthetic to be used is then poured out, thus avoiding the easy error of inadvertently administering an overdose of lignocaine. Progressive anaesthesia of the posterior pharyngeal wall, the fauces, the pyriform fossae and the larynx are then carried out, usually with the patient in the semi-recumbent position, and finally a small dose of diazepam is usually administered intravenously before the bronchoscopic procedure. Local anaesthesia of the larynx is contraindicated in patients in whom biopsies are being taken, because this prevents adequate postoperative coughing and expectorant of blood and other secretions.

TRACHEOSTOMY

Although tracheostomy may be performed as an emergency or lifesaving procedure, it is usually limited nowadays to patients requiring prolonged artificial ventilation or those undergoing laryngectomy as a result of neoplastic disease or trauma. Soft-cuffed, non-irritant endotracheal tubes have considerably reduced the incidence of tracheostomy in intensive care. The procedure, usually carried out under general anaesthesia except in severely ill or unconscious patients, involves making an aperture in the trachea, usually at the region of the second and third tracheal rings, with the creation of an anterior (Björk) flap attached to the skin to provide a ledge over which the tracheostomy tube is inserted. Anaesthetic complications which may arise from tracheostomy are largely limited to those concerned with the initial intubation of the patient—which will have been done already if they are receiving artificial ventilation. In patients with carcinoma or other obstructive lesions, extreme difficulty may initially be experienced in inserting an endotracheal tube, and this may require considerably pre-operative manipulation using extremely small uncuffed endotracheal tubes, introducers, etc. Tracheostomy may also occasionally be required before thyroidectomy in patients with a large retrosternal thyroid producing tracheal compression. This may result in a soft trachea postoperatively, which some surgeons prefer to protect with a temporary tracheostomy. Intra-operative anaesthetic management varies between a spontaneous respiration technique and IPPV. The former has the advantage that the patient breathes during the changeover period between endotracheal and tracheostomy tubes, which may help if the tracheostome is difficult to cannulate. It is essential before tracheostomy that the size of the tube required be available together with all the relevant connections, to allow reconnection to the anaesthetic equipment under the towels. If this is not done a vital part is invariably found to be missing. It is important also to have a range of tracheostomy tubes available, as in some cases a small internal diameter trachea is extremely difficult to predict. Once inserted, and before attachment to the ventilator, the tracheostomy tube should be sucked out to remove secretions and to allow the free passage of a suction catheter, thereby ensuring that it has not been misplaced into the anterior mediastinum, since only a few litres of air in the mediastinum may cause considerable cardiovascular embarrassment. Usually a cuffed tracheostomy tube is inserted and left in position for a few days before being replaced by a longer-term silver tube.

CHEST DRAINS

As already mentioned (p. 346), chest drains placed either at the apex of the lung to drain air or at the base of the lung to drain blood, are always connected to an underwater seal drainage bottle (*see* Fig. 35.3). The tubing from the patient is attached via a glass tube which passes under the surface of the water, the depth to which the tube is inserted in the water presenting a small resistance to expiration, usually of 3–4 cm. The initial level of he water in the bottle must be accurately recorded to allow the volume of blood collecting in the bottle to be measured. It is important also to ensure that the surface area of the water in the chest drainage bottle is large by comparison with the diameter of the chest tube, because considerable turbulence may occur as gas bubbles violently out of the chest during coughing or maximal expiration. In addition, if the drainage bottle is narrow, a small amount of fluid or blood draining from the chest will considerably raise the fluid level in the bottle and therefore the depth to which the chest tube is submerged and the resistance to expiration. On the other hand, if the tube is submerged to an inadequate depth, a large inspiration will draw up water, and then, when this is exhausted, air will be sucked up the tube.

POSTOPERATIVE THORACIC CARE

In most thoracic units, postoperative artificial ventilation is relatively rare, and patients are nursed on an intensive-care area within the normal thoracic ward. Experienced nursing care, together with oxygen, suction and the necessary equipment for emergency intubation and ventilation, should be on the spot. Postoperative respiratory failure may develop for several reasons, but should not be due to the patient being unable to manage on one lung, as this should have been detected at the time of operation (see above).

Pulmonary oedema, infection and, more commonly, postoperative pain leading to collapse and consolidation are the usual causes of respiratory failure in the immediate postoperative period, and of these the control of pain is probably the most important. Accurate volume replacement is also essential, particularly as many of the patients have concomitant cardiovascular disease. The development of atrial fibrillation, particularly where a lung tumour has involved the pericardium in the older age group of patients, is common, and intra-operative digitalisation is recommended in all thoracotomy patients over the age of 60, to prevent the development of fast postoperative atrial fibrillation, which may precipitate cardiac failure. Chest drains are usually left in position for several days until both air and fluid have stopped leaking. They are then clamped but left in place for a further 24 hours when the patient is examined by x-ray. If there has been no accumulation of air or blood, they may then be removed safely.

36 Anaesthesia for Open Heart Surgery

Technique of cardiopulmonary bypass. Pre-operative evaluation of patient. Anaesthetic technique. Postoperative management.

Thirty years ago cardiac surgery was limited to relatively simple operations such as the repair of small congenital defects. Its advance has been both rapid and spectacular; today complex intracardiac operations such as valve replacements, intricate microsurgery for coronary artery disease and even transplantation of the heart itself are established procedures.

A broad division can be made into 'closed heart' operations, such as pericardectomy or repair of patent ductus arteriosus, and 'open heart' operations in which normal ventilation and circulation are arrested.

This chapter describes the anaesthetic management of adult patients undergoing open heart surgery for the following conditions:

Valve replacements
Myocardial revascularisation
Congenital atrial and ventricular septal defects
Ventricular aneurysms
Tumours such as atrial myxomata
Heart transplantation

TECHNIQUE OF CARDIOPULMONARY BYPASS

If the patient's heart and lungs are arrested and bypassed, it is obvious that to sustain life one must substitute a pump (for the heart) and an oxygenator (for the lungs). These two pieces of apparatus together with the tubing, filters, reservoir and heat exchanger constitute the equipment required for cardiopulmonary bypass.

Pump

Mechanically driven rollers squeeze the tubing against a rigid semi-circular track and 'milk' the blood forward. The blood flow produced is usually 'non-pulsatile' but it can be modified to produce the more physiologically normal 'pulsatile' wave form which possibly improves tissue perfusion and oxygen uptake.

Oxygenator

This replaces the lung and its design must therefore mimic this organ, exposing a very large surface area of blood to allow oxygenation and carbon dioxide elimination. The three main types of oxygenators commonly used are:

1. Rotating disc oxygenator
2. Bubble oxygenator
3. Membrane oxygenator

The membrane oxygenator is the most anatomically and physiologically 'normal' as it has a semi-permeable membrane interface between blood and oxygen allowing gas exchange across the membrane. This type of oxygenator damages the blood less than the bubble oxygenator and its efficiency has been improved so much during the last decade that it is replacing the rotating disc and bubble oxygenators in general clinical use.

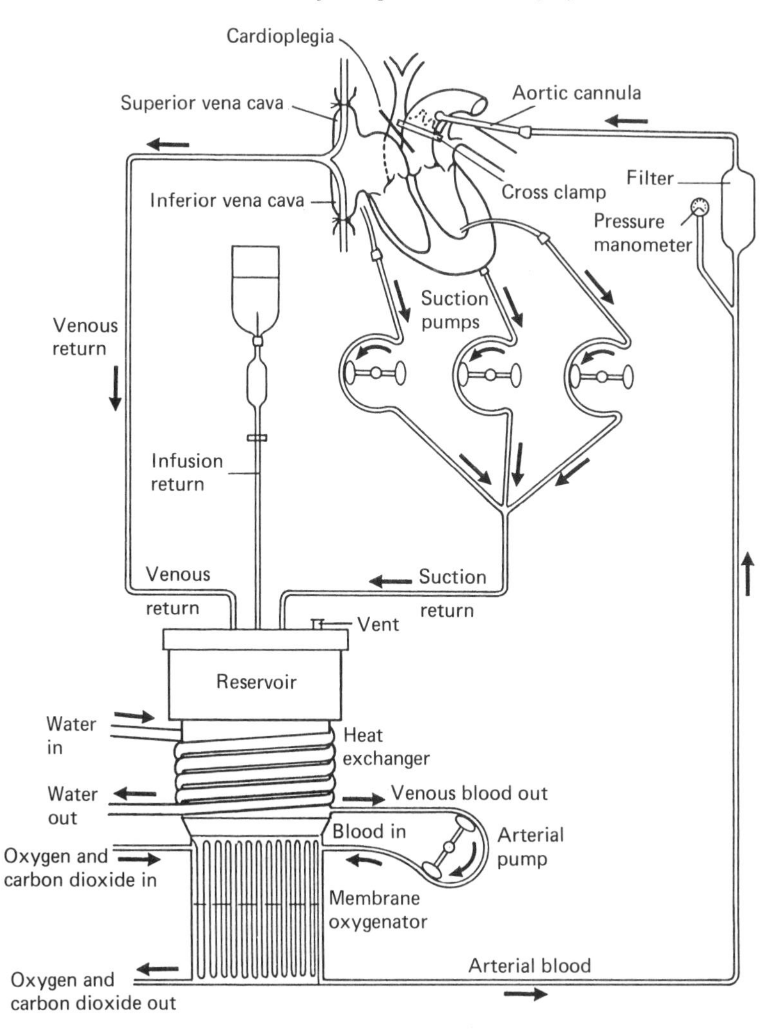

Fig. 36.1 Cardiopulmonary bypass circuit

Bypass Circuit

This is illustrated in Fig. 36.1. Venous blood bypasses the patient's heart by two cannulae placed in the superior and inferior vena cavae or by a single cannula into the right atrium. The venous blood is pumped through a heat exchanger and oxygenator and thence into a cannula in the ascending aorta or (less frequently) the femoral artery. For most types of cardiac surgery the ascending aorta is crossclamped below the aortic cannula and the arterial return from the oxygenator perfuses the brain, kidneys and vital organs and tissues of the body.

If the left ventricle is required to be kept undistended and empty during bypass a separate venting cannula is used. Hand-held suckers clear the operating area and blood from these suckers is returned to the oxygenator via a reservoir and micro-filter.

Priming the Circuit

Before the patient is connected, the bypass circuit must be primed with fluid. Modern practice is to use a 'bloodless' prime usually of Hartmann's solution (2·5–3·0 litres) with added sodium bicarbonate (1 mmol/kg). This produces considerable haemodilution during cardiopulmonary bypass but oxygen carriage is adequate and the reduced blood viscosity benefits organ and tissue perfusion.

PRE-OPERATIVE EVALUATION OF PATIENT

The patient is visited by members of the surgical, anaesthetic, physiotherapy and intensive care teams and the operation and postoperative period explained. It is particularly important that the patient is aware of postoperative artificial ventilation and physiotherapy. The severity of the heart disease is assessed from the history and clinical examination of the patient together with ancillary investigations such as ECG, chest x-ray, cardiac catheterisation, angiography, echocardiography, radionuclide imaging and laboratory tests (Table 36.1).

Pre-operative Drug Therapy

Most patients will be receiving a number of cardiac and related drugs, some of which may need to be increased, reduced or even stopped before surgery. Beta-adrenergic blocking drugs (e.g.

metroprolol, propranolol), calcium-channel blockers (e.g. nifedipine) and coronary vasodilators (e.g. glyceryl trinitrate) are continued up to the day of surgery.

Digoxin is usually stopped 36–48 hours before surgery but diuretics and potassium supplements are continued up to the day preceding surgery.

Aspirin should be stopped two weeks before the operation but dipyridamole (Persantin), which has a prophylactic action against coronary artery occlusion, should be continued.

Anticoagulants (e.g. warfarin) must be stopped two to three days before surgery to allow a normal prothrombin time. A raised prothrombin time can be corrected by infusions of fresh frozen plasma before or during the operation.

ANAESTHETIC TECHNIQUE

Premedication and Induction of Anaesthesia

The patients are premedicated in the usual way, although doses may be reduced in patients with low cardiac outputs. Pap-

Table 36.1 Laboratory investigations

Haematology	Full blood count	(Hb > 11 g/dl)
	Clotting profile	(Normal prothrombin time)
	Blood crossmatch	(Usually 6 units)
Biochemistry	Urea and electrolytes	(NB Danger of hypokalaemia in patients receiving long-term diuretics)
	Liver function tests	(Often abnormal in right-sided cardiac failure)
	Cardiac enzymes	(In patients undergoing coronary artery grafting)
Bacteriology	MSU and urinanalysis	
	Swabbing of nose, throat and perineum	
	HB Ag (Australia antigen)	
	HIV (human immunodeficiency virus) when indicated	

averetum or morphine are commonly used, usually in combination with hyoscine rather than atropine to prevent an excessive tachycardia. The oral doses of β-adrenergic blockers, calcium-channel blockers and coronary vasodilating drugs are given with the premedication to patients already receiving them pre-operatively. If there is undue anxiety, a small dose of oral diazepam (5 mg) or temazepam (10 mg) may also be given. Induction of anaesthesia is a critical time for many of these patients and the doses of i.v. induction agents may have to be reduced substantially. A defibrillator and resuscitative drugs must be available in the anaesthetic room. To obtain haemodynamic control before induction of anaesthesia, arterial and venous infusion lines are inserted under local analgesia and the ECG leads connected (Fig. 36.2). In no branch of anaesthesia is scrupulous attention to detail more important. The disconnection of an infusion line during an operation may have fatal consequences and *all* connections must be thoroughly checked before surgery. The aims of induction of anaesthesia are:

1. To avoid hypertension by producing a smooth loss of consciousness without coughing or straining.
2. To avoid myocardial depression with reduced cardiac output and hypotension.
3. To promote a mild peripheral vasodilatation and improve tissue perfusion.

The use of fentanyl (7 μg/kg) supplemented by the smallest sleep dose of thiopentone (1–2 mg/kg) after pre-loading the patient with 200–300 ml of crystalloid solution, will usually achieve unconsciousness with minimal cardiovascular disturbance. Muscle paralysis for intubation is produced with pancuronium bromide or vecuronium.

Anaesthetic Management During Surgery

The operation can be divided into three periods:

1. The pre-bypass period during which the sternum is split to allow access to the pericardium and heart with cannulation of the aorta and vena cava.
2. The bypass period.
3. The post-bypass period during which the patient must re-establish normal circulation.

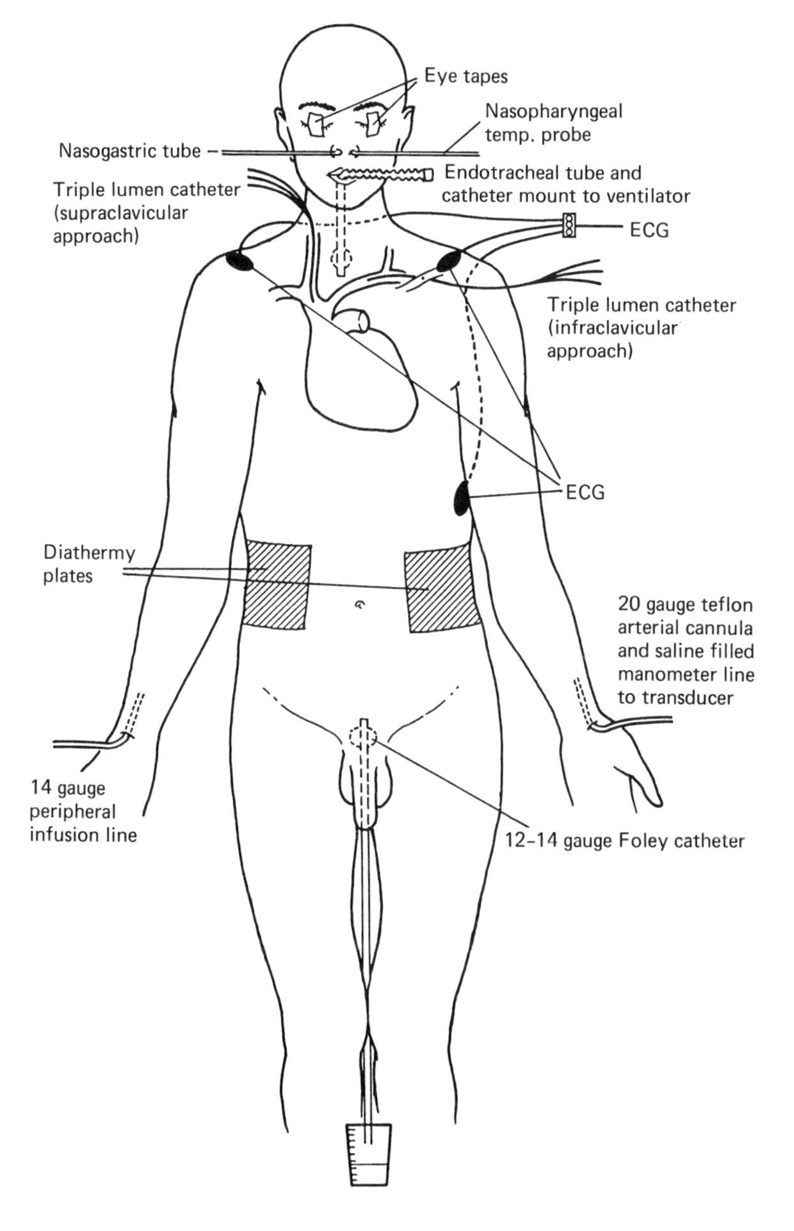

Fig. 36.2 Cannulation and monitoring before open heart surgery

Pre-bypass

The aim is to achieve anaesthesia with complete cardiovascular control. Both hypo- and hypertension may have serious consequences and meticulous attention must be paid to maintaining the arterial and venous pressure within set parameters. Accurate infusion or syringe pumps are necessary to infuse vasoactive drugs through a dedicated lumen of a triple lumen catheter inserted into the superior vena cava. One lumen is used to infuse drugs which will raise the arterial pressure (e.g. dobutamine, dopamine, adrenaline), the second lumen to infuse drugs which will lower the arterial pressure (e.g. sodium nitroprusside, glyceryl trinitrate) and the third lumen can be used for central venous pressure measurement. Anaesthesia is maintained with nitrous oxide and oxygen supplemented with inhalational agents (e.g. halothane or enflurane) and narcotic analgesics (e.g. fentanyl or morphine).

During bypass

Anaesthesia. Ventilation of the lungs is not required during cardiopulmonary bypass but they are kept slightly inflated with oxygen. Anaesthesia is maintained with narcotic analgesics and benzodiazepine drugs (midazolam, diazepam). During hypothermia metabolism of muscle relaxants and other drugs is reduced but care must still be taken to avoid awareness and respiratory movements.

Blood flow and perfusion pressure. An output from the arterial pump of 2·4 litres/minute/m^2 is required at 37°C with a 30% reduction for a 10°C drop in temperature. A perfusion pressure of 50–80 mm Hg is achieved by adjusting the pump flow between acceptable limits and the use of vasoconstrictor (e.g. metaraminol) or vasodilator (e.g. phentolamine) drugs.

Cardioplegia and myocardial preservation. To arrest the heart and protect the myocardium from hypoxic damage after aortic cross-clamping, the coronary vasculature is perfused with cold (4°C) cardioplegic solution containing potassium, magnesium and procaine in Ringer's lactate. An initial volume of 1000 ml is used supplemented by further infusions (500–1000 ml) every 30 minutes or if myocardial activity returns. Local cooling of the heart (to approximately 15°C) is achieved by ice-cold water or 'slush' placed in the pericardial sac.

Anticoagulation. This is carried out with i.v. heparin 2–3 mg/kg before cannulation of the heart. The activated clotting time is monitored and maintained at > 400 s by incremental heparin to the extracorporeal circuit.

Blood gas analysis. The supply of oxygen and carbon dioxide to the oxygenator is adjusted to produce normal blood gases. An increasing metabolic acidosis may indicate inadequate tissue perfusion requiring an increased pump flow or the production of peripheral vasodilation.

Potassium balance. Total body potassium is often reduced following long-term diuretics. On bypass, haemodilution, urinary loss and intracellular migration of potassium all contribute to a lowering of the plasma potassium concentration, which requires frequent monitoring and supplementation with potassium chloride. Conversely, patients receiving large volumes of cardioplegic solution into the pump circuit, and those on non-specific β-adrenergic blockers (e.g. propranolol) may develop high plasma potassium concentrations during bypass.

Urine output. This provides a good indication of tissue and organ perfusion. A diuresis is common during bypass due to the crystalloid fluid used in the prime.

Post-bypass

On completion of surgery and rewarming of the patient, the heart must be restarted and the lungs ventilated. Myocardial activity recommences as warm blood perfuses the coronary circulation. If there is ventricular fibrillation this must be corrected by internal defibrillation using 10–50 joules applied directly across the ventricles. Unsuccessful defibrillation may be due to potassium imbalance, hypothermia or overfull ventricles. As the heart ejects more vigorously, the venous return into the oxygenator is gradually reduced, thereby filling the heart. Finally the return to the oxygenator is stopped completely and the patient is 'off bypass'.

The immediate post-perfusion period is critical as the blood volume is restored to normal and the efficiency and contractility of the heart assessed. Falling arterial pressure with a rising central venous pressure indicates a failing heart requiring inotropic support with β-adrenergic agents, such as dopamine, dobutamine, isoprenaline or adrenaline (Chapter 14). Other inotropic agents such as calcium chloride, glucagon, ouabain or digoxin may also be necessary. Serious dysrhythmias such as heart block, ventricular extrasystoles, supraventricular tachycardia, atrial fibrillation, flutter or nodal rhythm may require pharmacological or electrical reversal to improve cardiac output (Chapter 19). Team work and experience are all important during this phase of the operation and constant reference to the ECG, arterial, venous and (when indicated) left atrial pressure is necessary to wean the heart off bypass and coax it into maximum efficiency. In extreme myocardial failure, coronary perfusion may be improved by using aortic counter-pulsation or 'balloon pump'.

When the circulation is stable, anticoagulation is reversed using protamine sulphate. Adequate reversal is confirmed using the activated prothrombin time estimation. After haemostasis is achieved, drains are positioned in the pericardium, mediastinum and, if inadvertently opened, in the pleural cavity. The chest is closed and the drains put on suction, blood loss being measured in graduated cylinders.

POSTOPERATIVE MANAGEMENT

After major cardiac operations all patients are routinely nursed either in a general intensive care unit or a specific postoperative cardiac ward. They are transferred to such a unit immediately after the operation and without reversal of muscle relaxation. Postoperative mechanical ventilation is used in almost all cases and continues for a few hours or overnight depending on the condition of the patient and the type of operation performed. It allows satisfactory sedation and analgesia to be given without the risk of respiratory depression and ensures adequate oxygenation during the period when the heart is recovering from surgery.

Blood pressure control is again of utmost importance in the immediate postoperative period. Hypotension can lead to inadequate perfusion of the coronary artery grafts while hypertension may exert dangerous pressure on suture lines. Meticulous care must be taken to ensure the arterial pressure is stable within set parameters by the use of vasoactive infusions administered by accurate infusion pumps.

Direct monitoring of arterial, central venous and often left atrial pressures is continued into the postoperative period to facilitate circulatory volume assessment and correct fluid balance. Particular attention is paid to blood loss and any co-agulation deficit corrected with fresh frozen plasma and platelet infusions.

Cardiac dysrhythmias are not uncommon during this period and these should be treated quickly as they impair cardiac output and graft perfusion. The type of sedation and analgesia used will depend on how imminent is extubation of the patient. Narcotic analgesics (e.g. morphine and fentanyl) with a benzodiazepine, e.g. midazolam (Hypnovel), can be used, but for an undepressed patient, prior to extubation, nitrous oxide or a propofol (Diprivan) infusion are preferred.

Most patients are easily weaned from the ventilator except those with chronic pulmonary hypertension or pre-existing pulmonary disease. They remain in the intensive therapy unit until they are metabolically stable with normal serum potassium levels and are independent of invasive monitoring.

37 Anaesthesia for Neurosurgery and Neuroradiology

Applied anatomy and physiology. Cerebrospinal fluid. Cerebral blood flow. General principles of neurosurgical anaesthesia. Posterior fossa craniotomy. Intracranial pressure. Emergency neurosurgical anaesthesia. Neuroradiology. Surgery of spine and spinal cord. Lasers. Postoperative neurosurgical care.

APPLIED ANATOMY AND PHYSIOLOGY

The skull is a rigid closed box, except in neonates and infants before the various component bones have fused together. This box contains the brain, blood and cerebrospinal fluid (CSF), and it is an important feature of neurosurgery that an increase in the space occupied by one of these must be compensated for by decrease in volume of one of the others. Failure to do this leads to a rise in intracranial pressure. The brain itself is composed of grey and white matter, the grey matter being the cerebral cells themselves and the white matter consisting of the nerve fibres and their surrounding myelin sheaths. The brain is surrounded by three meningeal layers, the pia, the arachnoid and the dura mater. The first of these layers is closely applied to the brain and between it and the arachnoid is the subarachnoid space containing the circulating CSF. This space is enlarged in parts of the brain to form ventricles, which contain both CSF itself and areas for secretion of this fluid, the choroid plexuses. CSF circulates in the subarachnoid space both surrounding the brain and the spinal cord and is reabsorbed by the arachnoid villi which lie in the superior sagittal sinus over the surface of the brain. It is essential that circulation of CSF is unimpeded because obstruction to the canals leading to and from the ventricles causes local accumulation of CSF and hydrocephalus.

CEREBROSPINAL FLUID

In normal man there are 120 ml of CSF, of which about 25 ml are in the spinal subarachnoid space. Its composition is similar to protein-free plasma. The functions of the CSF are both to buffer the brain against movements of the skull and to surround certain parts of the brain with a fluid capable of fluctuation in its concentration of ions, e.g. sodium, potassium and bicarbonate. Changes in CSF bicarbonate concentration may be responsible for alterations in respiratory rate and volume mediated by the chemoreceptors. Certain drugs can pass into CSF while others cannot, since its formation is one of selective secretion. The normal CSF pressure is about 120 mm water in the recumbent position.

CEREBRAL BLOOD FLOW

The brain is dependent for its blood supply on four main arteries: the two internal carotid arteries and the two vertebral arteries. These anastomose at the base of the brain, forming the circle of Willis (Fig. 37.1) which then gives off the anterior, middle and posterior cerebral arteries. Because of this anastomotic link the brain can survive with occlusion of one or even two of its main arteries. Under normal conditions the brain receives about 15% of the cardiac output and the cerebral circulation is able to regulate its own blood flow. This means that between mean

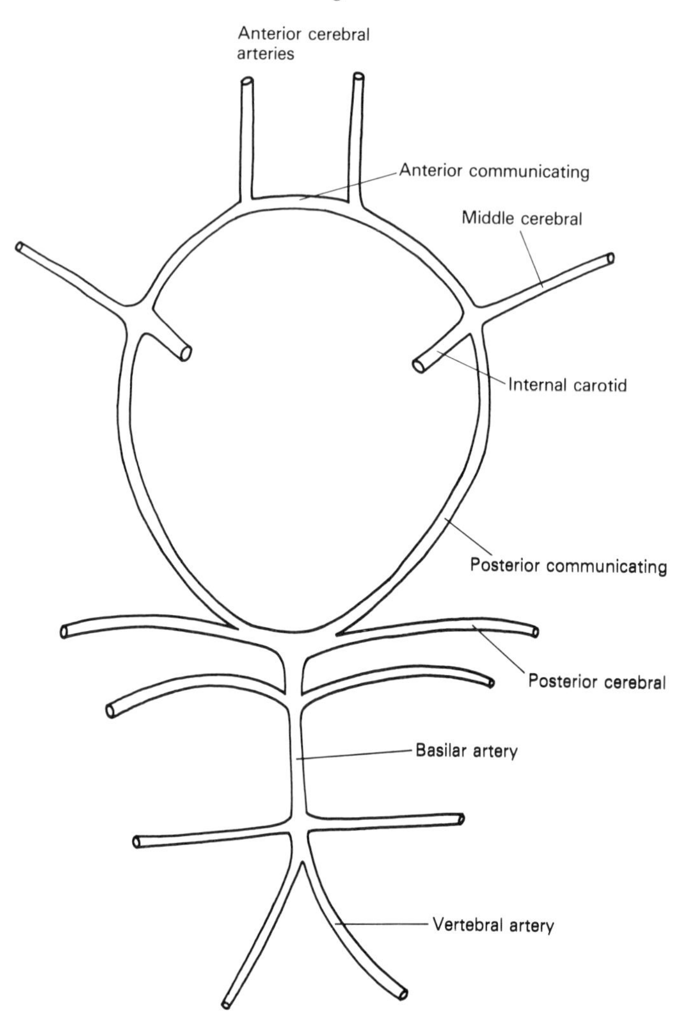

Fig. 37.1 Circle of Willis

arterial blood pressures of 60–140 mmHg the cerebral blood flow is maintained at a constant level by local alteration in the diameter of blood vessels. This process is known as autoregulation.

GENERAL PRINCIPLES OF NEUROSURGICAL ANAESTHESIA

Neurosurgical operations usually involve either the brain or spinal cord, operations on the brain requiring a craniotomy, i.e. removal of a flap of bone to gain access to the brain substance beneath. Operative treatment may range from the removal of either an intracerebral or extracerebral tumour to the clipping of an arterial aneurysm in the region of the circle of Willis, but anaesthesia for all these operations has many important factors in common. A smooth, uncomplicated anaesthetic technique is essential, avoiding increases in either venous blood pressure, carbon dioxide concentration or arterial blood pressure while at the same time avoiding a decrease in cerebral oxygenation. Most anaesthetists now tend to employ a technique using intra-operative analgesics such as fentanyl or phenoperidine, muscle relaxation using either pancuronium or curare, and IPPV. Volatile anaesthetic agents, particularly halothane, are contraindicated because, by producing cerebral vasodilation, they inevitably produce a rise in intracranial pressure. Many of these patients, particularly those with intracerebral tumours, already have high intracranial pressure and a further increase may severely compress the brain. Patients with raised intracranial pressure are prone to nausea and vomiting and for this reason some anaesthetists intubate the patients with a 'crash' technique using suxamethonium to avoid possible regurgitation. It is extremely important to ensure adequate fixation of endotracheal tubes and drips and to protect the eyes, all of which will disappear under the drapes during the operation. Monitoring of the ECG and blood pressure are essential at frequent intervals and, for this reason, direct arterial blood pressure and central venous pressure monitoring are often used (Chapter 23).

POSTERIOR FOSSA CRANIOTOMY

The posterior fossa approach is used for operations on the cerebellum and some surgeons prefer to have the patient sitting. This posture is also common for cervical laminectomy and poses several anaesthetic problems. Patients in the sitting position are prone to hypotension, which will inevitably result in poor cerebral perfusion. In the past, surgeons preferred to operate on a spontaneously breathing patient since many operations in the posterior fossa are in the region of the respiratory centre, and warning changes in respiratory pattern indicate to the surgeon that he is dangerously close to that centre. Air embolism may also be a problem since, when the skull is opened, many of the veins within the bone are held open and, if the venous pressure at this point is subatmospheric, air may enter the veins.

INTRACRANIAL PRESSURE

The main factors tending to cause a rise in intracranial pressure, together with the methods commonly employed to minimise them or to reduce intracranial pressure electively, are summarised in Table 37.1. The use of diuretics such as mannitol or frusemide is designed to deplete the intravascular fluid volume

Table 37.1 Causes of raised intracranial pressure and their treatment

Cause	Treatment
$\uparrow CO_2$	IPPV hyperventilation
Volatile anaesthetics (e.g. halothane)	Avoid these drugs
Coughing, straining	Smooth induction, muscle paralysis
Obstructed airway	Armoured endotracheal tube
Hypertension	Elective hypotension
Head-down position	Raise head

and subsequently reduce CSF production. Actual drainage of CSF may be accomplished either by lumbar puncture or by direct puncture of the cisterna magna or lateral ventricles.

EMERGENCY NEUROSURGICAL ANAESTHESIA

This is common for treating intracranial bleeding—usually as a result of trauma. Collections of blood may arise either extradurally, subdurally or intracerebrally and may accumulate either rapidly or slowly. Many of the patients presenting for anaesthesia will already be unconscious or semi-conscious and irritable as a result of raised intracranial pressure and cerebral compression. It is important to avoid long-acting opiate analgesics because these may mask the eye signs and the level of consciousness, which are used to follow the progress of cerebral trauma. The anaesthetic technique employed is one of muscle relaxation and ventilation preceded by emergency intubation with suxamethonium to avoid regurgitation in the patient with raised intracranial pressure. If the patient is unconscious the anaesthetic requirements initially may well be minimal and, indeed, decompression of intracranial haematoma through burr holes is often conducted under local anaesthesia. However, as the patient's brain is decompressed this may result in his level of consciousness lightening considerably and the anaesthetic may have to be deepened to prevent him waking up. Many patients with head injury require pre-operative neuroradiology and are subsequently kept asleep and taken to theatre for surgery to decompress the brain, usually by burr holes or craniectomy.

NEURORADIOLOGY

The introduction of the EMI (CAT) scanner has in fact removed the need for much neuroradiology. Nevertheless, anaesthesia is still required sometimes for two common neuroradiological procedures: carotid angiography and air encephalography.

Carotid Angiography

This is generally performed to outline the vascular system of the brain and involves injecting dye into one or both internal carotid arteries. Vertebral angiography is usually carried out using a femoral artery catheter inserted under local anaesthetic. The anaesthetic requirements are that the patient should remain still and analgesic and it is usually most satisfactory to ventilate the patients with a short-acting opiate such as fentanyl. Hyperventilation may improve the quality of the x-ray pictures by delaying the flow of dye through the cerebral vessels.

Air Encephalography

Air encephalography (AEG) is used to demonstrate the outline and size of the ventricular system of the brain. Air is injected through a lumbar puncture needle, usually in the spine, and rises to fill the ventricles. The patient is then positioned to allow the air to outline different portions of the ventricles as different x-rays are taken. Although a relaxant and short-acting analgesic technique is now often used for this procedure, some anaesthetists still allow the patients to breathe trichloroethylene spontaneously since this allows observation of their respiratory pattern. Air in the region of the fourth ventricle, and therefore the respiratory centre, may cause respiratory arrest and spontaneous ventilation is used as a safety indicator. It is extremely important in air encephaolography to anchor the apparatus and tubes adequately as the patients are often spun through 360° to position the air in the appropriate spaces in the brain.

Anaesthesia for Computerised Axial Tomography (CAT)

Although most patients tolerate this procedure without anaesthesia, restless, semi-conscious patients and children often need sedating or even a full anaesthetic to remain still throughout the procedure. Like other radiological investigations where the anaesthetist is required to leave his patient for a considerable time while x-rays are taken, a semi-remote control form of anaesthesia is preferable. Again it is usually found more satisfactory to ventilate the patient, although the procedure is often so short that while intermittent suxamethonium provides satisfactory muscle relaxation, the non-depolarising relaxants tend to last too long.

Anaesthesia for Magnetic Resonance Imaging (MRI) Scanning

The demand for general anaesthesia for this procedure is again small, but poses considerable problems, related particularly to the anaesthetic equipment used. Since the radiological technique uses an extremely powerful electromagnetic field, all apparatus must be made from non-ferrous metals. This includes the anaesthetic machine, cylinders and all parts of the anaesthetic circuit.

SURGERY OF SPINE AND SPINAL CORD

Several neurosurgical procedures involve surgery in the region of the spinal cord, usually either for the decompression of nerves as a result of prolapsed intervertebral discs or for the decompression of the cord when the spinal canal is occupied by tumour. In most instances—except when the cervical region is involved—patients should lie prone and an anaesthetic technique employing ventilation is essential since these procedures often take a long time. However, because raised intracranial pressure is not a problem it is often sufficient to ventilate the patient with a volatile anaesthetic agent unless this causes a fall in systemic blood pressure. As the spine is an extremely vascular area, hypotensive anaesthesia is occasionally used to decrease the bleeding and particularly the venous ooze in the area of the operation. This is also considerably reduced if the operation site can be placed above the level of the heart, this being another advantage of the patient being prone.

LASERS

Lasers are becoming increasingly used for tissue dissection and cautery, particularly in neuro- and ENT surgery. Their use may demand specialised anaesthetic techniques since the laser beam will burn through most substances such as endotracheal tubes. Theatre staff must wear eye protection during laser surgery. Their use in the treatment of laryngeal tumours demands specially designed equipment. Lasers must not be used in the presence of inflammable gases or vapours since the heat generated may ignite the gas producing an explosion.

POSTOPERATIVE NEUROSURGICAL CARE

Although many of the patients who have undergone spinal or cranial surgery are awake and conscious in the immediate postoperative period, some will still require active intensive treatment after their operation. This is particularly important in patients who still have raised intracranial pressure or when it is liable to rise, and in those who have undergone cerebral aneurysm surgery —when postoperative vasospasm is often a problem. Elective postoperative ventilation to control cerebral oxygenation and to produce a mild decrease of intracranial pressure is often employed, with continuous monitoring of both arterial and intracranial pressure. The latter is usually accomplished by placing a catheter within the ventricular system of the brain at operation. The patients are then treated with diuretics and possibly CSF drainage to control persistent rises in intracranial pressure. In the case of postoperative vasospasm, specific vasodilator therapy may be instituted to prevent local areas of cerebral ischaemia which may result in hemiplegia. In general, postoperative opiates are avoided in neurosurgical patients, codeine phosphate being used as an analgesic. They may also need an anti-emetic—for example, metoclopramide—to treat the nausea which is not uncommon after intracranial operations.

38 General Anaesthesia in Neonates and Children

Main differences between adults and children. Drugs in paediatric anaesthesia. Induction of anaesthesia. Maintenance of anaesthesia. Monitoring. General comment.

MAIN DIFFERENCES BETWEEN ADULTS AND CHILDREN

The most obvious difference is one of size, but both the anatomy and physiology of the neonate differ from that of the adult in several important respects, and these modify the anaesthetic care that the patients are given.

General Metabolism

The oxygen consumption of a resting adult is about 3 ml/kg/min. After the first week of life this figure for a neonate is about 9 ml/kg/min, or around three times that of the adult. This then slowly declines until around puberty when there is a brief spurt. This high oxygen consumption has a number of important anaesthetic implications:

1. Since oxygen is converted into carbon dioxide (CO_2) in the body the output of this gas per kg body weight is also three times that of the adult and in order to excrete this volume of CO_2 the

pulmonary ventilation of a neonate is correspondingly greater. This is achieved by trebling the respiratory rate, since the tidal volume is about the same (about 7 ml/kg). During anaesthesia the type of breathing circuit used, the gas flows into it and the amount of ventilation required must still enable the child to eliminate CO_2 efficiently.

2. If respiratory obstruction or arrest occurs during anaesthesia the oxygen reserves within the body are used up three times as quickly as in the adult—consequently a neonate will become seriously hypoxic in one-third of the time. There is much less margin for error.

3. Water and energy turnover are directly related to oxygen consumption, and are much higher in children. They are therefore much more susceptible to lack of food and water and become dehydrated and hypoglycaemic more rapidly.

4. Neonates have a high resting cardiac output in order to supply enough oxygen, carbohydrate and other molecules to the active cells of the body and to remove metabolites.

Respiratory System

The main anatomical differences between neonates and adults occur in the upper airway. The tongue is comparatively larger and tends to obscure the anaesthetist's vision during laryngoscopy, while the lower jaw is on the small side. The epiglottis is folded upon itself and is floppy, tending to fall down in front of the opening to the larynx and to hinder successful intubation. It is common practice to try to catch the epiglottis under the blade of the laryngoscope and thus open the way to the larynx.

Unlike the adult, the narrowest part of whose upper airway is the larynx, in the neonate and child up to about 8–10 years old the cricoid cartilage is the narrowest portion, smaller than both the larynx and the nasal passages. The cricoid is a circular ring, if an endotracheal tube is chosen an airtight fit may be obtained between the two, making it unnecessary to employ cuffed tubes. However, it is also very important not to use a tube that is too tight, since if prolonged and excessive pressure is put on the mucosa covering the inner surface of the cricoid it may become damaged, and after extubation may become oedematous and produce upper respiratory obstruction. The best fit is one which allows a slight leak when positive pressure is applied to the airway. The fact that the cricoid cartilage is narrower than even the nasal passages means that an airtight fit can be obtained with both oral and nasal intubation without using cuffed tubes, and this is made use of during long-term intubation in the intensive care unit, where nasotracheal intubation is often employed.

It is not always possible to judge accurately the correct size of endotracheal tube needed before it has been passed and tested for leaks. Three sizes of tube should therefore be prepared—the estimated correct size, one size above and one below. A rough estimate of the tube size can be made from the formula:

$$\text{Diameter (mm)} = \frac{\text{Age}}{4} + 4$$

Thus, for a 6-year-old child, the sizes that should be prepared are 5·5 mm ($\frac{6}{4} + 4 = 5{\cdot}5$) 5·00 mm, and 6·0 mm plain tubes. This formula may vary slightly for different types of endotracheal tube, a large variety being available, and does not apply to the very young (below about 4 years), for whom relatively large tube sizes are required. Nearly all neonates will accept a 3·0 mm without difficulty, though a 2·5 mm and 3·5 mm should also be available.

Following intubation many anaesthetists use an oropharyngeal pack. This has the advantages of reducing the air leak, greatly helping to stabilise the tube, and soaking up any secretions produced during anaesthesia.

The length of the endotracheal tube is important as well as the width since the neonatal trachea is only some 2·5 cm long, and there is therefore not much margin for error between a tube that is too short which may become displaced from the trachea, and one that is too long which will enter the right main bronchus. Nasal tubes need to be about 2 cm longer than oral tubes in the neonate.

Intubation

Intubation in the neonate is usually accomplished before induction of anaesthesia (awake intubation). This is entirely for safety reasons. Once a neonate is anaesthetised and paralysed, trouble may be experienced in keeping it well oxygenated because of difficulty in ventilating the lungs using a mask. If problems with intubation are also experienced, the child will rapidly become dangerously hypoxic. If it has not been paralysed, it can soon re-oxygenate itself by breathing oxygen from a mask after the laryngoscope has been withdrawn. Cyanosis frequently occurs during awake intubation due to coughing and breath-holding and it helps to avoid this if a small (size 6–8 FG) suction catheter is passed through the nose into the pharynx, and 0·5 litre per minute of oxygen delivered down the catheter. This provides a pool of oxygen in the pharynx for the child to breathe.

The main disadvantage of awake intubation is that it is more difficult to perform than in a well-relaxed baby, and is therefore more traumatic. Once the tube is in place it is quite well accepted by neonates, and anaesthesia can then be safely induced. It is commonly said that awake intubation can be used in the first three weeks of life, but in practice the limits are much wider than this. A large, day-old bouncing baby can be very difficult to intubate awake, whereas it may be quite easy in a sickly and underweight child of six weeks.

In children in whom awake intubation would be expected to be difficult and traumatic, it is better to use a relaxant after inhalational or intravenous induction of general anaesthesia.

The anaesthetist's assistant can be of great help in providing the right conditions for intubation, whether the child is awake or asleep. The child, including its arms, should be firmly wrapped in a swaddling cloth. The assistant stands on the right side of the patient and places his left hand behind the child's head. This enables him to control movements of the head, and also place it in the best position to make intubation easy. The laryngoscope is gently passed and the assistant uses his right hand to pass the tube to the anaesthetist. During insertion of the tube it is helpful if the assistant applies gentle backward pressure on the larynx thus helping to bring it into view. The correct anaesthetic circuit, plenty of adhesive tape, a small gauze pack and a small pair of Magill forceps should be available for use immediately after successful intubation.

Pulmonary ventilation

In neonates, as in adults, pulmonary ventilation is mainly diaphragmatic. In the neonate, however, the thoracic component is not nearly so powerful. There are two reasons for this. Firstly, the ribs are much more horizontal so that the possible lateral expansion of the chest is less. Secondly, and more important, the ribs are cartilaginous and therefore soft. In the event of respiratory obstruction (either partial or complete), or any other difficulty in respiration, instead of moving outwards to help respiration the rib cage is sucked inwards by the powerful action of the diaphragm, and this tends to decrease lung expansion, making the efforts of the diaphragm to suck air into the lungs less efficient. It is therefore especially important in this age group to use low-resistance (wide-bore) apparatus and endotracheal tubes, and to ensure that the airway is kept well open during anaesthesia so that there is as little resistance to breathing as possible. For these reasons many anaesthetists will intubate and ventilate all neonates during anaesthesia so that the work of breathing is taken over.

As well as having low resistance, the other important point about neonatal anaesthetic apparatus is that it should have a low dead space. In the normal neonate the tidal volume is about 20 ml, of which about 30–40% (6–8 ml) is dead space, so that only 12–14 ml of the inspired gases actually take part in gas exchange at each breath (the alveolar ventilation). If a piece of apparatus with a large dead space of, say, 10 ml is placed on the child's face, the total dead space (child + apparatus) will then amount to some 16–18 ml. Since the tidal volume is only 20 ml, the alveolar ventilation is therefore reduced to only 2–4 ml per breath.

Rendell-Baker apparatus (Fig. 38.1) consists of a wide-bore mask adaptor divided down the middle by a plate. Fresh gas flows in on one side of the plate, passes over the face of the child,

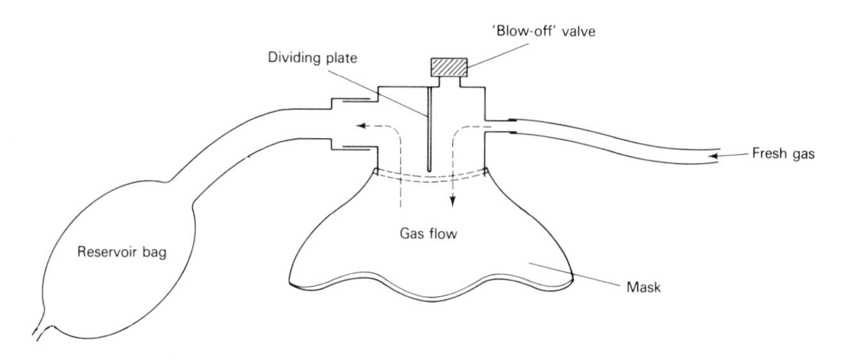

Fig. 38.1 Rendell-Baker apparatus

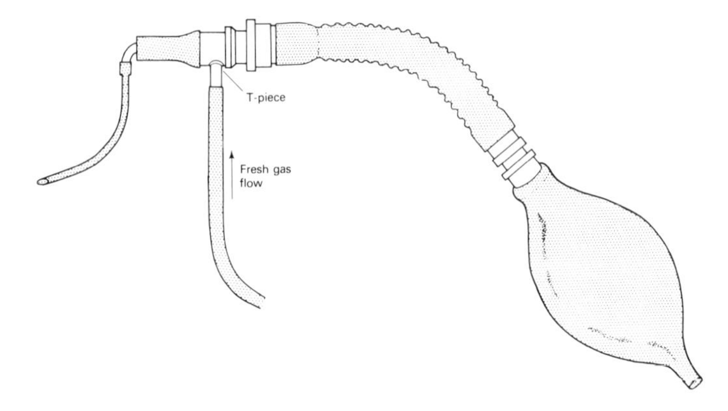

Fig. 38.2 Jackson-Rees modification of Ayre's T-piece (see also Fig. 9.4)

up the other side of the plate and out through a piece of wide-bore tubing into a small bag with an open tail. The child therefore inhales from a constant stream of fresh gas passing over its face, and the dead space is virtually zero. Three sizes of specially designed masks are provided for use with the apparatus, and it is excellent for short anaesthetics given without intubation with the child breathing spontaneously.

Ayre's T-piece (Fig. 38.2) is mainly used during endotracheal anaesthesia because it is small and can easily be fixed to a child's face. Fresh gas is provided through the side-arm and expired gas passes down the wide-bore tubing to a small bag with an open tail and thence into the atmosphere. The addition of the open-ended bag was suggested by Jackson-Rees, and enables artificial ventilation to be used. This is the Mapleson F system (Chapter 9). Inflation is accomplished simply by closing the tail and squeezing the bag, and expiration is allowed by releasing the bag and opening the tail. Specially designed paediatric ventilators can be attached instead of the bag, but mechanical ventilation is not as safe as manual. The apparatus dead space depends on the volume of the catheter mount, as can be seen from the diagram, and therefore during spontaneous ventilation this should be kept as small as possible. Light and convenient forms of the T-piece have recently become available.

The Rendell-Baker and Ayre's T-piece circuits are applicable particularly for the newborn to 3-years-old age group or up to 15–20 kg. Bigger children are better able to cope with the dead space and resistance problems presented by adult circuits.

Some anaesthetists like to humidify and warm the gases that are delivered from the anaesthetic machine. There are two reasons for this. Firstly, the normal humidifying function of the nose is bypassed during endotracheal anaesthesia, and dry gases entering the trachea have a detrimental effect on the tracheal and bronchial mucosa. Secondly, by providing warm gases the loss of heat resulting from the inhalation of dry gas at room temperature is avoided, and temperature maintenance is helped.

Heat Loss and Temperature Control

Up to about 3–6 months of age a baby is not able to control its temperature nearly as effectively as can an adult. This is due both to increased heat loss and a reduced capacity to increase its heat production. Both these factors are adversely affected by anaesthesia and surgery.

Sources of heat loss

A child has a greater surface area, weight for weight, than an adult, and therefore the potential for heat loss to the atmosphere is greater. Anaesthesia tends to produce skin vasodilation and thus increases heat loss from the skin. In the premature neonate the layer of subcutaneous fat is scanty, so the baby is only poorly insulated. Heat loss occurs because of evaporation from wounds and from exposed bowel or other organs. The infusion of cold intravenous fluids tends to lower the baby's temperature.

The infusion of cold intravenous fluids tends to lower the baby's temperature.

Sources of heat production

Shivering. Unlike adults, who can raise their heat production many times by shivering, newborn babies are unable to shiver.

Metabolism of brown fat. Situated around the scapulae and the back of the neck are deposits of brownish fat whose metabolism produces a considerable amount of heat. Metabolism of brown fat is triggered by the sympathetic nervous system in response to a cold environment, and the sympathetic system is effectively blocked by many anaesthetic agents such as halothane. Therefore the capacity to mobilise heat from brown fat is reduced by anaesthesia.

Carbohydrate metabolism. This is also increased in response to cold, and provides a ready source of heat production. Many neonates, however, have a tendency towards hypoglycaemia, and the increased use of glucose and glycogen to produce heat may accentuate this. Although the neonate cannot shiver, the metabolism of both brown fat and carbohydrate can increase its heat production some three times, but this is reduced by anaesthesia.

The harmful effects of allowing a baby's temperature to fall are as follows:

1. Difficulty in reversing relaxants and establishing breathing at the end of operation.
2. Hypoglycaemia.
3. Sclerema, or neonatal cold injury. This is a condition which appears postoperatively, in which the metabolism of subcutaneous fat alters and it becomes hard to the touch. This change can first be detected in the calves and forearms, and may spread to cover the whole body. Mortality is high in severe cases, and there is no effective treatment, so prevention is imperative. The three main predisposing factors are prematurity, an ill child and hypothermia.
4. Changes in electrolyte, water and acid-base status of the baby, due to reduced perfusion and the development of lactic acidosis.

Prevention of accidental hypothermia

In the unanaesthetised neonate the ambient temperature (e.g. in an incubator) should be kept at 32–34°C. During surgery the following precautions should be taken to prevent a fall in body temperature.

1. The operating theatre temperature should be raised to 'subtropical', especially with premature infants and when the operation entails the exposure of large areas of bowel or cut surface.
2. The child should be moved straight from the incubator or infra-red heat source onto a warm water mattress, and kept as well covered as possible during induction of anaesthesia. If anaesthesia is not induced in a warm environment temperature can easily fall 2–3°C. In premature babies and those in whom

induction of anaesthesia is expected to be prolonged this should all be done under an infra-red heater.

3. A water blanket set at 38–40°C should be placed between the child and the operating table. It is advisable to place a layer of gaugee or similar material between the child and the water-blanket as this prevents occasional burns on the baby's back.

4. The child should be covered with a layer of gaugee except for the operating site. The head as well as the body should be covered, because a neonate's head is large compared with its body, and much heat may be lost from its surface. One hand may be left uncovered for the anaesthetist to watch.

5. Some anaesthetists like to place a layer of baking foil or a 'silver swaddler' outside the gauze covering, as this reduces heat loss due to radiation. The baby is now effectively encased in a thermos flask!

6. All intravenous fluids and blood should be warmed.

7. Some anaesthetists like to warm the anaesthetic gases or a small humidifier may be incorporated in the circuit.

With these precautions, a serious fall in body temperature is rare. Above the age of about 6 months precautions should be reduced or the child may easily become hyperthermic.

Circulatory System

The resting cardiac output of the neonate is two to three times that of the adult, weight for weight. The resting pulse rate is variable, the normal ranging between about 110 and 160 beats per min. It may rise above 200 beats per min during crying. As the child grows older the variability becomes less and the average rate progressively declines. The systolic blood pressure is 80–90 mm Hg after birth, rising to 90–100 mm Hg at one year of age, and then slowly up to adult values as a late teenager. Again, there is much variability in the very young.

The blood volume of the neonate is about 85 ml/kg, so a 3 kg baby has about 250 ml blood. The haemoglobin is high, 18–20 g/100 ml consisting mainly of fetal haemoglobin, which progressively declines over 2–3 months to become replaced by adult haemoglobin. The total haemoglobin falls rapidly after birth, reaching a low point of 12–14 g/100 ml at 2–3 months of age, then slowly rising again to adult values (14–15 g/100 ml) at 1–2 years.

The principles of blood transfusion during surgery are the same as in the adult, namely that blood should be given if the loss exceeds about 10% of the blood volume, provided that the child is not anaemic. In a 3 kg neonate this amounts to a blood loss of about 25 ml. Measuring such small volumes of blood loss is difficult, and is normally done by swab weighing. At best this produces a somewhat inaccurate assessment of the loss—normally an underestimate due to evaporation—and the volume measured must be supplemented by a visual estimate of blood loss, including that in the sucker, on the drapes and elsewhere. It is advisable to be on the generous side when replacing operative blood loss.

All transfused blood should be warmed before being given, and if rapid transfusion is necessary, should be accompanied by calcium gluconate (0·1 ml of the 10% solution per 10 ml of blood) as neonates have a tendency to hypocalcaemia. Small volumes of blood in special 40 ml containers are available for neonatal transfusion.

Water and Electrolyte Balance

Water and electrolyte turnover in neonates is two to three times that of the adult, being closely related to the oxygen consumption. However, the ability of the neonate to deal with excesses or deficiencies in either is less than that of the adult, so more care has to be exercised in the amounts that are given or withheld. For instance, in adults it is customary to withhold all oral intake pre-operatively to reduce the risk of inhalation of stomach contents. Stopping fluids in an adult for 12 hours pre-operatively (i.e. overnight) does no appreciable harm, but if this is done to a neonate it has the same effect as withholding water from an adult for two to three times as long (i.e. 24–36 hours). Hence neonates and infants must not be starved for long periods and should be fed up to 4–6 hours pre-operatively. The final feed may be diluted (i.e. half-strength milk), though adequate water should be given. Similarly, feeds should be started as soon after operation as is practicable.

During operation a greater amount of fluid should be given (per kilogram) than to an adult. Provided that there is no fluid deficit before operation a suitable amount is 5–10 ml/kg/hour plus some extra to account for evaporation and other losses. When losses are high an amount nearer to 10 ml/kg/hour should be given. The solution used should contain some sodium and also some glucose or dextrose to provide calories and to prevent hypoglycaemia. A suitable fluid for general use is 4% dextrose with 1/5 normal saline, though this may have to be varied in some circumstances.

The normal response of adults to surgery is to retain fluid and sodium postoperatively, and neonates show much the same stress response. Some restriction of water and sodium intake is therefore desirable after surgery, as babies very readily become oedematous at this time.

Hypoglycaemia

In the first few days of life babies have a low blood sugar and low glycogen stores in the liver. This is because their stores are largely used up during delivery and take some days to be replenished, especially in ill babies who are not feeding properly. Severe hypoglycaemia (the signs of which are masked if the neonate is anaesthetised) may occur and cause brain damage. It may be necessary to estimate the blood glucose concentrations during anaesthesia and a simple method of doing this should be available. It may be necessary to administer 10% glucose to neonates.

DRUGS IN PAEDIATRIC ANAESTHESIA

Babies and children require relatively larger doses than adults to achieve the same effect. The main reasons for this are that (1) the higher metabolic rate results in the more rapid breakdown and excretion of drugs, and (2) the water content of the neonate (about 75%) is larger than that of the adult (about 50%), most of the extra being contained in the extracellular fluid. Hence any drug given is more diluted by body water, and a greater dose is required to achieve the same concentration at the receptor site.

The doses of most drugs may be estimated from the adult dose (more easily remembered than children's doses) by using the formula:

$$\text{Child's dose (mg/kg)} = \frac{\text{Total adult dose}}{50}$$

For example, the normal intubating dose of suxamethonium in the adult is 100 mg. Therefore:

$$\text{Child's dose} = \frac{100}{50} = 2\,\text{mg/kg}$$

There are some exceptions to this rule, the most important during anaesthesia being the non-depolarising relaxants (e.g. curare). During the first three weeks of extra-uterine life neonates are particularly sensitive to these drugs. A reduced dose must therefore be given until the response of the baby can be judged. In contrast, the neonate is resistant to the depolarising relaxant, suxamethonium, a higher dose being required to produce neuromuscular blockade.

Premedication

Anaesthetists vary widely in the premedication that they prescribe for children. The reasons for giving premedication at all are the same as for adults. Below a weight of about 10 kg it is usual to employ atropine alone in proportionately larger doses than would be given to an adult, mainly to suppress excessive secretions in the upper respiratory tract. Opiates are normally avoided in order to reduce the danger of severe respiratory depression, though this is only true in very young children and especially in the premature.

In older children intramuscular opiates in combination with atropine or hyoscine are commonly used, as is trimeprazine (Vallergan) 2–4 mg/kg and atropine given orally two hours pre-operatively. Oral diazepam and other benzodiazepines are also popular. In general, intramuscular drugs are more reliable than those given orally because of variability in absorption from the gastrointestinal tract, but have the disadvantage of having to be given by injection. The opiates especially give good postoperative analgesia, a property lacking in oral premedication, but are associated with a higher incidence of postoperative vomiting.

Emla cream, a recent product which helps to make intravenous induction less painful is discussed in Chapter 4.

INDUCTION OF ANAESTHESIA

It is a psychological advantage for a child (but not, as far as is known, for a neonate) if one parent is present at the induction of anaesthesia, though a few parents are upset by this. The incidence of behavioural changes once the child has returned home is less if someone he knows well is with him and he is aware of what is going on in the anaesthetic room, rather than being virtually unconscious. Most children are very composed and sensible if they know beforehand exactly what is going to happen to them at this time.

Induction itself can either be inhalational or intravenous.

MAINTENANCE OF ANAESTHESIA

A wide choice of techniques is available and used by different anaesthetists. In the neonate the tendency is to use a relaxant technique with artificial ventilation by hand using supplemented nitrous oxide to produce unconsciousness, but in older children a greater variety of methods is used. A typical sequence for a neonate undergoing laparotomy might be as follows:

1. Establish an open vein while keeping the baby warm.
2. Intubate while awake.
3. Administer nitrous oxide and oxygen and a small dose of a non-depolarising relaxant, and start artificial ventilation.
4. Give further doses of relaxant until the required effect is obtained. Anaesthesia is now maintained, giving more relaxant and anaesthetic if needed, until the end of surgery.
5. Give atropine and neostigmine to reverse the relaxant and re-establish spontaneous ventilation.
6. Withdraw nitrous oxide, give oxygen, and extubate when the baby awakens.
7. Transfer the baby back to the incubator as soon as possible.

MONITORING

Owing to their small size babies are not easy to monitor. The most useful single thing is to have a hand accessible, so that the radial pulse may be felt and the colour of the hand observed (a good light should be available).

A precordial (or oesophageal) stethoscope is useful. Through this any secretions in the respiratory tract can easily be heard, and the anaesthetist can note the intensity of the heart sounds. These become quieter if a fall in blood pressure occurs. The blood pressure may be measured using a narrow cuff (the width of the cuff should be equal to about two thirds the length of the upper arm). Several different methods are used to obtain the systolic pressure, including feeling the radial pulse, using a stethoscope or automatic blood pressure device, or using the flush technique. This latter involves squeezing the hand to exsanguinate it, blowing up the cuff, and then slowly letting it down; the point at which the hand flushes being the systolic pressure. Finally, the blood pressure may be measured by using a pressure transducer connected to an umbilical or radial arterial catheter. If this is available, blood can also be withdrawn from the catheter for measurement of blood gases and blood glucose.

The pulse rate is best measured using an ECG, and this facility should always be available for any neonatal operation. When very major blood loss is expected central venous pressure should also be monitored, and an estimate of the blood loss made as it occurs.

Transcutaneous oxygen measurement and pulse oximeters are very useful during major surgery, though each technique has its own deficiencies.

The temperature of the baby should be measured by using a rectal, oesophageal or nasopharyngeal probe, and it is useful to be able to measure the temperature of the water blanket or of the air enclosed in the child's coverings.

GENERAL COMMENT

Neonatal anaesthesia is demanding. For consistent success good teamwork is essential with meticulous preparation of the anaesthetic room, operating theatre and apparatus. There is very little room for error in these tiny patients.

39 Obstetric Anaesthesia and Analgesia

Obstetric anaesthesia. Pain relief in obstetrics. Awake caesarean section. The obstetric flying squad.

The first part of this chapter is concerned with anaesthesia for obstetric patients. This branch of anaesthesia is unique in that even elective operations carry a high degree of risk. The reasons for this are included in the 'Special considerations' section below. Despite these dangers, obstetric departments are often isolated and the anaesthetic help may temporarily be recruited from the midwives. Not all of these had anaesthetic training and the increased availability of skilled help for the obstetric anaesthetist would do much to increase the safety of obstetric anaesthesia.

The second part of this chapter briefly discusses methods of pain relief in obstetrics.

OBSTETRIC ANAESTHESIA

Physiological Changes in Pregnancy

Changes occur in most of the body systems. Some of the most important, from the anaesthetist's viewpoint, are outlined below.

Cardiovascular system
There is an increase in cardiac output from a non-pregnant level of about 4·5 litres/min to 6·0 litres/min. This is achieved by an

increase both in heart rate (to about 85/min at term) and in stroke volume. Many organs have an increased blood flow, but the biggest increase is to the uterus. In the last trimester of pregnancy, occlusion of the inferior vena cava by the gravid uterus tends to occur in the supine position. This is discussed in more detail below.

Respiratory system
Minute ventilation is increased by an increase in tidal volume of about 40% over non-pregnant values without an increase in respiratory rate. This meets the increased oxygen requirements and disposes of the increased carbon dioxide production of the growing uterus, fetus and placenta.The normal $P\mathrm{CO}_2$ at term is about 30 mmHg (4·0 kPa) compared with the normal 40 mmHg (5·3 kPa). This has important implications for the anaesthetist who must ensure that in pregnant patients he employs an anaesthetic technique capable of achieving these lower than usual $P\mathrm{CO}_2$ levels.

Blood volume and its constituents
Both the plasma volume and the number of red cells increase in pregnancy. However, the increase in the red cells is proportionately less so that there is a fall in the haemoglobin content of the blood to a level which should not be lower than 12 g/100 ml provided that the woman takes supplementary iron and folic acid. This is the so-called 'physiological anaemia' of pregnancy.

Special Considerations

A number of factors affecting obstetric anaesthesia—some of them unique to obstetric patients—deserve special mention.

1. The 'two lives' problem
The so-called placental 'barrier' is readily crossed by most pharmacological agents used in anaesthesia, including pethidine and the narcotic agents commonly used in premedication, the thiobarbiturates and other induction agents, the anaesthetic gases and volatile anaesthetic agents. The only frequently used drugs that do not cross the placenta in significant quantities are the muscle relaxants, with the possible exception of gallamine.

While the fetus is in utero, it relies on the placenta for its supply of oxygen and its excretion of carbon dioxide. At birth this facility is abruptly removed, and the newborn, by redistributing its circulation and expanding its lungs, has to fend for itself in obtaining oxygen and excreting carbon dioxide. Thus it has to initiate and maintain regular respiration and it is its ability to do this which is so readily adversely affected by depressant narcotic or anaesthetic agents.

Thus it is standard anaesthetic practice before obstetric anaesthesia not to give the mother any narcotic or sedative premedication. Induction is then carried out by a minimal dose of induction agent (e.g. sodium thiopentone 225–300 mg) and after intubation with suxamethonium; light anaesthesia is maintained with nitrous oxide and oxygen with only a trace of adjuvant until the baby is delivered. Thereafter, anaesthesia should be deepened to ensure that the mother is adequately anaesthetised.

2. Awareness in the mother

The possibility that a patient is not deeply enough anaesthetised is always a danger with muscle relaxant anaesthesia where the surgical operating conditions are achieved by the muscle relaxant rather than by depth of anaesthesia, as was the case when single agents, e.g. chloroform or ether, were used. The risk of awareness is therefore particularly high in obstetric anaesthesia, where in the interests of the fetus anaesthesia is deliberately kept as light as possible.

At present there is no complete solution to this problem, any additional safeguard against awareness in the mother attained by deepening the anaesthesia inevitably being achieved at the cost of a greater tendency to a depressed neonate. The best that the anaesthetist can do is to choose a technique which is known to have a low incidence of awareness allied to minimal depression of the newborn and to perform it meticulously.

3. Vomiting and regurgitation

The difference between vomiting and regurgitation is discussed in Chapter 26. Vomiting occurs only at a very light level of anaesthesia. With modern intravenous induction agents (unless these are given very slowly) the patient is taken down rapidly to a depth of anaesthesia well below the level at which vomiting occurs, but may become deeply enough anaesthetised for regurgitation to occur. The induction agent is immediately followed by a muscle relaxant. This is usually suxamethonium, which may cause strong enough twitching of the abdominal muscles to increase the intragastric pressure and facilitate reflux. It then paralyses the patient so that regurgitation is again more likely. An endotracheal tube is passed and once the cuff is inflated the patient's respiratory tract is secure against soiling by gastric contents until extubation at the end of the obstetric procedure.

There are several reasons why obstetric patients are likely to regurgitate. These factors are listed in Table 39.1, where they are considered in elective or emergency obstetric procedures. Examples of the former might be the insertion of a cervical circumsuture, while the latter nearly always implies that the patient is in labour.

Table 39.1 Factors facilitating reflux in obstetric patients

Danger factor	Elective obstetric procedures	Emergency obstetric procedures
'Big bump' problem	+	+
Heartburn problem	+	+
Full stomach problem	−	+

The 'big bump' refers to the gravid uterus, which in the second half of pregnancy occupies an increasingly large proportion of the abdominal cavity. It eventually occupies more space than any but the most enormous pathological tumours and in the recumbent position simply compresses the stomach against the diaphragm and tends to squeeze any gastric contents up into the oesophagus. This danger factor applies to both elective and emergency procedures, except possibly in women who are under 20 weeks pregnant, in whom the uterus is still relatively small, and in cases of retained placenta, where the uterus has already diminished in size.

Heartburn is a common symptom in pregnancy and implies reflux of acid gastric juice into the oesophagus due to incompetence of the gastro-oesophageal (cardiac) sphincter. The reason for this incompetence is not known for certain, but is believed to be partly hormonal. A weak sphincter is more likely to give way before the increased intragastric pressure caused by the gravid uterus, especially in the recumbent position. About

30% of women who complain of heartburn have a hiatus hernia, which can be demonstrated radiologically, but it is wise to consider all patients in the second half of pregnancy to be at risk from oesophageal reflux. Once again, both elective and emergency patients are at risk.

On the whole, pregnant women digest food adequately—otherwise they would reach term in a uniformly cachectic state! In labour, recent work has shown that digestion does continue, but two factors tend to cause delay in gastric emptying. The first of these is prolongation of labour, a duration of over 12 hours being likely to be associated with an increase in gastric contents. Secondly, the administration of pethidine or a narcotic causes a marked delay in gastric emptying.

In summary, all pregnant patients are at risk from inhalation of gastric contents, but patients in prolonged labour who have been given pethidine are particularly at risk because they have the added danger of gastric stasis.

Acid aspiration syndrome (Mendelson's syndrome)

In 1946 Mendelson, who was a New York obstetrician, described an asthma-like syndrome associated with a mottled appearance on the chest x-ray which he considered was caused by the inhalation of liquid acid gastric contents with a pH of less than 2·5. This hypothesis is now widely accepted and the clinical picture is referred to as 'Mendelson's syndrome'. The syndrome varies greatly in severity but can be fatal. It does not, of course, supplant the possibility of acute asphyxia caused by inhalation of solid or semi-solid gastric contents.

The logical prophylactic measure is to raise the pH of the gastric contents by administering alkali, and this is now routine in many maternity units. Until recently, the most popular alkali was the chalky Mist. Magnesium Trisilicate BPC, but it has been largely superseded by 0·3 molar sodium citrate which, while non-granular, is sometimes very short-acting. Whichever alkali is used, it should be given in a dose of 30 ml a few minutes before induction of anaesthesia, the former routine of giving it in 15 ml doses every two hours in labour having been abandoned. The search continues for a more palatable, longer-lasting, non-granular alkali.

It is sometimes thought that Mendelson's syndrome occurs only in obstetrics. This is not so. The term may be applied to acid aspiration occurring in any branch of anaesthesia, and the prophylactic use of alkali is slowly spreading to other conditions where patients are at risk from aspiration.

Nevertheless, all obstetric patients who are over about 20 weeks pregnant, whether for elective or emergency procedures, should be anaesthetised as for an intestinal obstruction, with pre-oxygenation, a rapid intravenous induction immediately followed by suxamethonium and regurgitation prevented by pressure backwards on a previously marked cricoid cartilage until an endotracheal tube is passed and its cuff inflated.

Treatment. This will consist (depending on severity) of parenteral steroids, bronchodilators, e.g. salbutamol (Ventolin), digoxin, antibiotics and symptomatic treatment of the respiratory state (again depending on severity) up to ventilation with 100% oxygen and positive end-expiratory pressure in the most serious cases.

4. Haemorrhage

Because of the nature of parturition, haemorrhage is an ever-present risk and remains one of the commonest causes of maternal mortality. When the placenta separates from the wall of the uterus in the third stage of labour, a raw and very vascular surface is exposed. Fortunately, the same contraction of the uterus that shears off the placenta also clamps down on the branches of the uterine artery which supply it by passing through the criss-cross syncytial arrangement of uterine muscle fibres. This arrests the haemorrhage and the retraction down of the uterus prevents further bleeding into its cavity.

Any anaesthetic agent that prevents the uterus from contracting down is likely to increase the incidence and severity of post-partum haemorrhage. Historically two agents, chloroform and di-ethyl ether were considered particularly to blame in this respect. However, these agents were always given in high concentrations with spontaneous respiration anaesthesia, and likewise the more modern, powerful volatile agents, e.g. halothane, enflurane and isoflurane, given in high concentrations may prevent uterine contraction. Fortunately, in the low concentrations in which they are used as adjuvants to nitrous oxide, oxygen and muscle relaxant anaesthesia these agents do not cause significant uterine relaxation. The other agent popular as

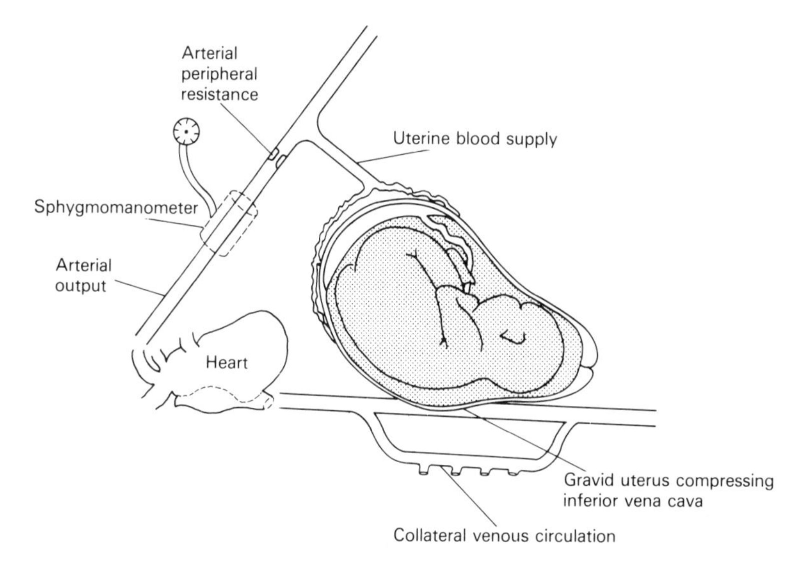

Fig. 39.1 Mechanism of venacaval occlusion

an adjuvant in obstetric anaesthesia is trichloroethylene, a powerful analgesic and amnesic agent which has little effect on uterine muscle tone.

It is a good rule to crossmatch fully two units of blood for all patients booked for elective caesarean section. For emergency caesarean sections and other obstetric emergencies, there should always be available un-crossmatched O Rhesus negative, Kell negative blood and for patients known to be Rhesus positive, O Rh +ve Kell negative blood.

5. Inferior venacaval compression syndrome

It has been known for 30 years that some women feel faint when lying on their backs in the last few weeks of pregnancy. It was thought that in this small group of women (about 5% of pregnant women) the inferior vena cava was being occluded by compression between the gravid uterus and the vertebral column. The heart, deprived of the major part of its venous return, could not maintain an adequate output, the blood pressure fell and the woman felt faint. More recently it has been shown that the inferior vena cava is almost completely occluded in all women in the last weeks of pregnancy when they are supine (Fig. 39.1). Venous return from the lower part of the body then reaches the heart by a collateral system of veins in the paravertebral region and in the epidural space. If this alternative pathway for the blood is well developed the woman lying supine behaves as if she had a patent inferior vena cava. If the collateral circulation is poor, the supine patient may feel faint within minutes. If the adequacy of the collateral system lies between these two extremes, the woman may be able to maintain her blood pressure, but only by compensatory vasoconstriction under the influence of the sympathetic nervous system. She is then particularly susceptible to the vasodilation associated with general anaesthesia and certain types of regional analgesia, e.g. epidural analgesia, and should never be left lying on her back. A rubber or inflatable wedge placed under one hip (usually the right) will usually suffice to roll the uterus off the vena cava and restore the venous return.

It should be realised that with moderate degrees of vena caval occlusion, where the mother is maintaining her blood pressure at a reasonable level by vasoconstriction, the fetus may be adversely affected by the constriction in the blood vessels supplying the placenta.

The alternative term 'aortocaval occlusion' is sometimes used and is justified in that at times, especially if the blood pressure falls, the aorta may also be compressed by the gravid uterus.

The older name, 'supine hypotension syndrome' should be reserved for severe degrees of vena caval occlusion where the blood pressure actually falls.

PAIN RELIEF IN OBSTETRICS

It is not necessary for the anaesthetic assistant to have a wide knowledge of this subject. The methods available are summarised briefly below.

Psychological

In its simplest form this includes the reassurance that can be given to the patient (especially the primiparous) by explaining the process of labour, the nature, origin and purpose of the pain she is likely to feel and the types of pain relief which will be available to her. More complex techniques include the teaching of special methods of breathing which the patient practises antenatally and then performs in response to the pains of labour. This is a form of conditioned response to the pain and acts largely by distraction.

Parenteral

Many drugs have been used in labour—the commonest by far, in the UK, being pethidine. This has the advantage that it requires no complicated apparatus and (with certain provisos) may be given by unsupervised midwives. Its disadvantages are that it is not always effective, it makes some patients nauseated and, if given in the period leading up to delivery, may depress the newborn baby so that it has difficulty in establishing respiration.

Inhalational

The only inhalational technique now approved by the National Boards for Nursing, Midwifery and Health Visiting in the UK for use by unsupervised midwives is the administration of Entonox (BOC), a pre-mixed combination of nitrous oxide 50% and oxygen 50% available in one cylinder or piped to the labour ward (Chapter 7). Although very popular as a method of analgesia, disadvantages include the difficulty in maintaining the technique for long periods, the fact that the patient needs practice to obtain maximum benefit, and that the women sometimes become drowsy and uncooperative, despite the short action of nitrous oxide.

Regional

Complete pain relief in the first stage of labour may be obtained by bilateral blockade of the 11th and 12th thoracic and 1st lumbar nerves. In the second stage of labour additional analgesia is required of the second to fourth sacral nerves.

Blockade of all these nerves by one injection can be obtained only by one of the central nerve blocks. These consist of lumbar or sacral epidural (caudal) analgesia and spinal analgesia. More peripheral blocks have to be bilateral and usually multiple.

The great advantage of the central blocks, especially continuous lumbar epidural analgesia by means of an epidural catheter, is that they can give many hours of complete pain relief, adding a new dimension to analgesia in labour. In addition they are, except in very large doses, virtually non-toxic to mother and fetus.

The main disadvantages of these blocks are that they require skill and experience to perform, they are potentially dangerous if not properly supervised on account of their detrimental effect on venacaval occlusion (see above) and they have a tendency to increase the forceps rate by obtunding the bearing-down reflex. However, with the advent of a more enlightened and less aggressive approach to the conduct of the second stage of labour, in many centres the incidence of forceps deliveries has returned to a level similar to that without the use of epidural analgesia.

Hypnosis and Acupuncture

These are mentioned only for completeness. While hypnosis, in particular, has been reported at times to be effective, both techniques tend not to be universally applicable or effective, may be time-consuming and require skills possessed by few practitioners. It is difficult to envisage their use becoming widespread for relieving pain in childbirth in the foreseeable future.

AWAKE CAESAREAN SECTION

Women are increasingly requesting to be awake for the delivery of their babies by caesarean section. Anaesthetists are keen whenever possible to accede to this request, because in addition to the obvious pleasure it gives to so many women, it also avoids the risks of Mendelson's syndrome and the condition of the newborn baby is usually excellent.

Caesarean section is the most major operation routinely carried out under regional anaesthesia in the UK, but not only is it not covered by light general anaesthesia, but also without pre-operative and preferably intra-operative sedation. It presents the anaesthetist with a considerable challenge, the main problems being the provision of good analgesia and the avoidance of hypotension.

Lumbar epidural or sometimes spinal block are used. Reference to Chapter 33 will reveal that a block up to T5 is required to prevent pain impulses travelling along the sympathetic nerves and even then vagal sensation and pain fibres from the lower surface of the diaphragm running to the cervical nerves will be unaffected. With gentle and careful surgical technique no pain may be initiated in either of these unblocked areas, but it does mean that perfect analgesia cannot be guaranteed.

Hypotension is avoided or minimised by adequate preloading with intravenous fluids, by careful attention to maternal posture (to avoid venacaval occlusion) and sometimes by the use of a vasopressor, ephedrine being the one usually preferred.

For these operations the highest standards of anaesthetic technique and nursing care in the anaesthetic room and theatre are required. The husband usually expects to come into the theatre to accompany his wife. If it can be arranged, a pre-operative visit by the anaesthetic nurse as well as by the anaesthetist is invaluable.

THE OBSTETRIC FLYING SQUAD

Although there has been a great decline in domiciliary midwifery in recent years, it is still possible that an obstetric emergency may arise in a patient's home. A much larger number of deliveries occur in general practitioner units which lack the obstetric and anaesthetic expertise to deal with a serious emergency. The choice then is between resuscitating the patient and always transferring her to the base hospital for definitive treatment, or despatching a skilled team with portable equipment from the base hospital to treat the emergency where she lies.

Which is the safest of these two choices is still debated, and in some parts of the UK there is no proper obstetric flying squad. In others a team usually consisting of a fairly senior obstetrician, anaesthetist and a midwife, with a comprehensive set of equipment travel in or with an ambulance to the emergency. The anaesthetic machine must be portable, robust and safe and for those competent in its use, the EMO vaporiser (Chapter 10) is outstanding in these respects. The anaesthetic can be based on a thiopentone-muscle relaxant–ether–air sequence, with only a lightweight oxygen cylinder being carried for supplementation. Other portable machines require the carrying of separate nitrous oxide and oxygen, or Entonox cylinders, perhaps with an Oxford Miniature Vaporiser for trichloroethylene supplementation (Chapter 10), but these machines are inevitably heavier and more complicated than the EMO system. Fortunately for those not conversant with the EMO, the majority of flying squad calls are now to cottage hospitals where there is a Boyle's machine available.

40 Local Analgesic Drugs

History. Definition. Pharmacology. Individual local analgesic agents.

HISTORY

For centuries the natives of Peru and Bolivia had chewed the leaves of a shrub, *Erythroxylon coca*, which lessened fatigue and appetite and numbed the tongue. These effects were due to the principal alkaloid, cocaine, contained in the plant.

In 1860 cocaine was isolated by Niemann and in 1884 Karl Köhler, a Viennese physician, noted its analgesic effect in the eye and published his results. Thereafter the use of local analgesia in its various forms developed quickly.

Dates of introduction of other particularly useful local analgesic drugs include: 1905—procaine; 1925—cinchocaine; 1948—lignocaine; 1963—bupivacaine.

DEFINITION

Local analgesics are drugs which block conduction when applied locally to nerve tissue. The block produced is completely reversible with no damage to nerve cells.

PHARMACOLOGY

Properties Desirable in a Local Analgesic

These are as follows:

1. They should have a rapid onset of action. The desired duration of action varies with the indication, e.g. a very long action would be ideal for postoperative pain relief, but a jaw made numb for many hours after a simple dental procedure would be tedious and inconvenient.
2. The systemic toxicity should be low.
3. They should be non-addictive, non-antigenic, non-irritant to tissues and should not interfere with wound healing.
4. They should be effective topically as well as when injected, although such versatility is not essential.
5. They should be soluble in water, stable in solution, and autoclavable at least once without loss of potency.

Sites of Application of Local Analgesic Drugs

Starting centrally and working peripherally, local analgesic solutions may produce the following types of analgesia:

Spinal block—where the injection is into the subarachnoid space.

Epidural block—where the injection is into the epidural space.

Nerve plexus block—where the injection is made into a nerve plexus, e.g. brachial plexus block.

Nerve block—where the injection is into a single nerve trunk, e.g. femoral block, ulnar block.

Local infiltration—where the injection is into the tissues, e.g. subcutaneous infiltration.

Intravenous regional (Bier's block)—where the injection is made into a vein of a limb whose circulation is occluded by a tourniquet.

Intra-arterial regional—where the injection is made into an artery of a limb whose circulation is occluded by a tourniquet.

Topical—where the drug is applied to skin or mucous membrane.

Intravenous infusion—seldom if ever used now to produce general analgesia, e.g. for burns dressings, although commonly used to prevent or treat ventricular dysrhythmias.

Mode of Action

In its resting state, the outside of the cell membrane of a nerve fibre is positively charged relative to the inside. When a nerve impulse is propagated along the nerve fibre, there is a sudden increase in the permeability of the cell membrane to sodium ions, which then flow into the interior of the nerve fibre and reverse the electrical polarity across the cell membrane so that the inside becomes positively charged with reference to the outside. This phenomenon is called 'depolarisation' and is fundamental to the transmission of the nerve impulse. It is this sudden increase in permeability of the cell membrane to sodium ions which in some way is interfered with by local analgesic drugs so that depolarisation is prevented and nerve fibre block occurs. The exact mode of action is unknown.

Chemistry

All local analgesic drugs of clinical interest belong to one main group, which has the following basic formula:

Aromatic group—intermediate chain—amino group

This main group of local analgesic drugs is divided into two subgroups depending on the method of linkage between the aromatic group and the intermediate chain. If this is an ester (-COO-) linkage the local analgesic belongs to the 'ester' group and if the linkage is an amide -HN.CO- linkage the drug belongs to the 'amide' group. Examples are illustrated on p. 402.

Most of the older analgesic drugs, e.g. procaine, cocaine and amethocaine, belong to the ester group. Most of the newer

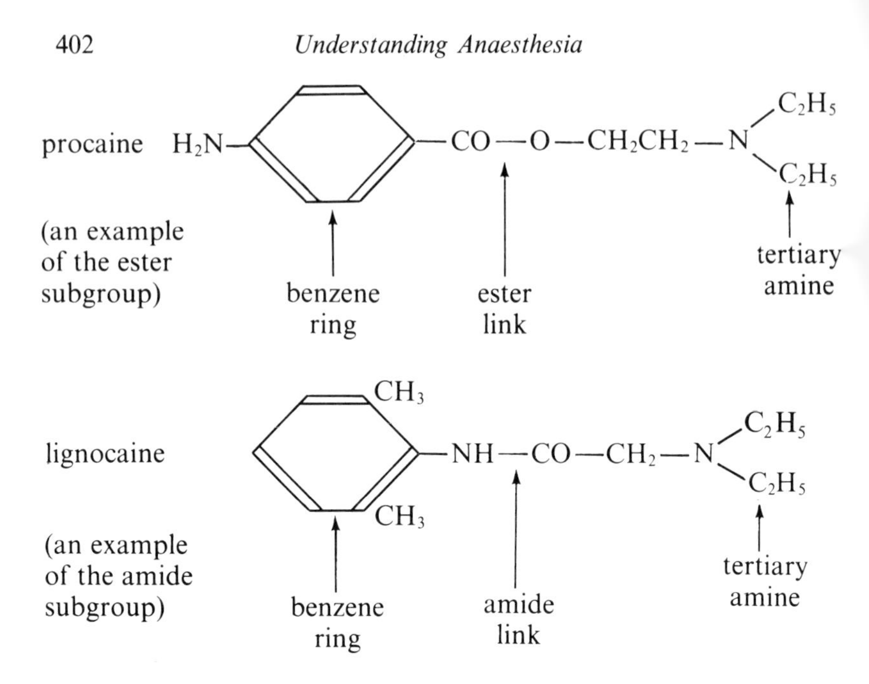

agents, e.g. lignocaine, prilocaine, mepivacaine, bupivacaine and etidocaine, belong to the amide group.

Metabolism and Excretion

The ester group of local analgesic drugs are hydrolysed in the plasma by the enzyme pseudocholinesterase (also involved in the breakdown of suxamethonium). Some of the breakdown products are metabolised further; some are excreted in the urine. The exception in this group is cocaine, which is largely detoxified in the liver, a small proportion being excreted unchanged in the urine. The amide group of agents are largely broken down in the liver, only a small fraction being excreted unchanged in the urine.

Toxicity

Toxicity means general systemic toxicity when absorbed into the circulation. In this, local analgesic agents differ from most drugs where toxicity is an exaggeration of their therapeutic effect. In the case of local analgesics, which are usually chosen for their local effect, the general toxic effects appear in other systems and do not have an obvious relationship to the local effect.

With the exception of those produced by cocaine, the toxic effects are similar for all local analgesic agents. They are mainly on the central nervous system, with secondary effects on other systems.

It has been customary to describe the central nervous system effects as stimulation first and then depression. It is now believed that the effect is purely depressant, the apparent stimulation being due to depression of inhibitory fibres revealing excitatory effects.

Clinically, the first sign is often numbness of the tongue and circumoral region. There may also be lightheadedness, dizziness and tinnitus. Anxiety and muscular twitching progress to generalised tonic and clonic convulsions as the stimulatory effects on the higher centres escalate. As the depressant effects follow, the patient becomes unconscious, while depression of the medullary vital centres leads to cardiovascular collapse and respiratory arrest. The cardiac effects may be augmented by direct depression of the myocardium by high blood concentrations of local analgesic drug.

It should be noted that the milder, premonitory excitatory signs are by no means always seen with the amide group of local analgesic agents. With lignocaine, in particular, the first sign of systemic absorption is often drowsiness, and this may be quite marked in old people.

Factors Affecting Toxicity

Systemic toxic effects appear when the concentration of local analgesic drug in the blood rises above a certain level, which varies for different agents. Thus most factors affecting toxicity do so by increasing the rate of absorption into the bloodstream, or sometimes by reducing the removal of the agent from it.

General factors

Age. It is a wise rule always to be particularly careful when giving any drug to the very old or the very young. Whether very young patients are particularly susceptible to the toxic effects of analgesic drugs is doubtful, but care must be taken on a dose/weight ratio. A technique for operating on congenital pyloric stenosis under local analgesia recommended a dose of 14 ml 0·25% lignocaine as the safe upper limit! Elderly patients are more liable to toxic effects than their body weight might indicate.

Sex. With the exception of the effect of body weight there is probably no difference between the sexes in their response to local analgesics. In the later months of pregnancy, however, smaller volumes of local analgesic drugs are required than are usual for the performance of spinal or epidural analgesia. In addition, when the patient is in labour it must be remembered that with at least one technique—paracervical block—it is possible to achieve higher blood concentrations of local analgesic in the fetus than in the mother.

Body weight. Blood levels of drug reached are approximately inversely proportional to body weight. Toxic doses, as usually recommended, apply to an average 70 kg person and should be adjusted accordingly.

General condition. The acutely ill or chronically debilitated patient is more susceptible to the toxic effects of local analgesic drugs.

Liver function. Most modern (amide) local analgesics are metabolised in the liver. The state of liver function will have no effect on the acute toxicity produced by a single, excessive administration of drug, but may affect the gradual build-up to toxic blood levels produced by repeated doses of the drug, as in a continuous epidural technique.

Local factors

Site of injection. Injection into particularly vascular areas is likely to lead to rapid absorption and high blood levels. Such areas include the head, neck and pelvic floor. Two other areas from which absorption can be alarmingly rapid are the upper respiratory tract and an inflamed urethra—when topical application is used.

Concentration of drug. This is a debatable factor but it is suggested that absorption down a concentration gradient will be faster from a more concentrated solution.

Use of vasoconstrictor agents. The addition to local analgesic injections of agents such as adrenaline, noradrenaline or octapressin slows their absorption from the site of injection and reduces the blood level achieved. Thus the toxic dose of the analgesic agent may be correspondingly increased, and its action is usually prolonged.

Use of hyaluronidase. This enzyme breaks down intercellular cement and increases the spread of injected fluid through tissues. It increases the area for, and therefore the rate of, absorption of injected local analgesic drugs, and so makes toxic effects more likely.

Regional techniques that require very large and potentially toxic doses of local analgesic drug, e.g. regional block for thoracoplasty, have now gone out of fashion. Toxic reactions due simply to a single overdose should no longer happen. The commonest cause today of toxic reactions is the inadvertent intravascular administration of the drug. Also potentially dangerous is the progressive increase in blood levels that may accompany repeated increments of an agent—as in a continuous epidural technique.

Treatment of toxic effects

If administration of the drug is continuing, it may be sufficient to stop, give the patient oxygen and watch carefully for any sign of worsening of the effects. If signs of excitation are more marked, it has been customary to recommend giving thiopentone slowly to prevent or abolish convulsions. However, it must be remembered that the condition is basically one of central nervous system depression, and that depressant drugs must be given with the utmost caution. Probably diazepam given slowly intravenously is less depressant, and therefore a better choice than thiopentone.

For established convulsions, suxamethonium will abolish the muscular aspect of the convulsion and allow intubation and ventilation with air or oxygen. If fits recur when the suxamethonium wears off, diazepam may be given. Cardiovascular collapse requires appropriate symptomatic treatment, which might include raising the legs, intravenous fluids and possibly a vasopressor. If cardiac arrest occurs, treatment is as described in Chapter 25.

Other Uses of Local Analgesic Drugs

Anti-dysrhythmic effect

The effect produced by local analgesic drugs on the cell membranes of nerve fibres whereby depolarisation is slowed or stopped also occurs at other cell membranes, notably those of cardiac muscle fibres. In this way, lignocaine may be particularly effective in preventing the abnormal contraction of ventricular muscle tissue seen in ventricular dysrhythmias, especially ventricular extrasystoles. If these are considered dangerous, a bolus injection of 1 mg/kg plain lignocaine is given, followed usually by an intravenous drip of lignocaine at a rate adjusted to suppress the ectopic beats.

Anti-convulsant action

At lower blood levels than those required to produce convulsions, some local analgesic drugs have an anti-convulsant action. Few would advocate their use for this purpose nowadays as other agents are safer and more effective.

Toxicity of Vasoconstrictor Agent

Confusion may arise from the statement that addition of a potentially dangerous agent like adrenaline makes local analgesics safer. This fact is entirely due to the slower absorption of the analgesic into the systemic circulation which occurs when a vasoconstrictor is added.

However, adrenaline *is* potentially toxic, and a maximum dose of 5 μg (0·5 ml 1:1000 adrenaline HCl) is usually recommended in a 70 kg man. Given into the tissues, this dose will normally produce no obvious effect on the cardiovascular system. If inadvertently given intravenously, the patient will probably suffer palpitations, a feeling of anxiety and possibly retrosternal discomfort. An ECG might show a ventricular dysrhythmia, but a fit patient would be unlikely to come to serious harm. An adrenaline concentration of 1:100 000 need never be exceeded for local infiltration and 1:400 000 gives excellent vasoconstriction. The systemic effects of adrenaline may be potentiated in patients on tricyclic antidepressants and its use should be avoided.

Local analgesic agents are commercially available with

adrenaline, usually in a concentration of 1:100 000 or 1:200 000. These are frequently used by surgeons (e.g. in plastic surgery and gynaecology) to reduce bleeding at operations under general anaesthesia. The presence of the local analgesic in these cases is usually unnecessary, and a cheaper alternative is to dilute the contents of an adrenaline ampoule in saline.

Noradrenaline is a safer alternative to adrenaline as it has less of adrenaline's powerful and stimulant effects on the myocardium. Its lack of popularity probably arises from its reputedly less powerful effect and risk of producing local sloughing of tissue.

Felypressin (octapressin) is a synthetic octapeptide with little cardiac effect. It has not gained popularity except in dentistry, where it is available in some cartridges of local analgesic.

It must be realised that a solution of local analgesic drug containing adrenaline may be toxic from the point of view of the local analgesic or the adrenaline, but the safety point may not necessarily be the same for each.

INDIVIDUAL LOCAL ANALGESIC AGENTS

Many drugs have been tried since cocaine was introduced. Of those still available commercially the choice differs somewhat from country to country. Only four will be discussed here: (1) cocaine because of its unique properties and side-effects, (2) lignocaine because it has become the classic agent against which new agents are compared, (3) bupivacaine because after more than ten years it remains the safest and most reliable of the agents with a longer action than lignocaine, (4) prilocaine for its unique ability to produce methaemoglobinaemia.

Cocaine

One of the ester group of drugs, cocaine is unique in several ways. It is the only naturally occurring local analgesic substance still in clinical use. It produces excitation of the central nervous system in low concentrations—the stimulatory effect on the higher centres being responsible for its addictive properties.

It is the only local analgesic agent which is a powerful vasoconstrictor, this action being the result of its potentiation of catecholamines. Its sympathomimetic action on the heart may cause ventricular fibrillation before the central nervous system effects can manifest themselves as convulsions. Although belonging to the ester group, it is mainly detoxified in the liver, the remainder being excreted almost unchanged by the kidneys.

It retains a place as a topical analgesic agent, mostly in ENT work. While potentially a very toxic agent, its powerful vasoconstrictor action prevents it from being absorbed rapidly and the maximum safe dose used in this manner is about 200 mg.

Lignocaine

Synthesised in Sweden in 1943, lignocaine (Xylocaine) was first used clinically in 1948. It has a rapid onset, good penetration in the tissues and can be used by any method of application. It is stable in solution and can be autoclaved more than once without losing potency. It belongs to the amide group.

Lignocaine has some local vasodilatory effect, while most other local analgesic drugs (apart from cocaine) have little or no effect. The toxic dose for a 70 kg man is 200 mg of the plain solution and 500 mg with adrenaline. Its use in the treatment of ventricular dysrhythmias has already been discussed. The toxic blood level is about 5 μg/ml.

Bupivacaine

Synthesised in 1957 and first used clinically in 1963, bupivacaine (Marcain) also belongs to the amide group. Early claims for a duration of action of 5–12 hours seem to be justified for peripheral nerve block and plexus blocks but not for epidural analgesia, where its action is usually about two hours. However, this is longer than can be reliably expected from lignocaine, and as blood levels in mother and fetus are also slower to rise than with lignocaine, it has become the agent of choice for continuous epidural block in labour.

Adrenaline has much less effect in prolonging the action of bupivacaine or in lowering the blood levels after injection than is the case with most local analgesic agents. The reason is not clear, but it is known that at some concentrations bupivacaine has some vasoconstrictor action of its own. Consequently the safe dose is taken to be the same whether given with or without adrenaline—150 mg.

Recently cases have been reported where the first sign of bupivacaine toxicity has been cardiac arrest due to ventricular fibrillation, which has proved particularly resistant to treatment. This has led to a reappraisal of its use in circumstances where high blood levels might be expected, especially during Bier's block, for which as a result prilocaine and lignocaine would now be the agents of choice.

Prilocaine

Another of the amide group, prilocaine (Citanest) was first used in 1959. It was claimed to be less toxic than lignocaine (toxic dose 300 mg plain; 600 mg with adrenaline) to which it is similar.

Unfortunately it was found that during its metabolism prilocaine produced a metabolite—o-toluidine which caused the conversion of haemoglobin to methaemoglobin, a form which takes no part in oxygen transport. While this tended to occur only when about 600 mg prilocaine had been used, these amounts could quite easily be used in continuous epidural analgesia in obstetrics, where the baby could also be adversely affected.

Because of this tendency to cause methaemoglobinaemia, this agent has largely disappeared from clinical practice, except in Bier's block and dentistry.

41 Local Analgesic Blocks

Principles of local analgesic blocks. Types of nerve block.

PRINCIPLES OF LOCAL ANALGESIC BLOCKS

No attempt will be made here to list the vast number of local analgesic blocks. Instead, some of the principles of local analgesic technique are discussed and some examples given of the commoner blocks.

Somatic nerves contain both motor fibres to skeletal muscle and sensory fibres carrying the sensations of pain, temperature, touch, position and proprioception. The sympathetic and parasympathetic nerves carry fibres to and from thoracic and abdominal viscera (e.g. the heart and bowel). Sympathetic fibres also pass to the sweat glands, to the erector pilae muscles affecting the skin hairs and, probably most important of all, to arterioles and venules throughout the body. The somatic motor fibres, which run from the spinal cord as the anterior nerve roots, are found at all levels of the spinal cord, as are the somatic sensory fibres which are attached to the spinal cord by the posterior nerve roots.

The sympathetic nerve fibres do not arise at all levels, but only in the thoracic and upper lumbar levels (Figs 41.1 and 33.2). They leave the spinal cord in the anterior nerve roots in company with the motor fibres, and pass out of an intervertebral foramen with the anterior primary ramus of the spinal nerve. The sympathetic fibres soon leave the anterior primary ramus as a white ramus communicans and after a few centimetres join a sym-

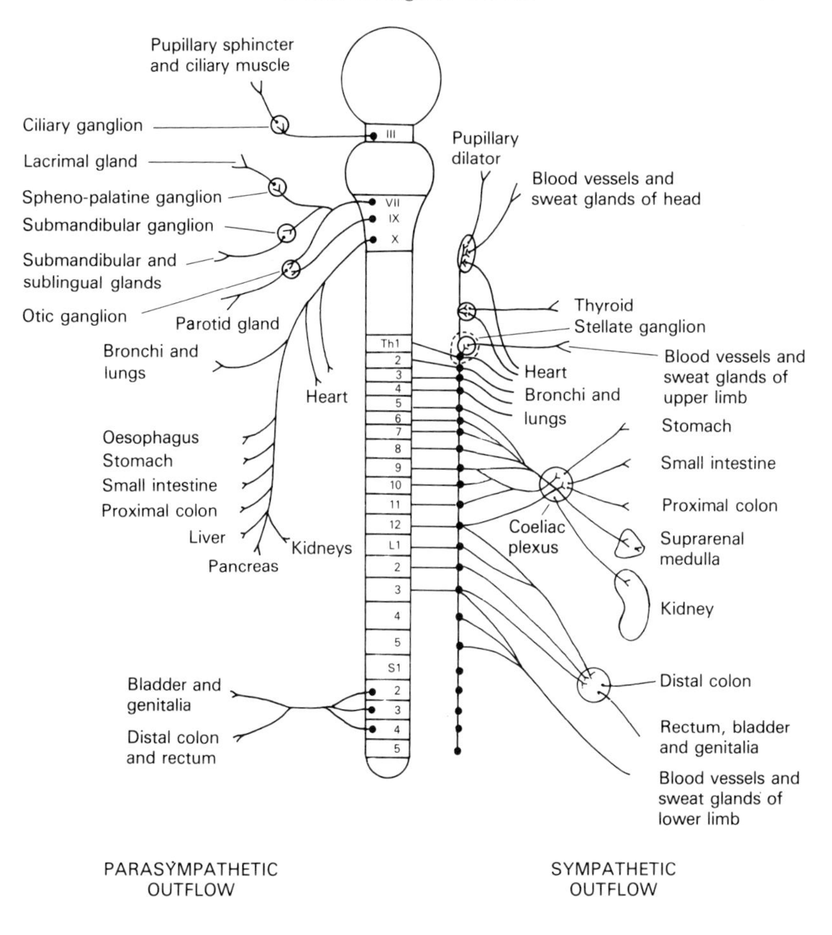

Fig. 41.1 Sympathetic and parasympathetic nervous systems

pathetic ganglion. These ganglia, of which there are some 24 on each side, lie anterolateral to the vertebral column and are joined by sympathetic fibres to form the sympathetic chain. Despite the limited outflow from the spinal cord, the sympathetic fibres are distributed to all parts of the body. The sympathetic ganglia are the sites where the preganglionic fibres from the spinal cord form synapses with postganglionic fibres. Most of the postganglionic fibres destined to supply vasoconstrictor fibres to limb blood vessels return to the spinal nerves via grey rami communicantes. Parasympathetic fibres (both efferent and afferent) are carried only in the vagus and 2nd, 3rd and 4th sacral nerves (Chapter 33).

It follows, therefore, that both spinal and epidural anaesthesia tend to block both the somatic and sympathetic nerve fibres. By carefully introducing a needle to the region of the sympathetic chain or ganglia, however, it is possible to produce a purely sympathetic block. It is not possible to produce the converse effect, i.e. a purely somatic block, by injecting more peripherally, as the sympathetic fibres to the blood vessels are distributed with the somatic fibres along the main nerve trunks. However, by common usage, these more peripheral blocks are often referred to as somatic nerve blocks.

Somatic nerve blocks are usually performed to enable some surgical operation or manipulation to be carried out, for post-operative pain relief or other painful conditions, e.g. fractured ribs.

Sympathetic nerve blocks have been carried out in a great many conditions with varying success. Vascular conditions probably provide the biggest group of indications. Damage to, thrombosis of, or embolism of a major vessel is associated with intense spasm in surrounding blood vessels which might provide a collateral circulation past the damaged vessel. Sympathetic block relieves this spasm and helps to restore arterial or venous circulation. Phenol may be used to produce a more prolonged block in more chronic vascular disease, e.g. where rest pain or incipient gangrene is associated with these conditions. A sympathetic block may also be used before amputation to improve the blood supply to the amputation site. Other indications include causalgia, phantom limb pain, and various types of visceral pain, e.g. angina, biliary and renal colic.

TYPES OF NERVE BLOCK

Somatic Nerve Blocks

Brachial plexus block

The upper limb is supplied by the brachial plexus which arises from the 5th, 6th, 7th and 8th cervical and the 1st thoracic nerve roots. It is the commonest of the nerve plexus blocks, although the multiplicity of techniques which have been described indicate that no method is perfect. Some of the advantages and disadvantages of three of the approaches which have achieved most popularity will be presented.

The interscaline approach. The injection is made into the plexus between the scalene muscles in the neck at the level of the 6th cervical vertebra. Advantages are that the method may be easier than others in obese patients, that it is effective for shoulder manipulations and it avoids the risk of a pneumothorax. Disadvantages include the possible injection into the subarachnoid or epidural spaces or into the vertebral artery, and phrenic nerve block may occur. The ulnar nerve is relatively difficult to block with this high approach.

The supraclavicular approach. The injection is made from above the clavicle down onto the plexus as it crosses the upper surface of the first rib. This approach has declined in popularity, because although it also gives analgesia for shoulder manipulation, it is the technique most likely to produce a pneumothorax. Spread to other nerves—phrenic, vagus, recurrent laryngeal and sympathetic nerves—can also occur.

The axillary approach. The injection is made into the axillary sheath round the brachial plexus by inserting the needle close to the axillary artery as high up as it can be felt in the axilla. The main advantages are that many of the complications of the other methods are avoided, e.g. the risk of pneumothorax, or subarachnoid or extradural injection, or spread to other nerves. Disadvantages are the difficulty of the technique in obese patients, its impossibility if the arm cannot be abducted, the failure to produce analgesia for shoulder manipulation and at times the failure of the block to include the musculocutaneous nerve.

Ulnar nerve block

This is included as an example of a single-nerve block. The ulnar nerve can easily be rolled over the posterior surface of the medial epicondyle of the humerus with the forefinger. This produces the familiar pain shooting down the inner aspect of the arm into the little finger and this part of the elbow is colloquially referred to as the 'funny-bone': 2–5 ml local anaesthetic injected here will produce analgesia of the little finger and the ulnar border of the ring finger. For brachial plexus block and ulnar nerve block suitable local anaesthetic solutions would be 1% lignocaine in 1:200 000 adrenaline or 0·25% bupivacaine plain or in 1:400 000 adrenaline.

Digital nerve block

The nerve supply to each finger (and toe) runs as a pair of digital nerves along each side of the digit. Excellent analgesia for operations on the distal part of the digit may be obtained by injecting a few millilitres of local anaesthetic at each side of the base of the finger or toe. The special consideration of this block is that the sole blood supply to the digit runs beside these nerves and if vasoconstrictor solutions are used gangrene of the finger or toe may occur. A similar block may be used in the penis for circumcision, so again only plain local anaesthetic solutions should be used.

Sympathetic Nerve Blocks

Stellate ganglion block

The cervical sympathetic chain normally consists of three ganglia —the superior, middle and inferior cervical ganglia. The inferior cervical ganglion is often fused with the first thoracic ganglion and in this case the combined ganglion is called the 'stellate ganglion'. Through this ganglion runs the entire sympathetic nerve supply to the head, neck and upper limb on that side. Stellate ganglion block may be useful in arterial and venous injuries to the upper limb, in arterial and venous thrombosis and of prognostic value before considering operation for the treatment of Raynaud's disease of the upper limb. It may also be of use in causalgia and Ménière's disease. Its use in strokes and in central retinal artery thrombosis has been abandoned because sympathetic block does not produce vasodilation of the cerebral blood vessels.

Lumbar sympathetic chain block

As there is no sympathetic outflow below the second lumbar segment, blockade of the sympathetic chain below this level affects the entire sympathetic nerve supply to the pelvis and lower limbs. Apart from its use in vascular conditions, causalgia, phantom limb pain, etc., as already described, lumbar sympathetic chain block has been used in renal colic and obstetric pain. However, it is not usually regarded as a continuous catheter technique and this fact limits its usefulness in these latter types of pain. For longer-term effect, aqueous phenol solution may be used instead of local analgesic in more intractable conditions.

Intravenous Regional Analgesia (IVRA; Bier's Block)

This technique was first described by August Bier in 1908 using procaine, and is often referred to by his name. It was reintroduced using lignocaine by Holmes in 1963 while working in Oxford. It has gained considerable popularity because very little skill is required, nor the knowledge of anatomy needed for many other analgesic blocks.

After inserting a needle or cannula, usually in the back of the hand, the limb is exsanguinated using an Esmarch's bandage or, in the presence of a painful lesion, simply by raising the limb. A pneumatic tourniquet which has been applied on the proximal part of the limb is then inflated to about 50 mmHg above arterial blood pressure and after removing the Esmarch's bandage local analgesic solution is injected via the indwelling needle into the exsanguinated limb. Many solutions have been used but the most popular are plain 0·5% prilocaine or lignocaine. About 40 ml solution are adequate for a man's forearm with proportionately less being used for a woman or child's upper limb. Analgesia begins quickly but may not be complete for up to 20 minutes. It begins proximally and works distally. Occasionally it may not extend to the fingers, but analgesia may be completed by injecting a few additional millilitres of local anaesthetic solution before removing the indwelling needle.

At the end of the operation the tourniquet is released and a considerable proportion of the local anaesthetic solution rapidly returns to the systemic circulation. The blood levels obtained may be high and toxic reactions have been reported. The proportion of local analgesic entering the circulation quickly is highest if the block has been maintained for a short time, and it is probably unwise to remove the tourniquet in under 20 minutes. The patient should be watched carefully for evidence of toxic effects, e.g. bradycardia or dysrhythmias. Probably the commonest toxic symptoms are auditory—either tinnitus or transient deafness. It has been suggested that toxic effects are less likely if the tourniquet is released and re-inflated to slow the release of analgesic solution into the systemic circulation. Thus the tourniquet may be released for five seconds every 30 seconds for five minutes.

In view of the possibility of a toxic reaction it is always a wise precaution to have an indwelling needle or cannula present in the other upper limb. It is also very important to test the apparatus for leaks before use.

Sooner or later most patients find the discomfort of the tourniquet intolerable. For this reason it is recommended that a second tourniquet be applied distal to the first tourniquet, it therefore being placed on analgesic skin. It can then be inflated to the same pressure as the proximal cuff, which is then released. Special double-cuff tourniquets have been designed for this purpose.

Intravenous regional analgesia may also be used in the leg, but even with a below-knee tourniquet the volume of solution required is greater and hence the risk of toxic reactions on release of the tourniquet more likely.

42 Spinal and Epidural Analgesia

History. Anatomy. Factors affecting spread of solutions in the subarachnoid space. Factors affecting spread of solutions in the epidural space, and epidural spaces. Complications of spinal analgesia. Complications of epidural analgesia. Uses of spinal and epidural analgesia. Contraindications to spinal and epidural analgesia. Intrathecal and epidural opiates. Drugs and equipment.

HISTORY

Spinals

1885 Corning of New York accidentally performed the first spinal while experimenting with cocaine in a dog.

1899 The first spinal for a surgical operation was carried out by August Bier of Germany.

1907 Barker of London described the importance of the curves of the vertebral column and the use of gravity in the spread of spinal solutions.

1940 Lemmon performed continuous spinal analgesia via a needle.

1946 Tuohy performed continuous *spinal* analgesia via Tuohy needle and ureteric catheter.

Epidurals

1901 Sicard and Cathelin of France performed the first epidurals by the sacral (caudal) approach.

1913 Heile of Germany tried epidural blocks via a lateral approach through the intervertebral foramina.

1921 Fidel Pages of Spain was the first to use the midline lumbar approach, relying on his sense of touch to detect the passage from ligamentum flavum to the epidural space.

1941 Hingson and Southworth of the USA performed the first continuous lumbar epidural via a needle.

1942 Manalan of the USA performed the first continuous caudal via a catheter.

1942 Hingson and Southworth performed the first continuous caudal via a needle.

1947 Manuel Martinez Curbelo of Havana carried out the first continuous lumbar epidural using a Tuohy needle and ureteric catheter.

ANATOMY

Bony Anatomy

There are 33 vertebrae grouped according to regions into seven cervical, 12 thoracic, five lumbar, five sacral (fused in the adult to form the sacrum) and four coccygeal (fused to form the coccyx).

A typical vertebra (Fig. 42.1a,b,c) consists of two main parts: (1) the weight-bearing vertebral body in front, attached to those above and below by intervertebral discs; and (2) the vertebral arch posteriorly, made up of the pedicles and laminae.

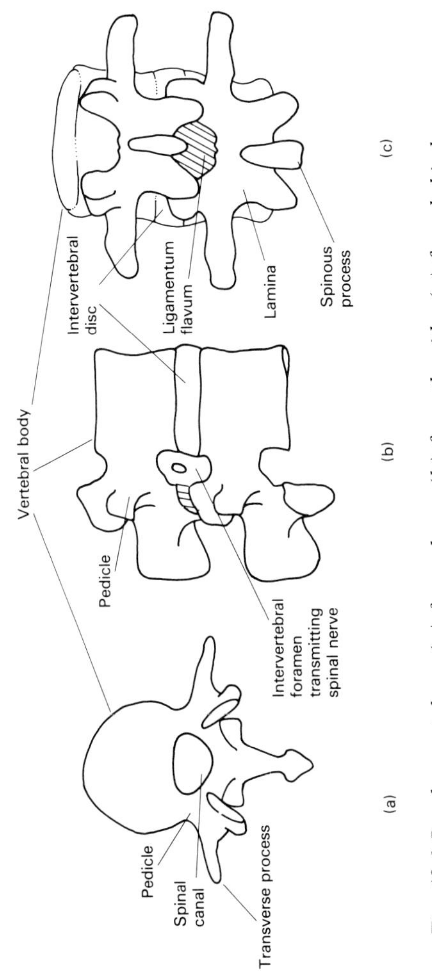

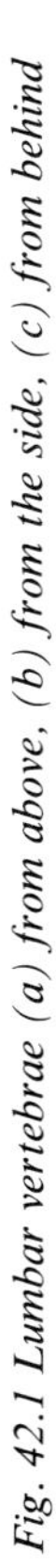
Fig. 42.1 Lumbar vertebrae (a) from above, (b) from the side, (c) from behind

The spinous, transverse and superior and inferior articular processes project from the arch. The lower and upper borders of the pedicles, helped by the adjacent bodies and disc and the superior and inferior articular processes, form the boundaries of the intervertebral foramina, through which the segmental nerves pass from the spinal cord.

Each lamina is joined to the one above and below by the fibro-elastic ligamenta flava. The vertebral foramen is formed by the vertebral arch and the posterior surface of the body. When the vertebrae are placed on top of one another the vertebral foramina become the vertebral canal, which houses and protects the spinal cord and membranes. At its upper end, the canal meets the skull at the foramen magnum and at its lower end it continues down into the body of the sacrum as the sacral canal and ends at the sacral hiatus.

The bodies, arches and processes have distinguishing features in the different regions of the vertebral column. One of the most

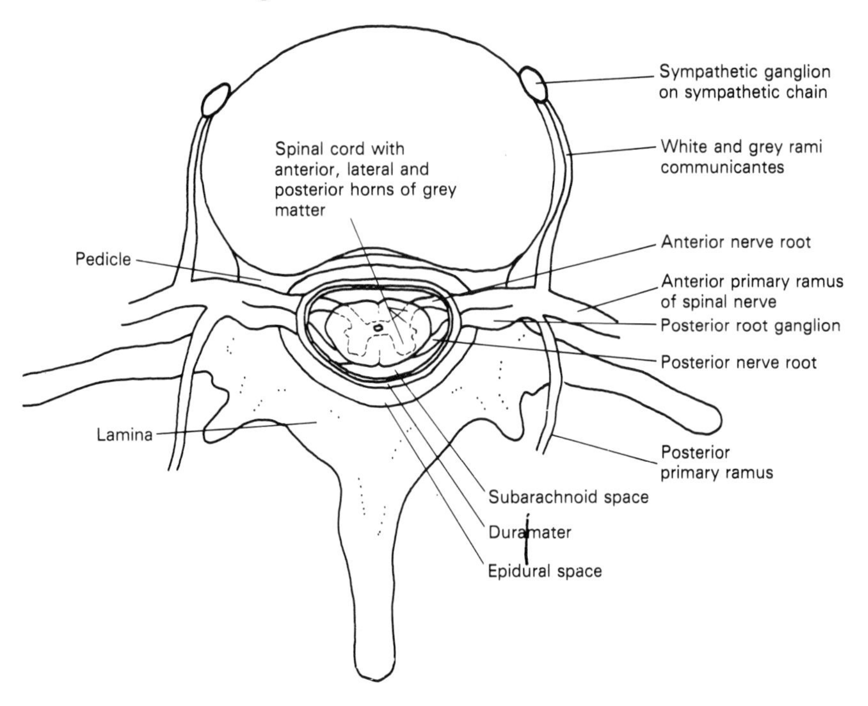

Fig. 42.2 Cross-section at level of upper lumbar vertebra showing spinal cord, subarachnoid and epidural spaces

important from the anaesthetist's point of view is the varying obliquity of the spinous processes in the thoracic and lumbar regions.

Spinal Cord and Spinal Nerves

The spinal cord begins at the level of the foramen magnum as the continuation of the medulla oblongata of the brain. It usually ends at the level of the upper part of the second lumbar vertebra, although in the newborn, and in some adults, it extends to the third lumbar vertebra. It gives off 31 pairs of nerves—eight cervical, 12 thoracic, five lumbar, five sacral and one coccygeal.

The grey matter of the spinal cord is roughly H-shaped (*see* Fig. 42.2). It contains the nuclei of the nerve cells, the anterior horns of the H containing the nuclei from which the motor fibres arise and the posterior horns containing the nuclei on which most of the sensory fibres end. In the thoracic and upper two or three

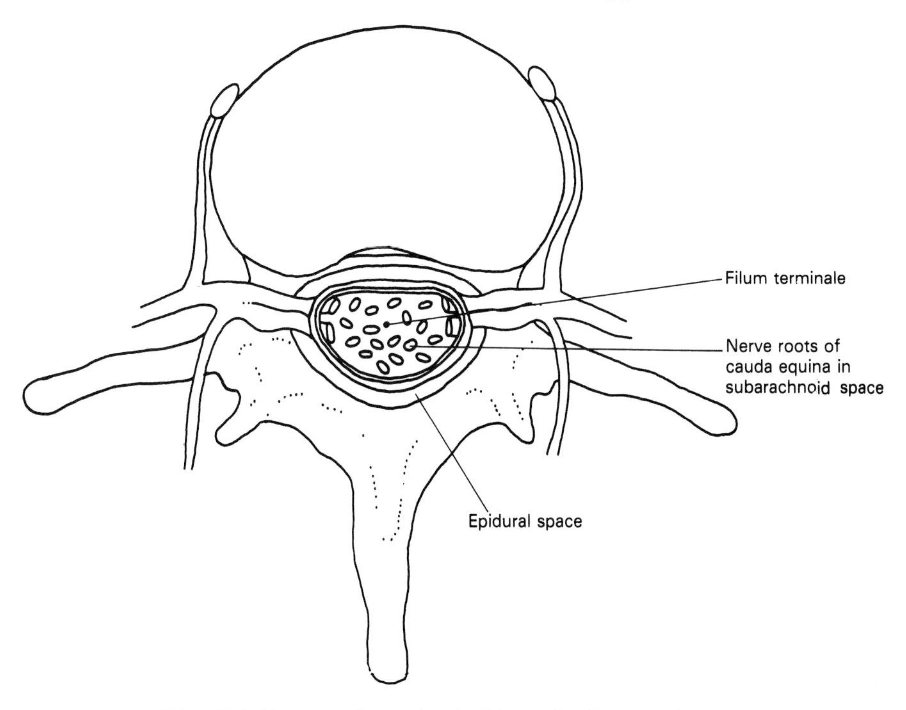

Fig. 42.3 Cross-section at level of lower lumbar vertebra

lumbar segments there are also small lateral horns in which sympathetic fibres arise.

Each spinal nerve is made up of an anterior root containing motor fibres derived from the anterior horns (and at some level sympathetic fibres derived from the lateral horns) and a posterior root containing sensory fibres passing inwards to the posterior horn.

A ganglion on the posterior root near the intervertebral foramen contains the nuclei of the sensory nerves. Just lateral to the ganglion the anterior and posterior roots fuse and their fibres intermingle to form a spinal nerve. Almost at once the nerve divides into the larger anterior primary ramus and smaller posterior primary ramus for distribution throughout the body.

The spinal nerves escape from the bony vertebral column through the appropriate intervertebral foramina, or in the case of the sacral and coccygeal nerves, through the anterior and posterior sacra foramina or sacral hiatus. The spinal cord having ended at L2, the nerve roots, especially the lower ones, have to pass downwards from their spinal cord origin to the point of emergence from their bony protection. The lower lumbar, sacral and coccygeal nerves thus form a bundle running vertically downwards in the subarachnoid space named, from its resemblance to a horse's tail, the 'cauda equina' (Fig. 42.3).

Subarachnoid Space

These are three fibrous membranes which surround the spinal cord. They are named from within outwards the pia mater, arachnoid mater and dura mater. The pia mater closely invests the spinal cord. The blood vessels ramify in this membrane before entering the cord. The arachnoid mater is separated from the pia mater by the subarachnoid space containing the cerebrospinal fluid (CSF). It is a delicate layer closely applied to the inner surface of the thick, fibrous dura mater. Usually when a needle pierces the dura mater it also passes through the arachnoid into the subarachnoid space.

The spinal subarachnoid space (which has a volume of about 25 ml) is in direct communication through the foramen magnum with the cranial subarachnoid space containing the CSF bathing the surface of the brain. It is therefore possible for solutions injected into the spinal subarachnoid space to gain access to the cranial nerves. The spinal subarachnoid space also communicates, though rather less freely, with the fourth ventricle of the brain by three openings in its roof. By this route it is possible for spinal solutions to reach the vital centres in the medulla.

Inferiorly the spinal subarachnoid space ends at the level of the 2nd sacral vertebra (Fig. 42.4), where it is within easy reach of a marauding caudal needle!

Epidural Space

The remaining space between the dura mater and the walls of the vertebral canal is the epidural space. Largely filled by fat and veins, it is traversed by the spinal nerves in their dural coverings. Its outer boundary is made up of the periosteum lining the bony parts of the vertebral canal with the ligamenta flava filling in the gaps posteriorly between the laminae. Superiorly the epidural

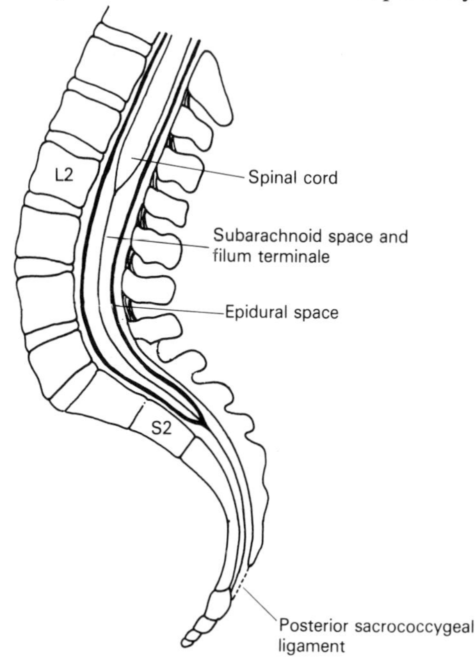

Fig. 42.4 Structures at lower end of vertebral column

space is limited by the attachment of both the periosteum lining the vertebral canal and the dura mater to the margin of the foramen magnum. (This periosteum and the spinal dura mater correspond to the two layers of intracranial dura mater.) This limits the upward spread of solutions injected into the epidural space.

Laterally, the epidural space is continuous with the paravertebral spaces which lie between the heads of the ribs in the thoracic region. As the pleura is one boundary of the paravertebral space, intrapleural pressure changes are transmitted to the epidural space.

Inferiorly, the epidural space ends where the posterior sacrococcygeal ligament roofs over the sacral hiatus (*see* Fig. 42.4). This is the point of entry for a needle when performing a sacral epidural or caudal.

The anterior (consisting of motor and, at some levels, sympathetic fibres) and the posterior (sensory) nerve roots of all the spinal nerves have to traverse both the subarachnoid and epidural spaces. Local analgesic solution injected into either of these spaces therefore produces a type of nerve block. In the case of the former space it is called a 'subarachnoid', 'intrathecal' or 'spinal' block and in the case of the latter it is called an 'epidural', 'extradural' or 'peridural' block.

After injection of solutions into the subarachnoid or epidural spaces, various factors affect the extent of their distribution and these differ in importance between the two spaces.

FACTORS AFFECTING SPREAD OF SOLUTIONS IN THE SUBARACHNOID SPACE

Specific Gravity and Posture

These two factors are considered together because they are interdependent. Different liquids have different densities. This is called the specific gravity (SG) and for each liquid this is calculated relative to the density of water at a given temperature. When two liquids are mixed, the one with the higher specific gravity sinks under the influence of gravity to the bottom of the container.

The CSF has an SG very similar to that of water. The simple salts of local analgesic solutions have specific gravities not usually very different from that of CSF but can be made heavier or lighter than CSF; heavier usually by adding dextrose to the solution, lighter usually by warming. A local analgesic solution with an SG higher than that of CSF is called 'hyperbaric'; if the SG is the same as CSF it is 'isobaric' and if lighter, 'hypobaric'. Traditionally, the great majority of spinal blocks have been carried out using hyperbaric solutions and the following comments on factors affecting the spread of solutions in the subarachnoid space refer to these solutions.

If a hyperbaric solution is injected into the subarachnoid space, it rapidly sinks in the CSF. With the patient in the lateral recumbent position, the vertebral canal is practically horizontal, and little movement of the injected solution occurs. However, if the patient is turned on his back, the effect which the curvatures of the spine will have on the injected solution becomes apparent. It is found that there is a cervical convexity forwards, a deep thoracic concavity forwards, a lumbar convexity forwards again and a small sacral concavity. The injection is usually made at the L2-3 or L3-4 interspaces, which are about the summit of the lumbar convexity. The injected solution thus divides into a portion which runs towards the sacrum and a part which runs down in the thoracic concavity. The first portion does nothing which has not already been done by the injected bolus spreading across the cauda equina. The upper portion, having reached the lowest part of the thoracic concavity (the mid-thoracic region), is prevented from spreading further cephalad by the slope leading up out of the cervical end of the thoracic concavity. This represents a built-in safety factor in spinal analgesia in that it is virtually impossible for a normal volume of spinal analgesic solution to spread much higher than the mid-thoracic level of the spinal cord unless the patient is left at all head-down on his side, or with the head much too far down in the supine position.

The other common posture for administering spinal analgesia is the sitting position. The patient may then be immediately laid down, or more commonly left in the sitting position for some minutes. With this latter technique, there is almost no analgesia above the level of insertion of the needle. Indeed, if the injection is made slowly enough, the analgesic solution may not even cut right across the cauda equina but, trickling down, anaesthetises only the lower sacral and coccygeal nerves. Because of the area rendered analgesic, this is termed 'saddle-block' analgesia, and provides excellent analgesia for operations on the urethra, anus and other perineal structures.

Volume

The extent of spread of solution is proportional to the volume injected, the local analgesic being 'fixed' by the nervous tissue. The range of volumes used for hyperbaric solutions is usually between 1 ml and 3 ml.

Rate of Injection

If the injection is made quickly, there is a tendency for turbulent currents to be set up in the CSF, and these spread the local analgesic more extensively. This factor has less influence on the spread of solutions in the cerebrospinal fluid since the almost universal adoption of small-bore spinal needles, which make very rapid injection impossible.

Barbotage

This technique is a more elaborate way of setting up turbulent currents. After injection of some or all the contents of the syringe, aspiration is rapidly carried out and followed by forceful re-injection. This manoeuvre may be repeated several times. The result tends to be a more widespread, but thinner distribution of the local analgesic. It is again difficult to make effective use of this factor with small-bore needles.

There is no particular, single technique to produce spinal analgesia to a particular level. Various combinations of posturing the patient before and after the injection and (particularly in the earlier days of spinal analgesia) different amounts of barbotage can produce identical results with different volumes of solution. Any individual anaesthetist will use a combination of these factors which experience has shown him will produce consistent results.

FACTORS AFFECTING SPREAD OF SOLUTIONS IN THE EPIDURAL SPACE

The site of action of local analgesic drugs injected into the epidural space is not known for certain, and it is possible that multiple sites are involved. From a clinical viewpoint, however, it is acceptable to consider that the local analgesic acts on the nerve roots in the epidural space in an area centred on the site of injection. This gives a segmental band of analgesia with epidural blocks, as opposed to the complete analgesia below the site of injection which occurs with spinal blocks due to the injection site being at the level of the cauda equina.

Volume

This is much the most important factor affecting the spread of epidural solutions. Spread tends to occur up and down the space from the site of injection, the degree of spread being proportional to the volume.

Gravity

The epidural space is filled primarily with semi-liquid fatty areolar tissue, but this is not true liquid like CSF. Thus SG has no effect on the spread of epidural solutions and no attempt is made to alter their baricity by adding dextrose. Gravity itself, however, tends to have some effect on the spread of epidural solutions, but to nothing like the same extent as intrathecal injections.

Site of Injection

While most epidurals are carried out in the lumbar region, the intention is to stop the needle well short of the spinal cord and it is accepted technique to carry out epidural block at any level. This has considerable advantages over the spinal technique if some high but restricted area of analgesia is required, e.g. to relieve the pain of fractured ribs.

Rate of Injection

Rapid injection may spread epidural solutions further, but again this is much less so than with spinal injections. In addition, many epidural injections are made through a catheter, which makes rapid injection impossible.

Concentration

It has been shown that a given volume of a more concentrated solution spreads further than the same volume of a lower concentration of the same drug. This is not a pronounced effect.

COMPLICATIONS OF SPINAL ANALGESIA

Effects on Cardiovascular System

The preganglionic sympathetic nerve fibres arise from the spinal cord between the 1st thoracic and 2nd or 3rd lumbar segments. Blockade of these nerves leads to dilation of the resistance and capacitance vessels. The reduction of peripheral resistance tends to cause a fall in blood pressure and the venous pooling to a fall in venous return, a reduction in cardiac output and further lowering of the blood pressure. With less extensive blocks, the blood pressure tends to be maintained by compensatory vasoconstriction in unaffected segments, but in general the reduction in blood pressure tends to be proportional to the height of the block.

A block to T1-T4 involves the cardio-accelerator sympathetic fibres with bradycardia and further depression of the blood pressure. Intravenous atropine will cure the bradycardia and help to restore the blood pressure.

Effects of Respiratory System

Most spinal solutions are powerful enough to produce at least partial motor paralysis in the nerve segments affected. Thus as the block spreads upwards, the intercostal muscles may be progressively affected, but the diaphragm with its C3, 4 and 5 innervation is unaffected until the block reaches the mid-cervical level. Fortunately, the spread of local analgesic solution to these higher levels is usually so thin that it is not strong enough to block the motor fibres. If the block were intense in the thoracic and cervical regions, all respiration might cease.

Respiration will also cease if local analgesic solution spreads up to the 4th ventricle where the respiratory centre may be affected directly.

Nausea and Vomiting

These distressing symptoms are often associated with restlessness and of course are seen only when supplementary anaesthesia has not been used with the spinal or epidural block. There are two main causes—hypotension and traction on hollow viscera. The latter causes pain and nausea because most intra-abdominal structures have some nerve supply from the vagus, which does not run in the vertebral canal and is therefore unaffected by spinals and epidurals. It is essential to diagnose the cause of the patient's symptoms before administering depressant sedative drugs.

Headache

Headache is probably never caused by a correctly performed epidural, but it is one of the commonest side-effects of spinal analgesia, or more simply of lumbar puncture. There are three possible causes.

Leakage of cerebrospinal fluid
There is normally a pressure of some 80–150 mm water in the subarachnoid space and a slightly negative pressure in the epidural space. This causes the CSF to leak through the dural hole caused by the needle and it will continue to do so until the hole heals over. It is thought that the loss of fluid allows movement of the brain within the skull and causes headache by traction on pain-sensitive structures in the basal blood vessels

and dura mater. The incidence of this type of headache, and its severity and duration are thus directly related to the bore of needle used. Spinal needles used today are almost always small bore, and headache is not usually a problem. On the other hand, the worst headaches tend to result from inadvertent dural puncture by a wide-bore epidural needle.

This type of headache is classically retro-orbital or may spread down the back of the head into the neck and is worse when the patient is upright—it nearly always disappears when lying flat or head-down. Treatment is directed towards keeping the patient well hydrated so that lost CSF is easily replaced and by methods which reduce, or stop, the flow of fluid through the hole in the dura so that the headache is eased and healing of the hole can take place. Thus the patient with a spinal headache should be kept recumbent for at least 24 hours and then sat up gradually. If the puncture is made during attempts at an epidural block, the epidural space should be located at an adjacent interspace and an epidural catheter connected to a drip of normal saline for the next 24 hours. This tends to reduce the pressure gradient across the dura so that the flow of fluid slows or stops and healing of the dural puncture is more likely to occur.

If this method is ineffective, an epidural 'blood patch' may be performed using the patient's own venous blood. A needle is inserted into the epidural space at the same interspace as that where the dural tap has been done; 10–20 ml blood is injected through the needle, which is then removed. The blood apparently acts as a patch over the epidural side of the hole in the dura mater. This technique has the extraordinarily high success rate of over 90%, but because the blood is a potential culture medium, the other more conservative methods should be tried first.

Meningitis

By definition, infection of the meninges is meningitis. With modern equipment and methods of sterilisation this most serious complication should not occur.

Meningism

This may mimic meningitis, but is an aseptic irritant reaction caused probably by blood in the CSF or antiseptic from the skin. Before the advent of modern pharmaceutical techniques, it was also caused by impurities in the local analgesic solutions.

Cranial Nerve Palsies

These are rare and like spinal headaches are probably caused by stretching of the cranial nerves by movement of the brain within the skull due to leakage of CSF, and so may occur after simple lumbar puncture. Most of the cranial nerves have been reported as being affected, but the commonest is the 6th cranial nerve (the abducent nerve) which supplies the lateral rectus muscle in the eye, paralysis of this muscle causing diplopia. These cranial nerve palsies usually recover spontaneously.

Other Neurological Lesions

A great variety of permanent lesions affecting the nerve roots, spinal cord or even brain have been reported following spinal analgesia. However, it has not been proved that these are caused by the local analgesic agent. Other possible explanations include contaminants of the local analgesic solution, a virus or other infection introduced by the needle, ischaemia of the spinal cord due to hypotension (especially if a vasoconstrictor is added to the spinal solution), or some unidentified coincidental cause (as these lesions may occur without lumbar puncture or spinal analgesia). Certainly, with modern analgesic solutions, series of many thousands of cases have been collected without any serious nerve lesions, and when used by anaesthetists who are familiar with the technique and in suitable cases, spinal analgesia must compare favourably for safety with general anaesthesia.

The 'Total' Spinal

If local analgesic solution reaches as high as the cranial subarachnoid space, not only are the respiratory muscles paralysed, but the patient also loses the use of the cranial nerves, so that apnoea occurs, there is profound hypotension and the patient becomes unconscious. The solution may also enter the fourth ventricle where it may directly paralyse the respiratory and vasomotor centres. The treatment involves ventilation, maintaining the blood pressure by raising the legs, administering intravenous fluids and possibly using vasopressors. Provided that this is carried out, the condition is self-limiting as the local analgesic loses its effect.

With the small volumes of local analgesic used as hyperbaric solutions this complication is seen only if the patient is left steeply head-down. It is more likely to occur if the needle pierces the dura mater unnoticed while attempting epidural analgesia and the larger (epidural) volume of solution is injected intrathecally.

COMPLICATIONS OF EPIDURAL ANALGESIA

Effects on Cardiovascular System

These are similar to those seen with spinal analgesia and are again caused by, and proportional to, the extent of sympathetic blockade.

Effects on Respiratory System

Nerve fibres are blocked by local analgesic solutions with a readiness which depends on their diameter. The fine sympathetic fibres are most easily blocked, pain and other sensations next and motor nerve fibres, which are the thickest, are the most difficult to block. Most local analgesic solutions in common use for epidural analgesia produce only partial motor block, so that a 'differential block' is achieved. Thus, even with a high block, respiration may be only slightly affected.

Backache

Some tenderness over the injection site for about 48 hours is common after epidural analgesia due to the relatively large bore of the needle. Epidurals should not cause long-term backache.

Haematoma

It is not unusual when performing an epidural to cause some bleeding into the epidural space by damaging an epidural vein.

This seldom causes any problem, but theoretically could produce pressure on nerve roots and require laminectomy.

Epidural Abscess

This could result from faulty technique or as a result of infection of an epidural haematoma by blood-borne bacteria. It is a serious complication usually requiring immediate laminectomy.

Retention of Urine

When an epidural catheter is inserted to produce prolonged analgesia, retention of urine may occur because of loss of bladder sensation.

Breakage of Catheter

When an epidural catheter technique is being employed, it is possible for a piece of catheter to break off and be left inside the patient's back. This is unlikely with modern, flexible vinyl plastic catheters. Much more likely is the shearing-off of the distal portion of the catheter on the bevel of the Tuohy needle if an attempt is made to withdraw the catheter through the needle.

Neurological Lesions

Slight motor or sensory weakness (usually a numb patch on one thigh) occasionally persists for days or weeks after epidural analgesia, especially where a catheter technique has been used to 'soak' the nerve roots repeatedly. Spontaneous recovery is the rule. More serious and prolonged neurological complications are even more rare than after spinal analgesia, many thousands of cases having been collected without serious nerve lesions. When they occur, they are usually of the anterior spinal artery syndrome type, and are probably the result of a period of hypotension.

Toxicity of Local Analgesic Solution

The possibility of exceeding the safe dose of local analgesic solution must be kept in mind when any nerve block is carried out. There is a reasonable margin of error with most epidural blocks, but there is danger of accumulation to toxic doses when repeated increments are given through an epidural catheter.

'Total' Spinal

(*See* p. 431)

Summary

This list of complications of spinal and epidural blocks may look formidable, but close scrutiny will show that most of them are either minor or short-term, and the more serious and longer-term ones can be almost completely avoided by scrupulous attention to technique and to sterility of equipment.

USES OF SPINAL AND EPIDURAL ANALGESIA

Operative

Both types of block may be used as the sole method of analgesia for surgical operations. This is particularly applicable to operations below the diaphragm, although vagus blocks may need to be added for some intra-abdominal procedures. The number of occasions on which these blocks are the technique of choice either alone or in conjunction with general anaesthesia has been drastically reduced by the advent of muscle relaxants. The extent to which they are used as the sole anaesthetic depends largely on public expectation. In the UK, most patients undergoing anything but very minor surgery expect to be put to sleep, but this is by no means so in all countries.

There undoubtedly remain some operations where spinal or epidural analgesia are the methods of choice. These consist of operations on the perineal structures or legs, especially in patients with severe cardiovascular, respiratory or metabolic disease. A 'saddle-block' spinal or caudal epidural has no adverse effect whatsoever on any of these systems.

Therapeutic

This group of indications consists of conditions where a longer duration of effect is usually required than can be obtained from a single dose of local analgesic agent. This means that a catheter technique is required for additional injections. In the past catheters have been used for continuous spinal analgesia, but this method has now been abandoned, and in most of the following conditions a continuous epidural technique is used.

Recently epidural opiates (see below) have been extensively tried, but while often effective and not causing numbness or hypotension, they may cause severe respiratory depression and also at times nausea and vomiting, pruritus and retention of urine. These side-effects have prevented their general acceptance.

Obstetrics
Numerically this is the commonest indication for epidural analgesia in the UK.

Postoperative pain relief
Superb pain relief may be obtained but hypotension has to be looked out for when local analgesic solutions are used.

Chest injuries
Again, excellent analgesia is obtained, and without affecting the level of consciousness. This may be particularly useful if there is an associated head injury.

Renal and biliary colic
These agonising types of pain can readily be abolished by a few millilitres of epidural local analgesic solution.

Back pain
Epidural injection of local analgesic solution, usually with an injectable steroid (Depo-Medrone) may be effective treatment for low back pain.

Hypotensive anaesthesia
Both spinal and epidural analgesia may be used to produce deliberate hypotension and reduce bleeding at certain operations. This indication has been less common since the introduction of pharmacological agents that produce more flexible control of blood pressure.

Acute arterial or venous thrombo-embolic conditions
Epidural analgesia may be used to produce vasodilation of the collateral circulation which tends to go into spasm when there is acute thrombosis or embolism of major arterial or venous channels.

Intractable pain
Intractable pain may be relieved by the injection of neurolytic solutions into the subarachnoid or epidural spaces. Spinal injections (e.g. 5% phenol in glycerine) are more effective than epidural injections for this purpose.

CONTRAINDICATIONS TO SPINAL AND EPIDURAL ANALGESIA

Bleeding Tendency

A haemorrhagic tendency due to either disease or anticoagulant therapy may result in an extensive epidural haematoma if an epidural vein is damaged by needle or catheter.

Skin Sepsis

Skin sepsis near the injection site is an absolute contraindication to spinal or epidural block.

Shock

Any patient whose circulating blood volume is depleted for any reason (e.g. haemorrhage, vomiting or diarrhoea) attempts to maintain his blood pressure by peripheral vasoconstriction. This attempt at compensation is impaired by a spinal or epidural block affecting the sympathetic outflow from the spinal cord, and a profound fall in blood pressure may result.

Absence of Patient's Consent

Although there are certain circumstances in which an anaesthetist may feel that a spinal or epidural block are in the patient's (or, in obstetrics, the baby's) best interests, he must never proceed if the patient refuses consent.

Demyelinating Conditions of the Spinal Cord

These conditions (e.g. multiple sclerosis) may be regarded as relative contraindications because the block may be blamed if there is a subsequent exacerbation of the condition. However, there is no evidence that there is a cause-and-effect relationship here and some anaesthetists would still perform these types of block in patients with these conditions after full discussion with the patient and after obtaining his consent.

Chronic Back Problems

These may also be considered as relative contraindications but, as indicated above, these cases are often treated by epidural block so it is quite reasonable to perform these techniques on a consenting patient.

INTRATHECAL AND EPIDURAL OPIATES

The discovery in the past few years of specific opiate receptors in the brain and in the substantia gelatinosa of the spinal cord, and of naturally occurring opiate-like substances (opioids), has led to much speculation and investigation into the possible uses of intrathecal and epidural opiates. The potential advantages of opiates used in this way are that they might relieve pain without the complications of motor block, sympathetic block or even of numbness. The situation is far from clear and is likely to remain so for some time but the following points seem to be emerging:

Spinal opiates seem to be more effective than epidural opiates, probably because of their injection in closer proximity to the spinal cord. They have, however, been less investigated than epidural opiates because the subarachnoid space is not regarded as suitable for a continuous catheter technique.

There is a wide variation in the efficacy of epidural opiates in different types of pain. They seem to be more effective in post-operative and traumatic pain than in obstetric pain and do not provide analgesia for surgical manoeuvres.

Respiratory depression may occur and occasionally may be extreme. The cause of this is uncertain at present, but as very small doses of opiates sometimes have this effect it may be that they are in some way gaining direct access to the respiratory centre in the floor of the fourth ventricle of the brain.

DRUGS AND EQUIPMENT

These will be mentioned only briefly as they are best learned in the anaesthetic room or classroom.

Drugs

While the standard solution of 0·5% plain bupivacaine has been quite extensively used as a spinal solution (it acts as an isobaric or marginally hypobaric solution), there is now only one solution in the UK specifically manufactured for spinal use *and* approved by the Committee on Safety of Medicines. That is 0·5% bupivacaine in 8% dextrose marketed by Astra Pharmaceuticals Ltd as Marcain Heavy.

A wider range of epidural solutions is available. These include:

0·5%	plain bupivacaine (Marcain)
0·5%	bupivacaine in 1:200 000 adrenaline
0·25%	plain bupivacaine
0·25%	bupivacaine in 1:400 000 adrenaline
0·75%	plain bupivacaine
1·5%	plain lignocaine
1·0%	lignocaine in 1:200 000 adrenaline

It should be remembered that the toxic dose of 1·5% plain lignocaine is only 13–14 ml in a person of 70 kg.

Needles

Many different spinal needles have been designed but are now being replaced by disposable needles. These are available in sizes down to 26 G and even finer reusable needles are made. The main requirement of a spinal needle is that it should have a short bevel so that the entire orifice can easily be accommodated in the subarachnoid space. With the finer needles a transparent hub is an advantage as it allows much earlier detection of cerebrospinal fluid in the hub.

Disposable epidural needles are also becoming increasingly popular and may be part of a complete disposable epidural pack. The most frequently used pattern of needle is the Tuohy needle which has its bevel pointing laterally to increase the ease of introduction of the plastic catheter. The most common size used in the UK is 16 G for adults, but 17 G and 18 G are also available. Whatever size is chosen, it is vital if a catheter is to be inserted that it will pass through the needle.

Double-Needle Spinal/Epidural Technique

This technique is gaining popularity in some branches of anaesthesia. Essentially it implies the insertion of an epidural needle into the epidural space in the usual way. A fine spinal needle, with a shaft long enough to protrude a few millimetres beyond the tip of the epidural needle is then introduced through it into the subarachnoid space. After injection of the spinal solution, the spinal needle is removed, and a catheter introduced into the epidural space before the epidural needle too is removed. The patient is then positioned appropriately for the spread of the spinal solution.

The advantages of this technique are that it provides the speed and reliability of the spinal technique, while the epidural catheter can be used to modify the extent of analgesia if the spinal technique is not perfect and can also be used to provide post-operative pain relief. The epidural needle also acts as a guide leading the fine spinal needle almost to the subarachnoid space.

43 Treatment of Chronic Pain

Assessment of patient. Methods of pain relief. Treatment of back pain. Spinal and extradural techniques—analgesics, opioids, neurolytics. Counter-irritation. Central nervous modification of chronic pain.

With the establishment of pain clinics the relief of chronic pain has recently become an important new sub-speciality of anaesthesia. A great many patients suffer varying degrees of chronic pain, which may be caused in several ways, e.g. postoperatively, post-traumatically, from neoplastic disease, for spinal disorders and from infections such as herpes zoster (shingles). Although many patients with chronic pain may accurately describe both the nature and site of their pain, the fact that they have borne it for some time often means that a considerable psychological overlay is involved, and it is important to consider this aspect of pain relief as well as the more definitive use of analgesic techniques.

ASSESSMENT OF PATIENT

In ideal circumstances, considerable time needs to be taken to assess the patients adequately and if necessary to admit them to hospital for further examination and tests. Those with disabilities and severe pain may take a long time to undress, and a busy outpatient clinic is not the place to examine them. It is necessary to obtain a detailed history of the factors causing the pain and those which aggravate it, together with its frequency, duration, nature and the mechanical factors or drugs which relieve the pain.

Much chronic pain results from previous treatment, either surgical or medical, so detailed knowledge of operations performed and treatment attempted is also important, together with the results of previous physical examination. Current drug therapy and possible allergies to analgesics and other agents employed in the past must also be sought, together with an evaluation of the underlying psychological influences in each particular case. These may include family pressures and, in some cases, the fact that litigation by the patient is in process as the result of an accident.

Examination of the patient may show the degree of physical impairment, and particularly what movements or activities cause the pain. Trigger areas and other sensitive spots which spark off cyclical pain may also be sought. It may be possible to evaluate the degree of the patient's over-reaction or under-reaction to his particular pain, which may help in future treatment, although accurate measurement of pain is at present unavailable and one has to rely on qualitative impressions.

Sometimes patients will present to a pain clinic having not been investigated before or examined for the existence of underlying pathology which may cause their particular pain. Laboratory tests, x-ray examinations and ECGs may be necessary to exclude underlying treatable conditions as a cause of the pain, and it is important not to overlook these by attempting simply to remove the pain.

METHODS OF PAIN RELIEF

As there are so many factors both producing and influencing chronic pain, many different methods of relief may be employed. These range from locally applied techniques such as heat, massage, physiotherapy, ultrasound and counter-irritation, to local analgesic techniques—either alone or combined with anti-inflammatory agents—and finally to specific neurolytic techniques designed to destroy nerves. Pain is a vicious circle which if interrupted may result in permanent pain relief. The central nervous factors modifying the degree and nature of the pain are often amenable to treatment with sedatives and anti-depressants.

Mechanical Methods of Pain Relief

Many patients in chronic pain benefit considerably from physiotherapy, which may include the use of heat, cold or vibration to modify pain and to restore mobility to painful joints. To produce good results it is essential that there is a close liaison between physiotherapists and anaesthetists treating patients in chronic pain. It is also important, before referring the patient to the physiotherapy department, to have adequate radiological and clinical evidence of the patient's lesion.

Local Nerve Blocks

The use of local anaesthetic techniques is an essential part of treatment within a pain clinic. Since local anaesthetics work only for a relatively short time, it is often possible to use them for diagnostic as well as therapeutic benefit. Painful or tender areas, as well as trigger points which may precipitate pain over a more diffuse region, are all amenable to injections of local anaesthetics; if this achieves satisfactory analgesia, then either a repeat block or the use of a neurolytic agent where a specific nerve is involved may have a more permanent effect. Pain in the distribution of a particular cutaneous nerve is relatively easy to treat provided that the nerve is accessible to local anaesthesia. However, referred pain (e.g. shoulder tip pain from diaphragmatic irritation) should not be forgotten. Disseminated cancer may also produce specific nerve pain, which is treatable by local anaesthesia.

In some patients it may be necessary to anaesthetise the nerve as it leaves the spinal cord, either by injecting local anaesthetic into the CSF (spinal block) or by an extradural technique. If local nerve block is successful, in most cases this can be followed by treatment designed to produce permanent nerve damage.

Nerves may be destroyed either by injection of neurolytic substances (e.g. phenol, chlorocresol and alcohol) or by using heat (diathermy), cold (cryosurgery), or by permanent surgical section. Local injection of neurolytic agents is usually a less complicated procedure more applicable to out-patient treatment, although diathermy and cryosurgery are, nowadays, both more widely used. If the nerve is attacked in its course along a limb, these locally applied neurolytic techniques do not destroy the cell body but merely the axon of the nerve, and regeneration is sometimes possible. This may result merely in a return of the pain, or may sometimes produce hypersensitivity of the area, worse than the original pain. Some types of pain are more suitable for local nerve blocks than others, and this must be considered when the method of pain relief is being contemplated.

Sympathetic Nerve Blocks

Deep-seated burning pain, phantom limb pain and areas of hypersensitivity are all often resistant to conventional nerve blocks, and sympathetic blockade is sometimes necessary to produce relief. The sympathetic nerves leave the spinal cord and join the sympathetic chain lying along the anterolateral borders of the vertebral bodies. Local injections in this region may produce sympathetic nerve block, which can also be achieved by intravenous injection of a dilute solution of guanethidine into an isolated limb, in a similar way to Bier's block (Chapter 41). Sympathetic blockade of the arm is best produced by stellate ganglion block.

TREATMENT OF BACK PAIN

Many patients present to a pain clinic with low back pain. Most have already received specialist investigation and treatment in other units, particularly orthopaedic and neurosurgical, and therefore come to the clinic as a last resort. By this stage many already have considerable psychological overlay and any planned course of treatment must take this into account. In some cases specific nerve involvement can be demonstrated and may be treatable locally, particularly by injection of specific lumbar or sacral nerves as they leave the spinal cord, but many patients may be suffering from a more diffuse pain which is difficult to treat. This may arise from the sacro-iliac or intervertebral joints and recent methods of treatment of low back pain have concentrated on this. Lumbar extradural anaesthesia with large doses of local anaesthetic mixed with long-acting steroids may also be successful in breaking down adhesions in the extradural space which give rise to pain. Nevertheless, the treatment of chronic low back pain is often laborious and sometimes unsuccessful.

SPINAL AND EXTRADURAL TECHNIQUES—ANALGESICS, OPIOIDS, NEUROLYTICS

If local anaesthetics, administered either extradurally or spinally, provide satisfactory, but temporary analgesia, it may then be necessary to use a more prolonged technique. This would be either intermittent or continuous infusion of opioids or a neurolytic technique.

Opioids administered either spinally or extradurally are becoming very popular in the treatment of some forms of back pain although the analgesia produced is usually not as profound as that achieved with local anaesthetics. Long-term infusion techniques using tunnelled spinal or extradural catheters have recently been developed to provide a continuous infusion over a prolonged period.

Most of the neurolytic techniques require precise application of the agent to the affected nerve root and therefore are unsatisfactory when used extradurally. Specific intrathecal (spinal) nerve blocks are more commonly employed. Hyperbaric solutions of phenol or chlorocresol are used and after lumbar puncture the patient is positioned so that a small puddle of the neurolytic agent lies over the nerve to be destroyed. This technique is particularly useful with severe lesions resulting from spread of cancer, when the results are often excellent and the occasional loss of accompanying motor function or bladder control is less important to patients with only a short life expectancy.

COUNTER-IRRITATION

Counter-irritation is used every day to alleviate pain, e.g. when rubbing a child's limb to remove the pain from a bruise, or applying local heat or cold to relieve backache. Transcutaneous nerve stimulation is an alternative method of producing pain relief, by counter-irritation of the skin overlying the painful area. Counter-irritant creams or lotions, and acupuncture may also help to alleviate pain in this way and it is important to explore every avenue of possible relief in patients suffering chronic pain.

CENTRAL NERVOUS MODIFICATION OF CHRONIC PAIN

Some psychological factors influence the degree and duration of pain. Anxiety and depression not only occur as a result of prolonged intractable pain, but may also influence the success of treatment such as nerve block. Many patients benefit from simultaneous analgesia and sedation or antidepressant therapy, and sometimes from such drugs alone. Diazepam and lorazepam in relatively small doses may be of considerable benefit to patients in helping them to tolerate severe pain, the intensity of which depends on its interpretation. Some patients get severely depressed during long illnesses and the use of tricyclic antidepressants (e.g. amitriptyline or imipramine) may be of considerable benefit. In many cases a single dose of antidepressant at night ensures a good night's rest and, as the effect is long-lasting, continues into the following day without causing drowsiness.

Adequate and caring conversations with the doctors and nurses concerned may also help. Patients who feel that they have been sympathetically treated often improve considerably by comparison with patients who become antagonistic towards the staff looking after them, implying that no one is doing any good for them and no one really cares about their pain either. Unfortunately this is not infrequent in patients suffering from chronic pain, and must be guarded against if treatment is to be successful.

44 Parenteral Nutrition

Protein. Carbohydrate. Fats. Vitamins. Ionic requirements. Suggested intravenous feeding regimens. Problems of parenteral nutrition. Assessment of parenteral feeding.

Parenteral nutrition is now extensively used both in intensive care units and pre-operatively in malnourished patients, although it is sometimes used in addition to oral feeding to increase calorie intake (hyperalimentation). It is important that parenteral feeding be considered as the sole source of the patient's calories and calculated accordingly.

A 70 kg man requires about 3000 calories per 24 hours, usually administered in 3000 ml intravenous fluid. As a general rule, therefore 1 ml fluid must contain 1 calorie. The normal diet is a balance of protein, fat and carbohydrate together with amino acids and electrolytes, which the body is able to conserve or excrete as necessary. A parenteral feeding regimen must therefore aim at reproducing normal food intake despite the fact that the gut is being bypassed. In general, parenteral feeding should only be employed in those patients with impaired intestinal absorption, nasogastric (enteral) feeding being preferable whenever possible. The individual requirements of an intravenous feeding regimen are best considered under their separate headings.

PROTEIN

The daily protein requirement to balance urinary loss is about 1 g amino acid per kg bodyweight, containing the equivalent of

10–15 g nitrogen per day for a 70 kg person. In order that the amino acid supplied to the body may be fully incorporated into body protein, 200 calories in the form of carbohydrate are required for every 5 g nitrogen supplied. Although several amino-acid solutions are available the most important are as follows.

Vamin

Vamin either supplied as an amino-acid solution containing 9 or 14 g nitrogen or combined with glucose which is added to provide the total daily requirement of amino acids, carbohydrate and electrolyte in one solution. The energy yield of Vamin Glucose is 650 calories per litre.

Aminoplex

This is produced either as Aminoplex 5, 12, 14 or 24 depending on the number of utilisable of nitrogen g/l. Aminoplex 5 is intended as a total intravenous feed in one bottle, providing the daily requirements of amino acids, electrolytes, carbohydrate and calories. Aminoplex 5 yields 1000 calories per litre. It is a solution of L-form amino acids with added calories in the form of sorbitol and ethanol. The sorbitol has been shown to produce considerable metabolic acidosis in patients fed for several days on the regimen, and most patients on prolonged intravenous feeding are better given a balanced regimen rather than a single solution. Aminoplex 14 and 24 provide a high level of nitrogen input in the form of amino acids in a low fluid volume. The calorie yields are low but the nitrogen content is about 14 and 24 g/litre respectively.

Synthamin 14

This is another amino-acid solution containing a similar amount of nitrogen to Aminoplex 14, and the two solutions are used in similar circumstances. Synthamin is also supplied combined with glucose and electrolytes as A and B bags depending on the glucose concentration.

CARBOHYDRATE

The most widely used carbohydrate source in parenteral feeding is dextrose, in concentrations ranging from 10 % to 50 %. In normal circumstances carbohydrate metabolism yields about 4 calories per g (glucose), and therefore a litre of 20 % dextrose, containing 200 g/litre, will yield about 800 calories. For this reason, any dextrose concentration below 10 % is inadequate, since the fluid volume required to yield adequate calories will be too large. Most pharmacies now stock litre bottles of glucose with added electrolytes similar to Glucopex 1200 (30 % glucose) or 1600 (40 % glucose) which yield 1200 and 1600 calories per litre respectively.

Recently it has been recognised that administering intravenous dextrose alone does not result in the sugar passing intracellularly where it is needed for metabolism. This function is insulin-dependent, and patients being parenterally fed on dextrose need insulin added. This may be accomplished in three ways, either by using a sliding scale base, usually on four-hourly urine or blood sugar testing, by adding insulin to the intravenous solution or by using a separate infusion of insulin. Insulin, however, is adsorbed on to the plastics of the intravenous solution container and giving set, and the amount reaching the patient therefore varies. Administration of glucose and insulin will also result in potassium passing intracellularly, and it is important not to allow the patient to become hypokalaemic.

Fructose is another carbohydrate source which was popular for a time, largely in the belief that insulin was not required to help in the passage of fructose into cells. This has now been proved incorrect and the vogue for fructose is declining. It is still sometimes administered in conjunction with amino-acid solutions, where it produces the same calorie yield as another carbohydrate source. Sorbitol is also used as a carbohydrate source, particularly in Aminoplex 5.

Ethanol may be used as a carbohydrate source and yields 7 calories per g as opposed to 4 calories per g for the other sugar solutions. The amount of ethanol which may be given daily is limited and it cannot therefore be used to supply the total carbohydrate requirements.

FATS

Intralipid, as either a 10 % or 20 % solution, is the only fat source used to any extent at present. As fat yields 9 calories/g.

Intralipid is a good source of energy, a litre of 10 % yielding 1000 calories and 20 % 2000 calories. When Intralipid was introduced certain problems were encountered with the high viscosity producing micro-aggregation in small vessels that was similar to fat embolism. This has now been overcome and Intralipid should be considered an essential part of any intravenous feed regimen. It should be remembered, however, that blood samples should not be taken while Intralipid is running because considerable inaccuracies may occur on auto-analysers used in many hospitals for electrolyte determination.

VITAMINS

It is important that both the fat-soluble and water-soluble vitamins are administered regularly in the form of Multibionta, Solvito and Vitalipid or Parentrovite A and B. These can conveniently be added only to isotonic fluid solutions such as dextrose or saline in the case of water soluble vitamin preparations, or to Intralipid for the fat soluble vitamins.

IONIC REQUIREMENTS

In addition to producing an adequate calorie intake, patients still require their normal intake of sodium, potassium and other trace elements such as magnesium, zinc and calcium. Some glucose and protein containing solutions contain various amounts of sodium and potassium and some of the trace elements, but it is important to determine the amount of sodium and other ions being administered to check that this is neither inadequate nor excessive. The specific requirements for fluid and electrolytes have already been discussed in Chapter 2. The overall daily requirements of individual ions are as follows:

Sodium	70–150 mmol per 24 hours
Potassium	60–80 mmol per 24 hours
Calcium	1000–1500 mg per 24 hours
Phosphate	1000 mg per 24 hours

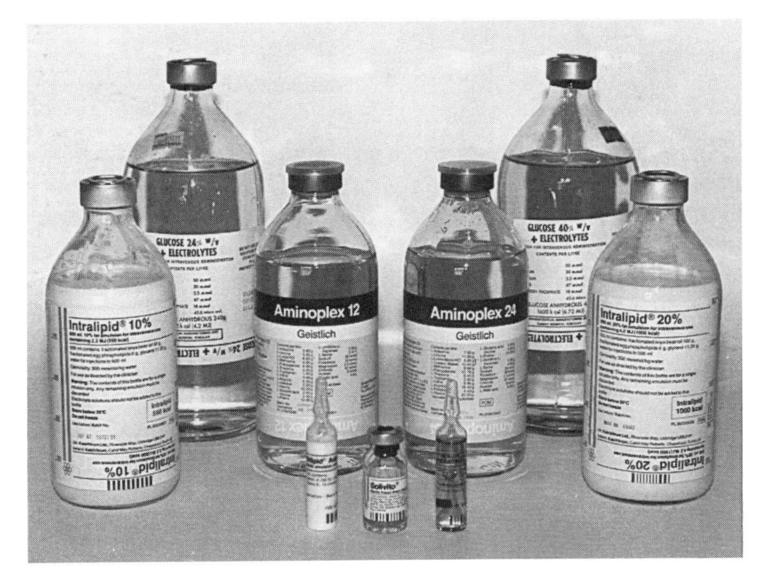

Fig. 44.1 Balanced range of parenteral feeding solutions

SUGGESTED INTRAVENOUS FEEDING REGIMENS

Although it may appear convenient to administer intravenous feeding consecutively in bottles, this is far from the normal way in which we obtain food. Serious metabolic imbalance may result from administering protein for four hours followed by dextrose for four hours followed by fats for four hours. Parenteral feeding is best accomplished by the simultaneous administration of two or more solutions through a central venous line, controlled by drip counters. Many hospital pharmacies have a sterile preparation area where a composite 24 hour, 3 litre bag can be made to match the requirements of a particular patient. These bags are sterile and, as with all parenteral feeding solutions, should *not* have anything added to them. If it is not possible to obtain a 3 litre bag or indeed to use the Synthamin A and B bag system then most parenteral feeding solutions are obtainable in either 500 ml or 1000 ml bottles (Fig. 44.1) and a satisfactory fluid and calorie input which is versatile enough to allow addition of electrolytes and vitamins is best achieved as follows.

	Line A	*Line B*
0–8 h	500 ml of Aminoplex 12	500 ml 30 % dextrose
8–16 h	500 ml 20 % Intralipid	500 ml 5 % dextrose or normal saline
16–24 h	500 ml of Aminoplex 12	500 ml 30 % dextrose

Obviously this regimen can be adapted to suit individual requirements by substituting one bottle for another, depending on whether one wishes to include a high nitrogen, a high calorie or high electrolyte input. It has several important advantages.

Firstly, that dextrose, a carbohydrate source, is given simultaneously with the amino-acid solution, the two being necessary for efficient utilisation of amino acids. Simultaneous administration of insulin will be necessary to permit glucose to pass intracellularly.

Secondly, the regimen may be adjusted so that Intralipid is not running in the morning when blood is taken for urea and electrolyte determinations.

Thirdly, a single bottle of isotonic 5 % dextrose or normal saline allows addition of both vitamins and added electrolytes where these are needed. Although Aminoplex 12 contains a considerable amount of sodium and some potassium, it is often necessary to supplement the potassium intake in particular. Most pharmacies will make up isotonic electrolyte solutions containing trace elements if these are required for intravenous feeding. The overall regimen provides just under 3000 calories in 3 litres of fluid, although this may be adjusted as necessary.

An alternative intravenous feeding regimen, particularly if it is required for only one or two days postoperatively, is simply to give 3 litres of Aminoplex 5 over the first 24 hours, and 2 litres plus a litre of either dextrose 5 % of normal saline over the second 24 hours, to which additional electrolytes may be added if necessary. However, as already mentioned, this does not allow individual variations in calorie and amino-acid input and may produce a metabolic acidosis from the metabolism of sorbitol after prolonged use.

PROBLEMS OF PARENTERAL NUTRITION

If intravenous feeding is used scientifically and early, it often considerably reduces morbidity from major surgery. Indeed, it is often now used pre-operatively, particularly in patients who are malnourished as a result of their illness. Nevertheless, fluid overload may be a problem if one is particularly anxious to increase the calorie intake, although certain solutions such as 20 % Intralipid go some way towards removing this risk. Some solutions, such as those containing amino acids, are irritant and certainly cannot be given through a peripheral drip. A central venous feeding line which is not used for aspirating blood or for giving other drugs is essential to maintain absolute sterility. These lines are best introduced either through the antecubital fossa or into the subclavian or internal jugular vein under strictly aseptic conditions. Accurate monitoring of fluid and electrolyte balance is vital as these are difficult to correct if allowed to get out of control. Hypokalaemia may be a problem and as there is a limit to the amount of potassium which can safely be administered intravenously—even under ECG control—it is important to consider adequate potassium replacement early.

ASSESSMENT OF PARENTERAL FEEDING

Although frequent measurements can be made of fluid and electrolyte balance, one of the most important indices of the adequacy of parenteral feeding is the nitrogen balance. This is not normally undertaken but is simple and revealing in some circumstances. By collecting all the urine which the patient passes during a 24-hour period and measuring its volume and urea content the overall urea output per 24 hours can be measured. Then, as 100 mmol urea = 6 g urea = 3 g nitrogen = 20 g protein (normal nitrogen output 9/10 in the urine, 1/10 in the faeces), it is possible to assess both the daily protein output and whether this exceeds the daily protein intake. Protein intake is easily calculated when parenteral feeding alone is used, but when this is combined with nasogastric feeding, or indeed nasogastric feeding is used alone, it is important to know the protein content of the individual nasogastric diets which the diet kitchen is able to supply. Simple calculations can therefore prevent patients getting into dangerously negative nitrogen balance.

45 Humidifiers

Effects of anaesthesia and intensive care. Methods of humidification. Nebulisers.

The most important function of the nose is to warm and humidify inspired air or gases. It performs this task with remarkable efficiency considering that—assuming a minute volume of 8 litres per minute—an average person breathes in over 10 000 litres of air in 24 hours. Over a wide range of inspired air temperatures the nose is capable of raising the temperature of the inspired air to within less than 1 °C of body temperature.

As regards humidification, the alveoli function best when the air presented to them is almost fully saturated. Here, an important physical principle is involved—namely, that the amount of water vapour required to saturate air or a gas mixture fully increases with the temperature. Thus the clear air of a warm day changes to mist or fog in the evening as the temperature falls and the air is unable to contain the water vapour which precipitates out. In the morning as the temperature rises, the air once again becomes clear as the amount of water vapour that it is able to contain increases.

For comfort, room air should only be about half-saturated with water vapour. However, even if fully saturated it contains only about 2 volumes per cent of water vapour, while at body temperature (37 °C) air requires 6 volumes per cent of water vapour to be fully saturated. This task of adding large quantities of water vapour to the inspired air is remarkably well achieved by the nose and upper respiratory passages.

EFFECTS OF ANAESTHESIA AND INTENSIVE CARE

With most modern anaesthetic circuits (e.g. Magill circuit, Bain circuit, or a circuit with a non-rebreathing valve next to the face mask or endotracheal tube) the patient receives at each inspiration an almost completely fresh supply of dry gases from the cylinders or pipeline. These gases have nearly always arrived at room temperature by the time they reach the patient along the anaesthetic tubing, but they then have to be warmed to body temperature and fully saturated with water vapour by the respiratory passages.

When a face mask is used the nose can still perform its function adequately, but when an oropharyngeal airway is inserted a proportion of the inspired gases bypasses the nose so that warming and humidification are less effective. An endotracheal tube completely bypasses the upper respiratory tract, so warming and humidification have to be achieved in the lower respiratory passages. This is much less effective, especially if atropine or any other antisialogogue have been given. The drying effect may produce at least some degree of tracheitis, and it is becoming commoner practice to attempt humidification during anaesthesia, especially during longer intubated cases (see below).

With a circle anaesthetic system humidification is not quite so difficult because the patient does rebreathe his own expired gases to some extent. However, even in this arrangement the temperature of the expired gases rapidly falls to room temperature in the anaesthetic tubing so that much of the water vapour condenses out on the inside. On re-inspiration the air passages once again have to re-warm the gases to body temperature and re-saturate them with water vapour at this higher temperature.

The problem of humidification is much more serious in intensive care where spontaneous respiration or IPPR may be carried out for days or even weeks through an endotracheal or tracheostomy tube. Some form of artificial humidification is necessary to prevent a serious or even fatal drying up and crusting of secretions. The various methods used are described below.

METHODS OF HUMIDIFICATION

Direct Instillation of Water Droplets

This consists of the direct injection of water droplets into an endotracheal or tracheostomy tube. While simple, this method is rather crude and ineffective and at times may result in a picture similar to a mild degree of acid-aspiration syndrome. It should therefore have little place in modern intensive therapy.

Water-Bath

In its simplest form this consists of bubbling the gases through water in a bottle, as shown in Figure 45.1. This is most inefficient, for two reasons: firstly, the bubbles tend to be too large to become fully saturated with water vapour, and, secondly, saturation at best occurs only at room temperature, which means only partial saturation when the gases are raised to body temperature. The system tends to be made even less efficient by the cooling effect produced by vaporising the water.

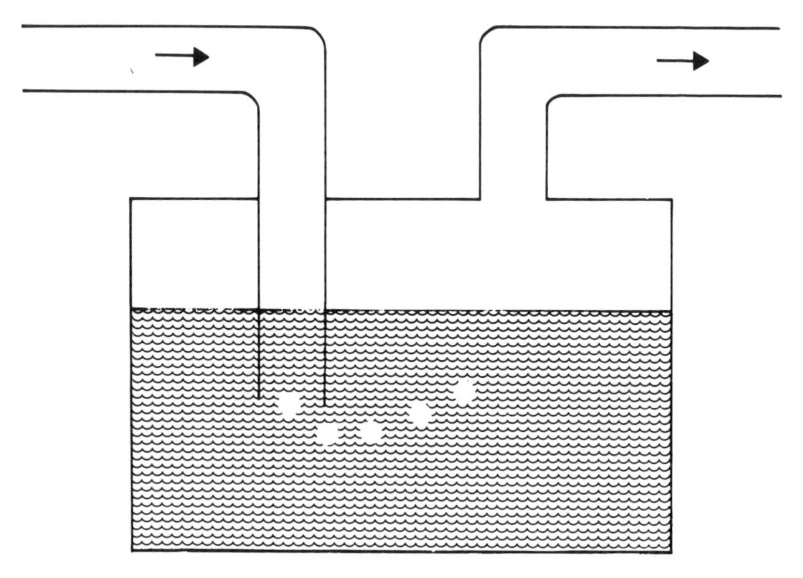

Fig. 45.1 Water bottle humidifier

The efficiency of this type of humidifier is greatly increased by breaking up the big bubbles into smaller ones so that they are more readily saturated and by adding a heater to the water-bath (Fig. 45.2). Because of the fall in temperature along the tube leading from the humidifier to the patient, for maximum efficiency the temperature of the water should be kept at about 55°C. However as air when fully saturated at body temperature contains less water vapour than when fully saturated at 55°C, some water vapour must condense out in the tube before it reaches the patient. Care must be taken either by positioning the humidifier below the patient or by using a water-trap to prevent pooling of water, which might spill into the patient's respiratory tract.

If the water temperature is kept near 60°C, sterility of the humidifier is maintained by a prolonged pasteurisation effect. This type of humidifier should have a thermostat as well as a thermometer and an automatic cut-out in case the temperature exceeds its setting. In some of these humidifiers it is also possible

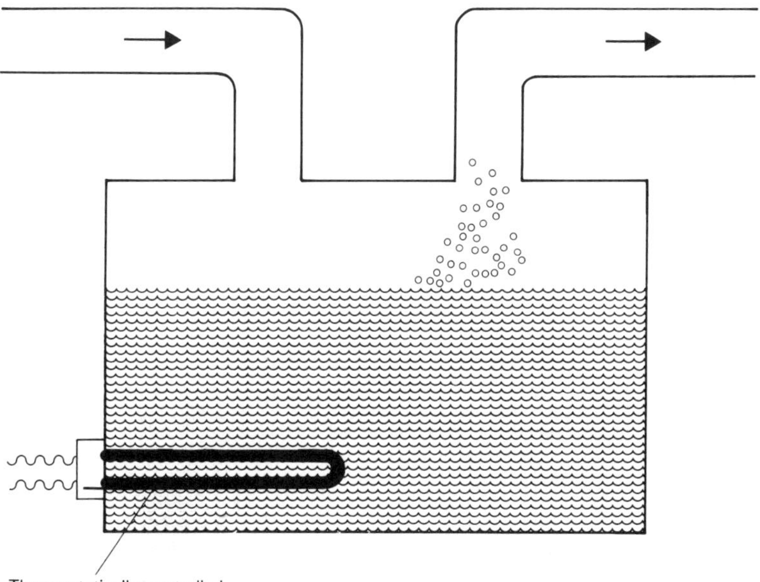

Fig. 45.2 Heated water bath humidifier

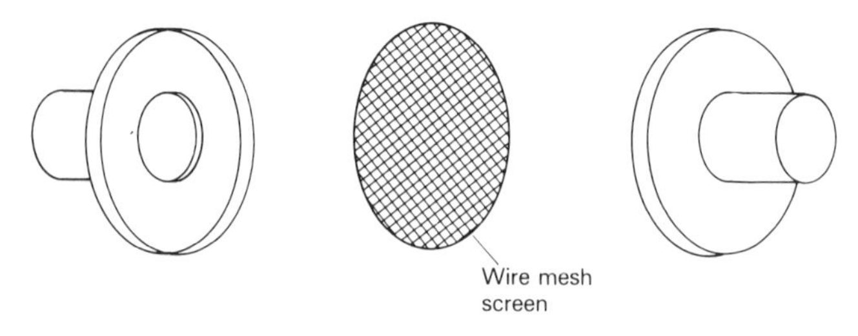

Fig. 45.3 Condenser humidifier ('artificial nose' or 'Swedish nose')

to override the thermostat so that the apparatus can be fully sterilised by boiling before being used in another patient.

These water-bath humidifiers are usually placed on the inspiratory side of a ventilatory system. Others—usually referred to as blower humidifiers—are intended for use when the patient is breathing spontaneously. In these circumstances the humidified air is blown past a T-piece inserted into the patient's tracheostomy or endotracheal tube.

Condenser Humidifiers, Heat and Moisture Exchangers (HMEs)

These lightweight pieces of apparatus (Fig. 45.3) are designed to fit into an endotracheal or tracheostomy tube. The functional part of the humidifier consists of a disc of wire mesh through which the patient breathes. As this disc is at a lower temperature than body temperature, some of the water vapour in the expired air condenses on it and at the same time warms the mesh by the latent heat of the condensation. When inspiration occurs, this moisture vaporises again, thus humidifying and warming the air or gases as they are carried into the respiratory tract.

This type of humidifier is by no means 100 % efficient, but it is compact and convenient and works reasonably well, especially if the room air is not too dry. The main disadvantage is that if the patient is coughing up sputum this becomes entangled in the wire mesh, which may have to be changed frequently to prevent severe obstruction to respiration. In addition, this part of the humidifier may act as a potent source of infection, and these pieces of apparatus are usually now made in such a way that the wire mesh can easily be removed for cleaning and sterilising. This

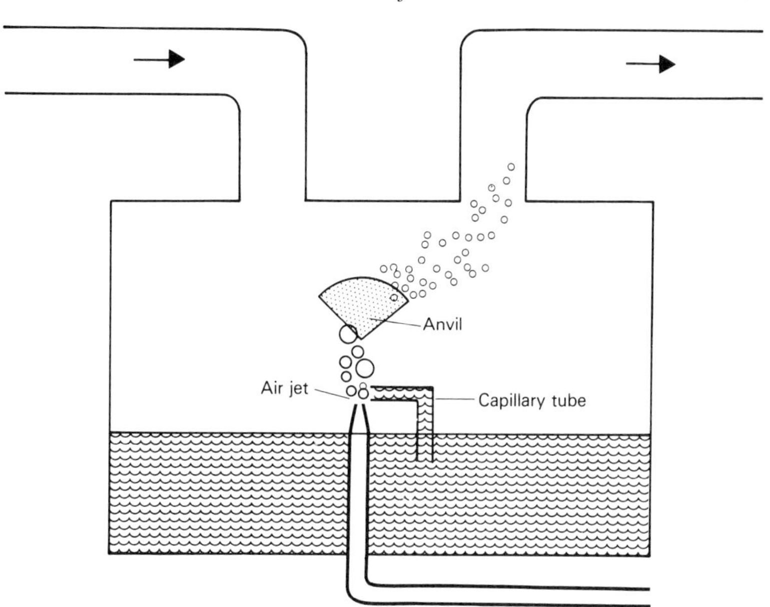

Fig. 45.4 Gas-driven nebuliser

should be done at least every three hours in intensive care situations.

Several manufacturers now make disposable condenser humidifiers with a variety of condensation materials, e.g. hygroscopic foam, corregated aluminium foil, and some are even made with a dead space small enough for paediatric use. They have become popular for use during longer anaesthetics, as well as in intensive care.

NEBULISERS

Gas Driven

Most examples of this type of nebuliser (Fig. 45.4) depend on the Bernouilli effect whereby gas blown at high pressure through an orifice causes a fall in pressure around the orifice. Fluid is drawn up a capillary tube to the area of the orifice where the fluid is

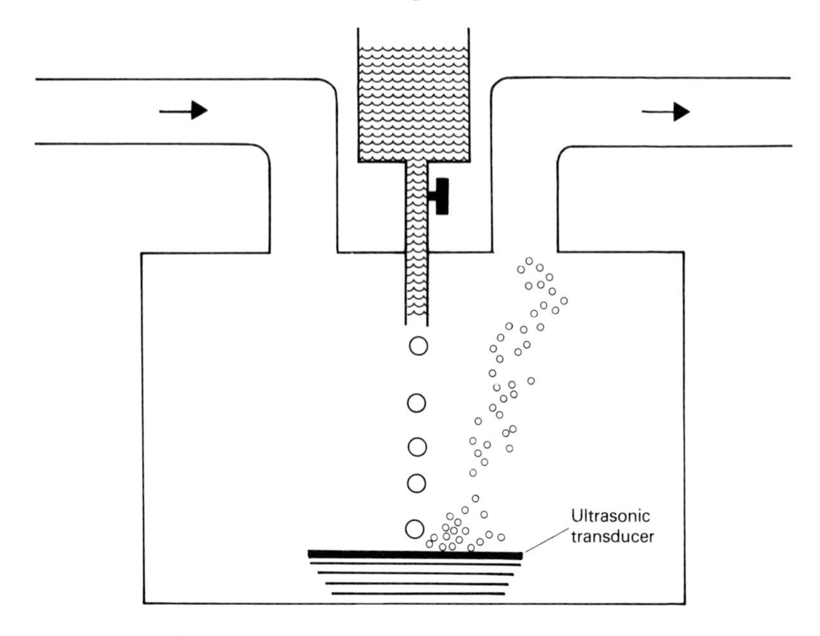

Fig. 45.5 Ultrasonic nebuliser with water dropping on the transducer head

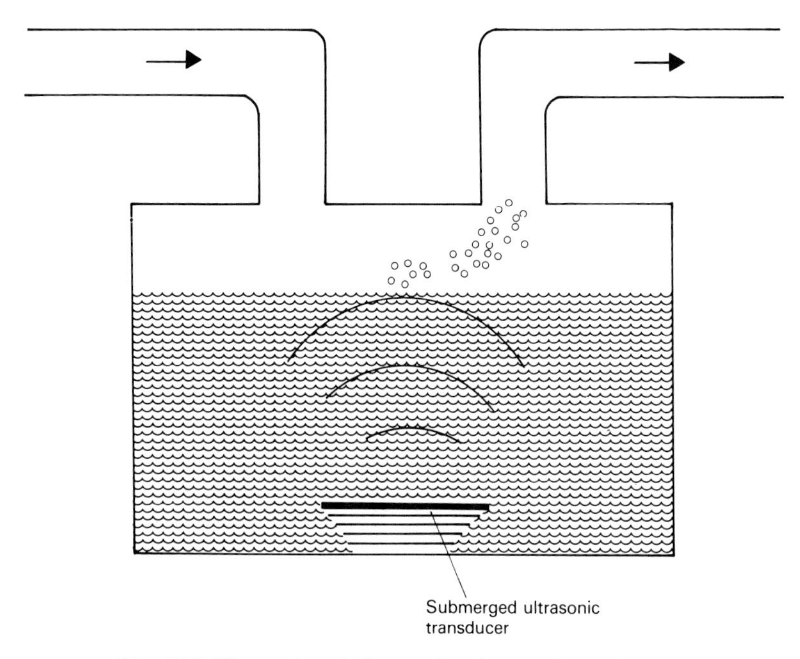

Fig. 45.6 Ultrasonic nebuliser with submerged transducer head

vaporised by the gas jet. The larger droplets can be filtered off by striking an 'anvil', or metal plate. The efficiency of this type of nebuliser can be increased by heating the liquid in the container. The Bennett Cascade humidifier is an example of a heated, gas-driven nebuliser, although it does not make use of the Bernouilli effect.

Spinning Disc Nebulisers

A rotating disc is mounted on a hollow shaft up which the liquid is drawn. As the liquid touches the disc it is thrown out by centrifugal force in a variety of droplet sizes.

Ultrasonic Nebulisers

In these nebulisers liquid is either dropped on to a transducer which vibrates at ultrasonic speed (Fig. 45.5), or liquid in a container covers the head of a transducer which vibrates at an ultrasonic frequency (Fig. 45.6). The size of the droplets depends on the speed of vibration.

With nebulisers of all types, the size of the droplets is important. If these are larger than 20 μm diameter they tend to condense out in the tubing of the apparatus or in the upper respiratory tract and are merely a nuisance. Droplets of 5–15 μm size deposit mostly in the trachea and larger bronchi which they help to keep moist. Droplets of 1 μm diameter pass on to the alveoli where they are deposited. Droplets of less than 1 μm diameter tend to be remarkably stable, passing into alveoli and out again. They may escape into the atmosphere, where they become an infection risk.

The droplets produced by the ultrasonic nebulisers tend to be largely in the 1 μm range so that, while they tend to be extremely efficient as humidifiers, overhydration of the patient is a possibility, especially in children.

46 Sterilisation of Anaesthetic Equipment

Definitions. Methods of sterilisation. Sterilisation indicators. Methods of disinfection. Filtration. Cleaning and sterilising anaesthetic equipment. Hepatitis B antigen. AIDS (acquired immune deficiency syndrome).

In recent years two developments have tended to reduce the extent to which anaesthetic nurses, operating department assistants (ODAs) and other theatre staff have been directly involved in maintaining and sterilising anaesthetic equipment. The first of these has been the introduction of theatre sterile supply departments (TSSUs) and central sterile supply departments (CSSDs). The second factor is the ever-expanding use of disposable equipment. While this originally applied mainly to simple items of equipment such as syringes and needles, now quite complicated packs (e.g. for setting up central venous lines or performing epidural blocks) may be entirely disposable.

Economic considerations make it impossible to provide fully sterilised anaesthetic apparatus in every case, even in those parts of the system through which rebreathing has occurred. Fortunately, although cross-infection between patients can occur by means of contaminated anaesthetic apparatus, it seems to be unusual except in the case of ventilators. Economy also leads to a tendency to try to reuse or resterilise equipment which is meant to be disposable. This should be done only with the utmost caution because certain materials, especially plastic and rubber, tend to deteriorate rapidly with repeated sterilisation.

Thus, although the standards of sterility in anaesthesia tend to be a compromise between what is desirable and what is economically practicable, it is essential that all those working with anaesthetic equipment should not only understand what standards of cleanliness and sterilisation are acceptable in everyday practice, but should also have some knowledge of the methods of sterilising such equipment.

DEFINITIONS

Sterilisation

This is the process by which all micro-organisms, including bacterial spores, are destroyed.

Disinfection

This is the process by which the vegetative forms of micro-organisms are destroyed, but not usually bacterial spores.

Pasteurisation

This is a process of disinfection by heat at temperatures of about 60–80°C.

Disinfectant

This is an agent, usually a chemical solution, used for disinfection. Sometimes heat is employed (see above).

Antisepsis

This is a process by which micro-organisms are destroyed on the surface of living tissues. Spores are not usually killed and, while some vegetative forms may also survive, they are usually reduced to low levels not normally harmful to health.

Antiseptic

This is a chemical agent, usually weaker than a disinfectant, used in antisepsis. It must be non-toxic and non-corrosive.

Fumigation

This is also a method of disinfection, but by exposure to the fumes of a vaporised disinfectant (e.g. formaldehyde).

Pyrogen

This is protein organic matter which is capable of producing fever and is sometimes found in sterile infusion fluids. It is produced by bacteria entering the fluid during distillation and storage. The bacteria are killed during sterilisation but the pyrogenic particles of protein are left behind.

METHODS OF STERILISATION

Heat Sterilisation

Moist heat: autoclaving
The autoclave is a special sterilising container from which the air is first removed and replaced by steam under pressure. As the pressure is increased, the temperature of the steam rises and the length of exposure required for sterilisation is reduced. For example, at a temperature of 134°C a period of three minutes is satisfactory, and at a temperature of 147°C only 30 seconds are required for sterilisation. Of course, the full autoclaving cycle takes longer than this.

The method is effective against spores as well as vegetative bacteria, provided that the items to be sterilised are packed in such a way that the steam can gain access to them. The steam penetrates paper, cardboard and fabrics, but unfortunately tends to dull sharp edges slightly and speeds the deterioration of rubber and plastic.

Dry heat
Theoretically dry heat in hot air ovens is a simple method of sterilisation, and sealed containers may be used. However, a long period of exposure is required (e.g. 160 °C for one hour) and it is difficult to ensure that all parts of the load have been held at the full temperature for the necessary time.

Gas Sterilisation

Two methods are available.

Ethylene oxide
This colourless gas is effective against both vegetative bacteria and spores. It has excellent powers of penetration, leaves most materials undamaged, and is useful for sterilising heat-sensitive materials and ventilator circuits, where a closed-circuit technique is used. Its disadvantages are that it is toxic to inhale, it is explosive, slow (up to eight hours) and needs considerable skill for correct use. It is also difficult to eradicate all traces of ethylene oxide from materials like rubber and plastics.

Low-temperature steam plus formaldehyde
In normal autoclaving, the pressure is raised above atmospheric to produce steam at temperatures above 100 °C. In this technique a subatmospheric pressure is produced in a purpose-built autoclave, and formaldehyde and then steam at 73 °C are added and the temperature held steady for two hours. This method is faster and cheaper than ethylene oxide and the formaldehyde is easier to get rid of at the end of the process.

Sterilisation by Irradiation

Gamma rays
Gamma rays from a radioactive source, usually cobalt-60 in a

dose of 2·5 megarads are used. This method gives good penetration of closed packs and is commonly used for disposable equipment. Glass tends to turn brown and may be damaged. Also damaged are some types of rubber and, if irradiated more than once, many other materials including metals, PVC, nylon, paper, wool and cotton.

Ultra-violet light

This method has only a limited application as it is effective only on the surface area exposed.

STERILISATION INDICATORS

Sterilisation indicators are important in that without them it is impossible to be sure which packs have been sterilised. Some of the commoner indicators are listed below.

Autoclave Tape

This adhesive tape incorporates a heat-sensitive stripe which turns dark brown when exposed to normal autoclave conditions. Two such types of tape are approved by the Department of Health and Social Security (DHSS) for the Bowie Dick Autoclave Test, in which the autoclave tape is buried inside a stack of towels and then examined for uniformity of colour change after autoclaving.

Sterilisation Indicator Panels

These panels are found on sterilisation bags and contain a stripe similar to autoclave tape.

Browne's Tubes

Various tubes are available for different sterilisation processes, e.g. autoclaving, hot air sterilisation. The liquid changes from red to green when sterilisation is complete.

Irradiation Labels

These are small adhesive discs which change from yellow to red when irradiation has taken place.

METHODS OF DISINFECTION

Disinfection by Heat (Pasteurisation)

Traditionally this term was used for the process of raising the temperature of a liquid (commonly milk, whose proteins would be denatured by boiling) to temperatures between 60°C and 80°C for periods of between a few seconds and about an hour. This treatment is sufficient to kill most bacteria and viruses, but not spores.

In hospital, pasteurisation is carried out either by hot water or steam.

Hot water pasteurisation
This is usually carried out in tank pasteurisers or washer pasteurisers. The former usually have a pre-set process timer. The washer pasteurisers are useful for simultaneously cleaning and pasteurising anaesthetic equipment, some being fitted with long metal spouts upon which tubing is mounted. The Scott's washer is an example.

Note: Boiling, now seldom used in hospitals, is only a method of disinfection, not sterilisation, as it cannot be guaranteed to be sporicidal.

Steam pasteurisation
This is carried out in the special autoclaves constructed for sterilisation with low-temperature steam plus formaldehyde (described above), but in this technique the formaldehyde is omitted. This method has become more popular with the

increased use of materials damaged or destroyed by higher temperatures.

Chemical Disinfection and Sterilisation

A wide variety of chemical disinfectants is marketed, one of the commonest used being 2 % glutaraldehyde (Totacide 28, Cidex). The makers claim that after careful cleaning, immersed instruments are disinfected in 10 minutes and sterilised in 10 hours.

FILTRATION

Bacterial filters for use on the inspiratory side of ventilators used in intensive therapy units have been available for some time. More recently it has become customary to inject solutions into the epidural space (at least when repeated injections through an indwelling catheter are given) through a filter which removes particles down to a diameter of 0·5 μm. This includes almost all the pathogenic bacteria.

CLEANING AND STERILISING ANAESTHETIC EQUIPMENT

Face Masks

These are usually made of antistatic rubber which may be boiled or autoclaved. However, both methods cause rapid deterioration of the rubber, and it is accepted practice simply to wash the mask with soap or cetrimide and rinse thoroughly. Pasteurisation of face masks and airways may be done in a Scott's washer.

Airways and Endotracheal Tubes

Ideally, these should be disposable, but because of the cost even the disposable varieties are commonly reused. It is important that they be thoroughly cleaned inside with a suitable brush.

Sterilisation is most commonly achieved by autoclaving, but this hastens the deterioration of plastic and rubber, the former becoming discoloured and harder, while the latter becomes softer.

Nylon-reinforced latex endotracheal tubes must not be compressed when hot because the nylon may be permanently deformed. Gamma-ray irradiation and ethylene oxide are also satisfactory means of sterilisation but have the disadvantages enumerated above.

Double-lumen tubes are usually sterilised by irradiation.

Laryngoscope Blades

After removal, laryngoscope blades may be boiled or autoclaved. It is common practice simply to scrub laryngoscope blades with soap and water between cases.

Corrugated Tubing and Reservoir Bags

These are usually made of antistatic rubber, which deteriorates rapidly on boiling or autoclaving. These items of equipment should be thoroughly washed and rinsed after every use, but in many hospitals are only cleaned at the end of every list. If a greater degree of sterility is required, then pasteurisation is usually carried out in low-temperature steam or a washer pasteuriser.

Ventilators

Various methods have been described for sterilising ventilators. Most are rather specialised, some are expensive and none are entirely satisfactory. They include the use of formaldehyde vapour, ethylene oxide, ultrasonic alcohol and ultrasonic hydrogen peroxide. The best solution is to design ventilators with patient circuits which are fully autoclavable.

Syringes and Needles

Reusable syringes and needles are much less used nowadays. Syringes are sterilised by autoclaving with the plunger removed from the barrel. Needles must be carefully washed through with a detergent and rinsed in water or in an ultrasonic washer. Finally they are blown through with high-pressure air before autoclaving.

HEPATITIS B ANTIGEN

This is the antigen (HBAg, Australia antigen) carried by the dangerous virus which can cause serum hepatitis. It is transmitted in the blood or secretions of patients who either have active hepatitis or who are symptom-free (or healthy) carriers. All hospitals should have a detailed policy for dealing with such patients requiring operation.

The virus is readily killed by autoclaving and the general policy with potentially contaminated instruments and materials is to autoclave or incinerate them. Of the chemical agents, hypochlorite is the most effective.

AIDS (ACQUIRED IMMUNE DEFICIENCY SYNDROME)

As in the case of serum hepatitis, the causative organism of AIDS is a virus. This has been given a number of different names, of which the commonest is HIV or human immunodeficiency virus. Not surprisingly, therefore, the Microbiology Advisory Committee to the Department of Health and Social Security, in a report which has also been approved by the Expert Advisory Group on AIDS (EAGA) has recommended that whenever practicable the same procedures are used in HIV as in hepatitis B contamination.

While these precautions should be adequate to prevent contamination with the AIDS virus, it must be realised that patients with established AIDS may be suffering from opportunistic infection by a wide variety of potentially pathogenic bacteria, against which more elaborate precautions may be required.

47 Pollution

Possible hazards. Scavenging systems. Summary.

It is only in recent years (as indeed is the case with more general environmental and atmospheric pollution) that serious consideration has been given to the possible hazards of pollution of the operating theatre atmosphere by gaseous anaesthetics. As soon as the problem was identified a great deal of evidence was accumulated, much of its conflicting and none of it conclusive. This chapter indicates some of the possible hazards, and what methods should be used to reduce the severity of pollution in the operating theatre.

POSSIBLE HAZARDS

Spontaneous Abortion

An increased incidence of spontaneous abortion among women working in operating theatres is the possible hazard for which there is the most convincing evidence, but even this is not certain.

Effect on Fetal Development and Infertility

Some surveys indicate an increased incidence of fetal abnormalities of a minor nature and an increased tendency towards involuntary infertility in women working in operating theatres. The evidence is not clear, but merits further investigation.

Cancer and Other Tumours

It has been suggested that there is an increased tendency to develop neoplasms among anaesthetists. One study from the USA indicated an increased incidence of tumours of the lymphoid and reticulo-endothelial systems (e.g. lymphosarcoma, Hodgkin's disease) among anaesthetists. However, this was not confirmed in a second, similar study.

It has also been suggested that there is an increased incidence of cancer in female anaesthetists, but again evidence is unconvincing.

Impaired Mental Performance

Another possible hazard among operating theatre staff is impairment of their mental function by traces of gaseous anaesthetics. While the concentrations of nitrous oxide and halothane in unscavenged operating theatres is not considered high enough to affect mental performance in other theatre staff, anaesthetists using unscavenged anaesthetic circuits may be exposed to high enough concentrations of these agents to be affected in this way. Even in the case of the spontaneous abortion question there is no justification for assuming a cause-and-effect relationship with trace concentrations of gaseous anaesthetics in the operating theatre atmosphere. It may well be that the special physical and emotional effort required in operating theatre work may be the true cause of the increased tendency to abortion. Indeed, in one Scandinavian survey the nurses exposed to the highest concentrations of anaesthetic vapours were not those with the highest incidence of abortion, the rate being highest in scrub nurses, next intensive therapy unit nurses, and finally anaesthetic nurses.

Although there is a lack of convincing evidence that atmospheric pollution by traces of anaesthetic agents has any serious effects on theatre staff, it is just as difficult to prove that it is has not. For this reason, because unscavanged systems at times expose anaesthetists to quite high concentrations of anaesthetic vapours, and because traces of gaseous anaesthetics may summate with other adverse factors (e.g. impaired physical health, fatigue or other poor environmental conditions to reduce mental performance), it is wise to minimise the amount of such vapours inhaled by staff working in these areas. The Council of the Association of Anaesthetists of Great Britain and Ireland has recommended the use of scavenging devices whenever they are available and the DHSS has issued a circular to the same effect.

SCAVENGING SYSTEMS

These may be passive or active.

Passive Systems

In these systems the gases are carried away by the patient's own expiratory effort. This adds to the expiratory resistance, the extent depending in particular on the length and diameter of the tubing and the number of acute bends it contains. More severe obstruction may occur if there is kinking of the tubing.

The system may either vent directly to the atmosphere at an external wall or roof, or into the hospital ventilation system. If the outlet is to the atmosphere, variations in pressure, either positive or negative caused by variations in the strength or direction of the wind must be checked for by ventilation engineers. It is also important that the outlet be fitted with an insect-proof wire mesh cover. If the system vents into the hospital ventilation, again it is necessary for engineers to test for the variations in pressure occurring at the outlet point. Other theoretical risks include the transfer of flammable anaesthetic gases into the ventilation systems and the possible deleterious effect of some anaesthetic vapours on lubricants used in that system.

The Cardiff Aldasorber is another type of passive scavenging system. The patient's expired gases pass through activated charcoal which absorbs volatile agents like halothane and ether, but not, unfortunately, nitrous oxide.

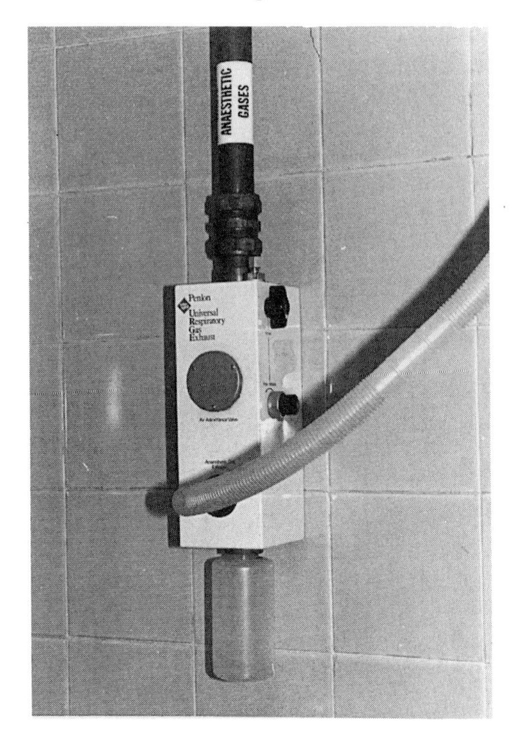

Fig. 47.1 Penlon Universal active/passive gas exhaust system

Active Systems

In these systems the expired gases are carried away by active suction provided by pump, fan or ejector. It is important that this suction is not applied directly to the patient's airway. If the hospital piped suction is used, the negative pressure supplied is about 1000 times too high! In addition, there are again potential hazards of flammable vapours in the main hospital suction pump and of those vapours on pump lubricants. For these reasons it is better to have a separate extraction system tailor-made for scavenging anaesthetic gases. For example, Penlon Ltd and the British Oxygen Company now provide a variety of active and passive systems (Figs 47.1 and 47.2).

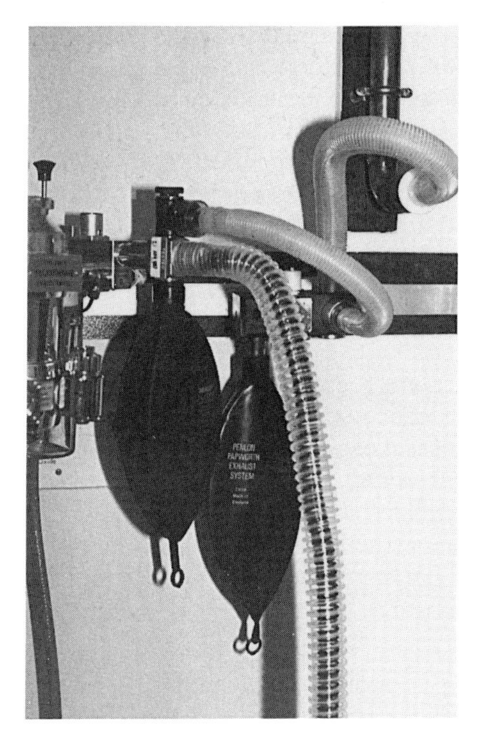

Fig. 47.2 Penlon Papworth active exhaust system

SUMMARY

At present the literature on the occupational hazards of anaesthesia provides reasonably convincing evidence only of an increased risk of spontaneous abortion among women working in operating theatres. Even then, there is no particular reason to believe that this is caused by trace quantities of anaesthetic gases. There is no convincing evidence of any other hazard. Nevertheless, it is now accepted that attempts should be made to reduce atmospheric pollution in operating theatres because it is also difficult to refute some association between atmospheric pollution and some adverse effects. All theatres and anaesthetic rooms should now be fully equipped with an approved and functioning scavenging system.

However, it should be realised that while these attempts to reduce pollution may lead to increased safety for the operating theatre staff, none of the methods do anything to add to patient safety. Some of the potential dangers of the various scavenging systems have already been mentioned. In addition, both active and passive systems increase the dangers of disconnection, misconnection and infection of the tubing. Also, the muffling effect of the lengths of expiratory tubing required reduces the anaesthetist's ability to hear when something is amiss with the anaesthetic—a useful safety bonus with old, noisy valves like the Heidbrink.

Finally, there are areas other than operating theatres where pollution may occur with anaesthetic gases and vapours and in some of these scavenging arrangements may be even more difficult to introduce. These include obstetric units (where patients may exhale large volumes of nitrous oxide), surgeries where dental anaesthetics are given, and recovery rooms.

48 Electrical Safety

Abnormal electric currents. Prevention of explosions.

Since several individual gases and anaesthetic agents are inflammable, it is essential that the potential sources of ignition, usually electric sparks, be minimised in operating theatres. In modern anaesthetic practice almost the only inflammable agents now used are ether and cyclopropane, both extremely explosive when combined with oxygen. In many theatres, however, neither agent is commonly used and as a result electrical safety is to a certain extent neglected. Electric sparks not only cause ignition of inflammable gas mixtures either inside or outside the body, but may also produce burns.

ABNORMAL ELECTRIC CURRENTS

Abnormal electric currents may arise in three important ways.

Static Electricity

Static electricity builds up when two dissimilar materials in contact with one another are pulled apart, for example a nylon shirt next to the skin. It commonly occurs when one substance which does not conduct electricity is in contact with one that does. Important non-conductors are rubber, plastic, wool, cotton and nylon. To allow the flow of static electricity to earth it is important that all rubber on anaesthetic and operating equipment (e.g. anaesthetic circuits, trolley tyres, operating table and stool tops) should be made of conducting rubber with antistatic properties. Such rubber is widely used by theatres and is black due to the inclusion of conducting carbon. All routinely used rubber anaesthetic equipment is antistatic. It is also important that the floor of the operating theatre be a good conductor so that static electricity will flow away when conductive equipment comes into contact with it.

Electric Current

Normal flow of electricity occurs intra-operatively, both intentionally—when diathermy is used to produce coagulation or cutting—and unintentionally—due to faulty electrical equipment such as x-ray machines or electric motors producing sparks. Surgical diathermy is a low voltage, high frequency current which produces heat and therefore coagulation at the tip of the diathermy forceps. It is essential that the current should be conducted away from the patient through a large earth electrode, thereby reducing the intensity of the current and preventing burns occurring under the electrode. If the earth is not attached to the patient, current will be conducted through the patient's body, passing into whatever conductive surface he is touching. If this area of contact is small, high current density may result in electrical burns. It is also a possible for other electrical equipment (e.g. ECG leads) to act as earths in the absence of a normal diathermy earth, and this is dangerous.

It is essential that all electrical apparatus in theatre should be frequently inspected for poor connections and other faults. All monitoring apparatus is now patient-isolated, which means that leads from the patient do not come into direct contact with apparatus within the machine, thereby minimising risks of abnormal currents flowing.

Heat

If intense enough, heat produced by hot surfaces or wires (e.g.

resectoscopes and endoscope bulbs) is also a potential source of ignition of inflammable gases.

PREVENTION OF EXPLOSIONS

Apart from minimising the ignition risk in operating theatres and avoiding the use of inflammable anaesthetic agents whenever possible, several methods for minimising the explosion risk in theatre are essential.

1. The use of antistatic materials, both in clothing, blankets, anaesthetic and surgical equipment and the soles of footwear.
2. The provision of an adequately conductive theatre floor.
3. Maintenance of a humid atmosphere within theatre, as static sparks occur much more commonly in a dry atmosphere. Relative theatre humidity should not fall below 50 %.
4. Ensuring that diathermy equipment is safe and that the earth electrode is correctly applied.
5. The avoidance of the use of diathermy when inflammable gases such as ether or cyclopropane are being used.
6. If explosive anaesthetics are essential, their administration should be stopped five minutes before diathermy is to be used. Other electrical equipment should not be used within 25 cm of apparatus containing flammable gas. Cardiac pacemakers and ECG machines are often inadvertently kept in close proximity to the anaesthetic machine.

With modern equipment, explosions in theatres are rare, but their effects, particularly when occurring close to or even in the airway of a patient, may be severe or even fatal. Ether is still used as the agent of choice in certain circumstances, particularly in children or in patients suffering severe bronchospasm, and great care is essential whenever this agent is being employed, particularly if an ether/oxygen mixture is used rather than ether/air, the former being considerably more explosive.

Appendix

Normal biochemical values. Output of electrolytes in urine. Haematological values. Normal respiratory values. Physiological gas tensions. Normal blood gas/acid–base values. Body water. Conversion factors.

NORMAL BIOCHEMICAL VALUES

Sodium	133–144 mmol/l
Potassium	3·2–5·1 mmol/l
Chloride	96–109 mmol/l
Bicarbonate	18–29 mmol/l
Urea	2·5–7·5 mmol/l
Creatinine	35–123 μmol/l
Calcium	2·1–2·65 mmol/l
Phosphate	0·7–1·4 mmol/l
Alkaline phosphatase	20–110 IU/l
Acid phosphatase	0–5 IU/l
Bilirubin	0–20 μmol/l
Total protein	62–80 g/l
Albumin	30–45 g/l
ALT (SGPT)	< 35 IU/l
AST (SGOT)	< 45 IU/l
LDH	200–500 IU/l
Amylase	70–300 IU/l
Sugar (fasting)	3·4–6·2 mmol/l
Osmolality (plasma)	275–295 mosm/l

OUTPUT OF ELECTROLYTES IN URINE

Sodium	100–250 mmol/24 h
Potassium	35–90 mmol/24 h
Chloride	170–250 mmol/24 h
Urea	300–400 mmol/24 h

HAEMATOLOGICAL VALUES

Haemoglobin	Male	14–18 g/100 ml
	Female	12–16 g/100 ml
	At birth	17–20 g/100 ml
Haematocrit (PCV)	Male	42–52 %
	Female	37–47 %
White cells		4000–10 000 cells/mm^3
Neutrophils		40–75 %
Eosinophils		1–6 %
Basophils		0–1 %
Lymphocytes		20–50 %
Monocytes		2–10 %
Platelets		150 000–400 000/mm^3

NORMAL RESPIRATORY VALUES (70 kg man) (Chapter 2)

Vital capacity	4800 ml
Functional residual capacity	2400 ml
Residual volume	1200 ml
Total lung capacity	6000 ml
Tidal volume	600 ml
Dead space (anatomical)	2 ml/kg (140 ml)
Alveolar ventilation	4200 ml/min
Forced expiratory volume in one second (FEV_1)	> 85 % of vital capacity
Oxygen consumption at rest	240 ml/min
Carbon dioxide production at rest	192 ml/min
Respiratory quotient (RQ)	0·8

Composition of Air

Nitrogen 78 %
Oxygen 21 %
Carbon dioxide 0·03 %
Argon 0·93 %
+ rare gases

PHYSIOLOGICAL GAS TENSIONS (Chapter 2)

	Inspired air	*Alveolar gas*	*Arterial blood*	*Mixed venous blood*
Nitrogen	610	573	573	617
Oxygen	150	100	100	40
Carbon dioxide	—	40	40	46
Water vapour	—	47	47	47

NORMAL BLOOD GAS/ACID–BASE VALUES

pH 7·36–7·44
$P\text{CO}_2$ (36–45 mmHg) 4·5–5·8 kPa
Standard bicarbonate 22–26 mmol/l.
Base excess ± 3 mmol/l.
$P\text{O}_2$ (80–100 mmHg) 10·5–13.5 kPa
Oxygen saturation 80–100 %

BODY WATER (Chapter 2)

	Male (litres)	*Female*
Total body water	45	30
Intracellular	30	18
Extracellular	15	12
1. Intravascular	3	3
2. Interstitial	12	9

Water intake/24 hours

	Male	*Female*
Liquid	1800 ml	1500 ml
Food	800 ml	700 ml
Metabolic	400 ml	300 ml
	3000 ml	2500 ml

Water output/24 hours

	Male	*Female*
Skin	700 ml	500 ml
Lungs	500 ml	400 ml
Faeces	100 ml	100 ml
Urine	1700 ml	1500 ml
	3000 ml	2500 ml

CONVERSION FACTORS

Weight Pounds to kilograms—multiply by 0·454
Kilograms to pounds—multiply by 2·205
Rough guide—6 kilograms = 1 stone

Volume Pints to litres—multiply by 0·568
Litres to pints—multiply by 1·760

Temperature Centrigrade to Fahrenheit $°F = °C \times 9/5 + 32$
Fahrenheit to Centigrade $°C = (°F - 32) \times 5/9$

Pressures 1 atmosphere = 760 mmHg
1 kilopascal (kPa) = 7·6 mmHg
100 kilopascal (kPa) = 760 mmHg = 1 bar
mmHg to kPa divide by 7·6
kPa to mmHg multiply by 7·6
1 kPa ≡ 10 cmH_2O
1 bar ≡ 10^5 newtons/metre^2 (N/m^2)
1 kPa/cm^2 ≡ 14·22 lbf/in^2 (p.s.i.)
1 mmHg ≡ 133·3 newtons/metre^2 (N/m^2)
1 mmH_2O ≡ 9·81 newtons/metre^2 (N/m^2)

Solutions A 1 % solution contains 1 g/100 ml
i.e. 10 mg/ml

Recommended Reading

Atkinson R.S., Rushman G.B., Lee J. Alfred (1987). *A Synopsis of Anaesthesia*. 10th edn. Bristol: John Wright & Sons Ltd.

Braimbridge M.V. (1981). *Post-operative Cardiac Intensive Care*. 3rd edn. Oxford: Blackwell Scientific Publications.

Bromage P.R. (1978). *Epidural Analgesia*. Philadelphia: W.B. Saunders Co.

Brown T.C.K., Fisk G.C. (1979). *Anaesthesia for Children Including Aspects of Intensive Care*. Oxford: Blackwell Scientific Publications.

Bryn Thomas K. (1975). *The Development of Anaesthetic Apparatus*. Oxford: Blackwell Scientific Publications.

Bullingham R.E.S. (1981). Synthetic opiate analgesics. *British Journal of Hospital Medicine;* **25/1:** 59–65.

Burn J.H. (1975). *Autonomic Nervous System for Students of Physiology and Pharmacology*. 5th edn. Oxford: Blackwell Scientific Publications.

Campbell D., Spence A. (1985) *Anaesthetics, Resuscitation and Intensive Care*. 6th edn. Edinburgh: Churchill Livingstone.

Davenport H.T. (1986) *Anaesthesia in the Elderly*. London: Heinemann Medical.

Davenport Horace W. (1974). *The ABC of Acid-Base Chemistry*. 6th edn. Chicago and London: University of Chicago Press.

Eltringham R., Durkin M., Andrewes S. (1983) *Post-anaesthesia Recovery*. Springer-Verlag

Emery E.R., Yates A.K., Moorhead P.J. (1984). *Intensive Care*. London: English Universities Press.

Eriksson E. (1979). *Illustrated Handbook in Local Anaesthesia*. 2nd edn. London: Lloyd-Luke.

Feldman S.A., Crawley B. (1977). *Tracheostomy and Artificial Ventilation in Treatment of Respiratory Failure*. 3rd edn. Baltimore: Williams & Wilkins Co.

Ganong W.F. (1985). *Review of Medical Physiology*. 12th edn. Los Altos, California: Lange Medical Publications.

Gray T. Cecil, Nunn J.F., Utting J.E. (1980). *General Anaesthesia*. 4th edn. London: Butterworths.

Green J.H. (1976) *An Introduction to Human Physiology*. 4th edn. Oxford: Oxford University Press.

Harrison M.J.G., Horsburgh A.G., Wake P., Mansfield Averill O., Snell M.E., Croft R.J. (1980). Vascular surgery. *British Journal of Hospital Medicine;* **24/2:** 108–140.

Hill D.W. (1980). *Physics Applied to Anaesthesia.* 4th edn. London. Butterworths.

Howell R.S.C. (1980). Piped medical gases and vacuum systems. *Anaesthesia;* **35:** 676–698.

Hunter A.H. (1976). *Neurosurgical Anaesthesia.* 2nd. edn. Oxford: Blackwell Scientific Publications.

Kaplan J.A. (1979) *Cardiac Anaesthesia.* New York: Grune & Stratton.

Katz J., Kadis L.B. (1981). *Anaesthesia and Uncommon Diseases.* 2nd edn. Philadelphia: W.B. Saunders Co. Ltd.

Latimer R.D. (1971). Central venous catheterisation. *British Journal of Hospital Medicine;* **5/1:** 369–376.

Lee J. Alfred., Atkinson R.S. (1985). *Macintosh's Lumbar Puncture and Spinal Analgesia.* 5th edn. Edinburgh: Churchill Livingstone.

Lipton S. (1977). *Persistent Pain: Modern Methods of Treatment.* New York: Grune & Stratton.

Macintosh R., Bryce-Smith R. (1962) *Local Analgesia: Abdominal Surgery.* 2nd edn. Edinburgh: E. & S. Livingstone Ltd.

Macintosh R., Mushin W.W., Epstein H.G. (1987). *Physics for the Anaesthetist.* 4th edn. Oxford: Blackwell Scientific Publications.

Macintosh R., Ostlere M. (1967). *Local Analgesia: Head and Neck.* Edinburgh: E. & S. Livingstone Ltd.

Maurer I.M. (1985). *Hospital Hygiene.* 3rd edn. London: Edward Arnold.

Mehta M. (1973). *Intractable Pain.* Philadelphia: W.B. Saunders Co. Ltd.

Mollison P.L. (1987). *Blood Transfusion in Clinical Medicine.* 8th edn. Oxford: Blackwell Scientific Publications.

Morrow W.F.K., Morrison J.D. (1985). *Anaesthesia for Eye, Ear, Nose and Throat Surgery.* Edinburgh: Churchill Livingstone.

Mushin W.W., Rendell-Baker L., Thompson P.W., Mapleson W.W. (1980). *Automatic Ventilation of the Lungs.* 3rd edn. Oxford: Blackwell Scientific Publications

Parbrook G.D., Davies P.D., Parbrook E.O. (1985) *Basic Physics and Measurement in Anaesthesia.* London: Heinemann Medical.

Rollason W.N. (1980). *Electrocardiography for the Anaesthetist.* 4th edn. Oxford: Blackwell Scientific Publications.

Rosen M., Latto I.P., Ng W.S. (1981). *Handbook of Percutaneous Central Venous Catheterisation.* London: W.B. Saunders Co. Ltd.

Rosenberg P., Kirves A. (1973). Miscarriages among operating theatre staff. *Acta Anaesthesiologica Scandinavica (Suppl.)*; **53:** 37–42.

Sabbawala P.B., Strong M.J., Keats A.S. (1970). Surgery of the aorta and its branches. *Anaesthesiology;* **33:** 229–255.

Scurr C., Feldman S. (1982). *Scientific Foundations of Anaesthesia.* 3rd edn. London: Heinemann Medical.

Smith G., Aitkenhead A.R. (1985) *A Textbook of Anaesthesia.* Edinburgh: Churchill Livingstone.

Spence A.A., Knill-Jones R.P. (1978). Is there a health hazard in anaesthetic practice? *British Journal of Anaesthesia;* **50:** 713–719.

Stoddart J.C. (1976). *Intensive Therapy.* Oxford: Blackwell Scientific Publications.

Sykes M.K., Vickers M.D., Hull C.J. (1981). *Principles of Clinical Measurement*. 2nd edn. Oxford: Blackwell Scientific Publications.
Vander A.J., Sherman J.H., Luciano D.S. (1975). *Human Physiology: The Mechanism of Body Function*. 2nd edn. New York: McGraw-Hill.
Vickers M.D. (1975). Pollution of the atmosphere of operating theatres. *Anaesthesia;* **30:** 697–699.
Vickers M.D. (1978). *Medicine for Anaesthetists*. 2nd edn. Oxford: Blackwell Scientific Publications.
Vickers M.D. Schnieden H., Wood-Smith F.G. (1984). *Drugs in Anaesthetic Practice*. 6th edn. London: Butterworths.
Ward C.S. (1985) *Anaesthetic Equipment: Physical Principles and Maintenance*. 2nd edn. London: Baillière Tindall.
White G.M.J. (1960) Evolution of endotracheal and endobronchial intubation. *British Journal of Anaesthesia*; **32**, 235–246.
Willatts S.M., Walters F.J.M. (1986) *Anaesthesia and Intensive Care of the Neurosurgical Patient*. Oxford: Blackwell Scientific Publications.
Wolfson L.J. (1962). *Anaesthesia for the Injured*. Oxford: Blackwell Scientific Publications.
Wylie W.D., Churchill-Davidson H.C. (1984) *A Practice of Anaesthesia*. 5th edn. London: Lloyd-Luke.

Index